Plant Science Research and Practices

New Developments in Medical Research

nova
Medicine & Health
New York

Plant Science Research and Practices

A Closer Look at Photosynthesis
Vijay Kumar Dalal, PhD (Editor)
Amarendra Narayan Misra, PhD (Editor)
2023. ISBN: 979-8-88697-815-5 (Hardcover)
2023. ISBN: 979-8-88697-861-2 (eBook)

Vitis Products: Composition, Health Benefits and Economic Valorization
António Manuel Jordão (Editor)
Renato Vasconcelos Botelho (Editor)
2021. ISBN: 978-1-53619-982-6 (Hardcover)
2021. ISBN: 978-1-68507-041-0 (eBook)

More information about this series can be found at
https://novapublishers.com/product-category/series/plant-science-research-and-practices/

New Developments in Medical Research

The Dangers of Psychoactive Substances
Denise J. Burton (Editor)
2023. ISBN: 979-8-88697-705-9 (Softcover)
2023. ISBN: 979-8-88697-712-7 (eBook)

An Innovative Program at Alfaisal Medicine:
A Brief History and Guide to Success
Paul Ganguly, MBBS, MD, FACA (Editor)
2023. ISBN: 979-8-88697-638-0 (Softcover)
2023. ISBN: 979-8-88697-703-5 (eBook)

More information about this series can be found at
https://novapublishers.com/product-category/series/new-developments-in-medical-research/

Arpita Roy
Editor

Antidiabetic Plants

Properties and Applications

nova
Medicine & Health
New York

https://doi.org/10.52305/KBPH8734

NOTICE TO THE READER

The Publisher has taken reasonable care in the preparation of this book but makes no expressed or implied warranty of any kind and assumes no responsibility for any errors or omissions. No liability is assumed for incidental or consequential damages in connection with or arising out of information contained in this book. The Publisher shall not be liable for any special, consequential, or exemplary damages resulting, in whole or in part, from the readers' use of, or reliance upon, this material. Any parts of this book based on government reports are so indicated and copyright is claimed for those parts to the extent applicable to compilations of such works.

Independent verification should be sought for any data, advice or recommendations contained in this book. In addition, no responsibility is assumed by the Publisher for any injury and/or damage to persons or property arising from any methods, products, instructions, ideas or otherwise contained in this publication.

This publication is designed to provide accurate and authoritative information with regards to the subject matter covered herein. It is sold with the clear understanding that the Publisher is not engaged in rendering legal or any other professional services. If legal or any other expert assistance is required, the services of a competent person should be sought. FROM A DECLARATION OF PARTICIPANTS JOINTLY ADOPTED BY A COMMITTEE OF THE AMERICAN BAR ASSOCIATION AND A COMMITTEE OF PUBLISHERS.

Library of Congress Cataloging-in-Publication Data

Names: Roy, Arpita, editor.
Title: Antidiabetic plants: properties and applications / Arpita Roy.
Other titles: Plant science research and practices
Identifiers: LCCN 2023030061 (print) | LCCN 2023030062 (ebook) |
ISBN 9798886979572 (hardcover) | ISBN 9798886979824 (adobe pdf)
Subjects: LCSH: Diabetes--Alternative treatment. | Herbs--Therapeutic use.
| Materia medica, Vegetable.
Classification: LCC RC661.H4 A685 2023 (print) | LCC RC661.H4 (ebook) |
DDC 616.4/6206--dc23/eng/20230706
LC record available at https://lccn.loc.gov/2023030061
LC ebook record available at https://lccn.loc.gov/2023030062

Published by Nova Science Publishers, Inc. † New York

Contents

Preface

Diabetics is one of the chronic diseases of metabolism that account for approximately 2.8% of the world's demography. It is up surging across every continent in the world. Treatment to prevent this disease is an important challenge for researchers. Conventional drugs for the treatment of this disease improve insulin sensitivity. Increased insulin production results in a decrease blood glucose level. However, they have additional side effects and do not always provide satisfactory results. The WHO estimates that approximately 80% of the world's population rely on traditional medicine for primary health care and many plants have ethnomedical claims of usefulness in the treatment of diabetes and other chronic diseases worldwide, and have been employed empirically in antidiabetic, antihyperlipidemic, antihypertensive, ant inflammatory, and antiparasitic remedies. Plants are a key source for potential lead candidates' discovery, which can play an essential role in drug discovery and drug development projects. Plants are an alternative source to overcome this problem, as they contain various phytocompounds that show protective effects against diabetics.

This book provides systematic information about different plants and their active compounds, as well as their mode of action in the prevention and treatment of diabetes.

Chapters 1 and 2 discuss the antidiabetic plant-derived compounds of Indian origin. It reported that approximately 288 plant species recognised for their hypoglycaemic effects. As per their botanical name, family, and type of active substances, the plants are described in the chapter.

Chapter 3 discusses the antidiabetic plants from African region. It reported that the plants most researched are those in the Asteraceae and Lamiaceae families, and West Africa has a greatest number of these species that act as antidiabetic agents.

Chapters 4 and 5 discuss plant-based compounds for diabetic management and reported studies of different compounds that were isolated from a wide range of plants which exhibit α-amylase and α-glucosidase inhibitory activities.

Chapters 6-10 discuss the role of Aloe Vera, Momordica charantia, Zanthoxylum armatum, Ocimum sanctum, and Azadirachta indica in diabetes management. The potential benefits of all plants have been reported.

Chapters 11 and 12 discuss the conservation strategies for antidiabetic plants. There are several challenges to the conservation of antidiabetic plants, including threats from habitat degradation, overexploitation, and climate change. The potential of using legal and policy instruments to protect these plants and the need for more research and data collection to understand their ecology and use. It proposes some recommendations for improving conservation strategies for antidiabetic plants. In general, these chapters provide a comprehensive overview of the conservation strategies for antidiabetic plants and identify gaps in current efforts.

Chapter 1

Antidiabetic Plant-Derived Compounds with an Indian Origin

Usha Kiran Rout[1]
Chita Ranjan Sahoo[1,2,*]
Debdutta Bhattacharya[1]
and Rabindra Nath Padhy[2]
[1]ICMR-Regional Medical Research Centre (Department of Health Research, Ministry of Health and Family Welfare, Govt. of India), Bhubaneswar, India
[2]Central Research Laboratory, Institute of Medical Sciences and Sum Hospital, Siksha 'O' Anusandhan (Deemed to be University), Bhubaneswar, Odisha, India

Abstract

India is known as the world's largest botanical garden because it produces the most therapeutic herbs. With the expansion of traditional medicine over the past few decades, green, biofriendly, affordable, and generally safe plant-based medications have transitioned from the peripheral to the main drug development. The most informative survey of the literature on antidiabetic herbal remedies comes from information from the collective literature on more than 288 plant species recognised for their hypoglycemic effects. In this plant chapter, antidiabetic plants of Indian origin have been discussed.

Keywords: medicinal plant, bioactive compound, diabetes phytocompounds

---

[*] Corresponding Author's Email: chitaranjan.biotech@gmail.com.

In: Antidiabetic Plants
Editor: Arpita Roy
ISBN: 979-8-88697-957-2

Introduction

Traditional remedies have been used for a long time and play an essential role in alternative therapies. Traditional medicines have less adverse effects than modern remedies. Around 75-80% of the world's population still relies on traditional remedies. Various medicinal plants are beneficial in the treatment of diabetes around the world and have been used experimentally as antidiabetic and antihyperlipidemic treatments. However, research on novel anti-diabetic drugs derived from natural plants remains appealing, including phytoconstituents with alternative and safe effects in the treatment of diabetes mellitus (Tran et al., 2020).

In ancient times, Vyas and Purohit estimated that around 70,000 plant species have been used as herbal medicine throughout history. Ayurveda originated in India and is the oldest (almost 5000 years old), serving as an alternative to the medical system. Furthermore, Susruta Samhita and Charaka Samhita contain enormous information about traditional medicine (Jain et al., 2019). For 1000 years, the traditional Indian health system has used a variety of therapeutic plants in herbal remedies. Traditional remedies are heavily on medicinal plants, minerals, and organic compounds. Most Indian traditional medicine practitioners create and administer their formulations. The WHO lists 21,000 plants that are used for medical reasons across the world. There are 2500 different species in India, among which 150 are used economically. India is the world's largest producer of medicinal plants known as the botanical garden. Ethnobotanical data indicate that 800 plants have antidiabetic properties (Kayarohanam, 2015).

Although synthetic antidiabetic drugs used with insulin are the primary method of regulating diabetes, they do not completely reverse the course of its problems and aggravate it by exhibiting significant adverse effects (Alam et al., 2022). This is the driving factor behind the search for alternative sources of antidiabetic drugs. Despite the substantial improvement in the treatment of diabetes with oral hypoglycemic medications over the past three decades, the result of treatment does not completely cure the patient (Patil et al., 2011). Numerous drawbacks to existing medications are found, such as toxicity, drug resistance (reduced effectiveness), and other side effects.

Due to the numerous restrictions associated with the use of existing synthetic antidiabetic medications, the search for additional antidiabetic therapies from natural sources is reported. Presently, focussing on all the obstacles, the main alternative found that the shift from synthetic to herbal treatment, which can best be described as "return to nature" is the call of the day (Kumar et al., 2019). In this chapter, a detailed description of Indian medicinal plant species with their phytocompounds is reported for their antidiabetic effects.

Diabetes and Therapeutic Strategies

Diabetes mellitus is an anomalous endocrine disease characterized by abnormal carbohydrate, lipid, and proteins. These abnormalities lead to abnormal insulin production, secretion, and action (Kayarohanam, 2015). Globally, around 422 million people are affected by diabetes. Its prevalence has increased from 6.4% to 9.3% in 2019 (Saeedi et al., 2019). The frequency is expected to increase to 10.2% by 2030 and 10.9% by 2045. Diabetes is expected to be the seventh leading cause of death by 2030, according to the World Health Organisation. Type 1 and Type II are the two main types of diabetes disease. Type 1 diabetes is caused by a near-total insulin deficiency or lack of insulin. Type 2 diabetes is a diverse set of diseases defined by varying degrees of insulin resistance, decreased insulin secretion, and increased glucose production. Prediabetes and gestational diabetes are two more types of diabetes. Gestational diabetes refers to glucose intolerance during pregnancy. Most women regain normal glucose tolerance after giving birth, but there is a significant risk of developing type 2 diabetes later in life.

Uncontrolled hyperglycemia and hyperlipidemia cause acute and long-term problems in both type 1 and type 2 diabetes. (Subramoniam, 2016). Acute complications of diabetics cause ketoacidosis and hyperglycemic hyperosmolar state (HHS). Ketosis is caused by increased fatty acid release from adipocytes, as well as a shift toward the production of ketone bodies in the liver. In the liver, these fatty acids are normally metabolised to triglycerides or VLDL. However, hyperglucagonemia affects liver metabolism and favours the synthesis of ketone bodies. Diabetic ketoacidosis is typically caused by both insulin deficiency and excess glucagon production. It is also triggered by high levels of catecholamines, cortisol, and/or growth hormone. People with type 2 diabetes with polyuria and weight loss are at risk of HHS. Chronic diabetes complications are classified as vascular or nonvascular. Microvascular problems include neuropathy, retinopathy, and nephropathy, while macrovascular complications cause peripheral arterial disease, coronary artery disease, and cerebrovascular disease (Subramoniam, 2016).

Table 1. Indian medicinal plant and its antidiabetic activities

Sl No.	Plant Species	Common name	Family	Phytochemical properties	Activity
1.	*Abrus precatorius*	Jequirity bean or Rosary pea	Fabaceae	Alkaloids, Cyclitols, Saponins, Fluoroacetate, Terpenes, Flavonoids	Modulation of insulin
2.	*Acacia arabica*	Babool	Fabaceae	Alkaloids, Cyclitols, Saponins, Fluoroacetate, Terpenes	Decreasing serum glucose level
3.	*Acacia catechu*	Catechu	Fabaceae	Epicatechin	Antidiabetic action
4.	*Acacia modesta*	Phulai	Fabaceae	Flavonoids and phenolic acids	Glucose uptake employing α-amylase inhibition
5.	*Acalypha indica*	Indian Copperleaf	Euphorbiaceae	Alkaloids, Cyclitols, Saponins, Fluoroacetate, Terpenes, Flavonoids	*Lower increased blood glucose*
6.	*Acanthopanax senticosus*	Siberian Ginseng	Araliaceae	Phenolic compounds such as syringin and eleutheroside E	*Suppressed glucide absorption by inhibition of intestinal α-glucosidase activity*
7.	*Achillea millefolium*	Common yarrow	Asteraceae	Flavonoid	Reduces blood glucose
8.	*Achyranthes rubrofusca*	Devil's horsewhip	Amaranthaceae	triterpenoid saponins, ketosteroids, and ketosteroids and polysaccharides	*Improvement in beta cell function, insulin resistance, glucose (re)absorption, and glucagon-like peptide-1 homeostasis*
9.	*Acorus calamus*	Sweet flag	Acoraceae	Asarones, β-Asarone	The expression and secretion of glucagon-like peptide-1 (GLP-1) is related to its hypoglycemic effects
10.	*Adansonia digitata*	Baobab tree	Malvaceae	Vitamin-C, Steroids, Flavonoids	α-amylase inhibitor

Sl No.	Plant Species	Common name	Family	Phytochemical properties	Activity
11.	*Adiantum capillus-veneris*	Maidenhair fern	Pteridaceae	Flavonoids	*Reduces blood glucose*
12.	*Adina cordifolia*	Haldina	Rubiaceae	Flavonoids, alkaloids, terpenoids, tannins, gums and carbohydrates	Control glucose level
13.	*Afzelia africana*	Lengue	Fabaceae	Flavonoids, proanthocyanidins, tannins, phenols and alkaloid, terpenoids	Potentiation of insulin from β cells
14.	*Ailanthus excelsa*	Tree of heaven	Simaroubaceae	Phenolic components, ailantic acid, sitosterol, and Quassinoids	reduced blood glucose level
15.	*Alangium salvifolium*	Sage-leaved alangium	Cornaceae	Alangine, ankorine, tubulosine, alangicine, salsoline	Hypoglycemic
16.	*Albizzia lebbeck*	Woman's tongue	Fabaceae	Alkaloids, anthraquinones, essential oils, flavonoids	Decreasing blood glucose
17.	*Allium cepa*	Onion	Liliaceae	Quercetin and allicin	Stimulate the production of insulin
18.	*Allium sativum*	Garlic	Amaryllidaceae	Flavonoids	Enhance glucose tolerance
19.	*Aloe ferox*	Bitter aloe	Asphodelaceae		Lower fasting blood glucose levels.
20.	*Aloe vera*	Aloe vera	Asphodelaceae	Alkaloids and aromatic compounds	Decrease the blood glucose
21.	*Alpinia galanga*	Thai ginger	Zingiberaceae	α-fenchyl, β-pinene	Inhibits enzymes in carbohydrate metabolism, that is α-amylase and α-glucosidase
22.	*Alstonia scholaris*	White cheesewood	Apocynaceae	Picrinine	α-glucosidase inhibitor
23.	*Amaranthus tricolor*	Elephant-Head Amaranth	Amaranthaceae	Ascorbic acid and flavonoids	Antihyperglycemic activity

Table 1. (Continued)

Sl No.	Plant Species	Common name	Family	Phytochemical properties	Activity
24.	*Anacardium occidentale*	Cashew	Anacardiaceae	beta-carotene, lutein, zeaxanthin, alpha-tocopherol, gamma-tocopherol, thiamin	Lower blood glucose level
25.	*Andrographis paniculata*	Bitterweed	Acanthaceae	Diterpenoids, flavonoids, and polyphenols.	Decreasing hepatic glucose production
26.	*Anthocephalus cadamba*	Kadam	Rubiaceae	Linalool	*Glucose lowering efficacy*
27.	*Aphanamixis polystachya*	Pithraj Tree	Meliaceae	Terpene and alkaloid	Lower glucose level
28.	*Argyreia nervosa*	Woodrose	Convolvulaceae	Ergoline alkaloids such as ergine	Increasing insulin secretion
29.	*Artemisia parviflora*	Himalayan wormwood	Asteraceae	β-caryophyllene, camphor, germacrene D, artemisia ketone, 1,8-cineole	Reduce blood glucose
30.	*Artocarpus heterophyllus*	Jackfruit	Moraceae	Prenylflavonoids, hydroxycinnamic acids and glycosides	Hypoglycemic, α-amylase inhibitor
31.	*Azadirachta indica*	Neem	Meliaceae	Nimbolide, azarirachtin, and gedunin	α-glucosidase and α-amylase inhibitor, hypoglycemic
32.	*Barleria prionitis*	Vajradanti	Acanthaceae	Alkaloids, flavonoids, glycosides, phenolics, and saponins	Decreased blood glucose
33.	*Barringtonia acutangula*	Mango-pine	Lecythidaceae	Triterpenoids,	Suppression of transfer of glucose
34.	*Basella rubra*	Red Ceylon Spinach	Basellaceae	Phenolic compounds	Possess insulin mimetic action
35.	*Bauhinia thoningii*	Camel's foot tree	Fabaceae	Flavonoids and tannins	Reduction in blood glucose

Sl No.	Plant Species	Common name	Family	Phytochemical properties	Activity
36.	*Begonia roxburghii*	East Himalayan Begonia	Begoniaceae	Alkaloids and carbohydrates	Alteration of glucose metabolism;
37.	*Berberis aristata*	Dāruhaldhi	Berberidaceae	Triterpenes	Lower blood glucose
38.	*Blepharis molluginifolia*		Acanthaceae	Apigenin, Flavonoid, alkaloids, phenolic	Antidiabetic activity
39.	*Boerhavia diffusa*	Punarnava	Nyctaginaceae	Alkaloids, flavonoids, tannins and anthraquinones	Modulates abdominal glucose
40.	*Boswellia ovalifoliolata*	Indian frankincense	Burseraceae	Monoterpenes, diterpenes, triterpenes, and tetracyclic triterpenic acids	Protective effects on diabetic complications
41.	*Brassica juncea*	Indian Mustard	Brassicaceae	Esters, alcohols, ketones, acids, nitriles, aldehydes, phenols, hydrocarbons	Decreasing hepatic glucose production
42.	*Brassica rapa*	Field mustard	Brassicaceae	Polyphenols	Antidiabetic efficacy
43.	*Buddleja asiatica*	Dog tail	Scrophulariaceae	6-O-(3”,4”-dimethoxycinnamoyl) catalpol	Production and intestinal absorption of glucose
44.	*Butea frondosa*	Flame of the forest	Fabaceae	Alkaloids, flavonoids, phenolic compounds, steroids	Significant reductions in blood glucose
45.	*Caesalpinia bonducella*	Gray Nicker	Fabaceae	Alkaloids, flavonoids, phenolic compounds, amino acids, glycosides, steroids	α-amylase inhibitor
46.	*Caesalpinia ferrea*	Leopard Tree	Fabaceae	Butanedioic acid	Reduction of blood glucose levels
47.	*Cajanus cajan*	Pigeon pea	Fabaceae	Flavonoids and stilbenes	Maintain blood glucose and cholesterol
48.	*Calamus erectus*	Viagra palm	Arecaceae	α-asarone, α-cedrene, (E)-methylisoeugenol	α-glucosidase and α-amylase enzyme inhibition

Table 1. (Continued)

Sl No.	Plant Species	Common name	Family	Phytochemical properties	Activity
49.	*Calamus tenuis*		Arecaceae		Anti diabetic property
49.	*Callicarpa arborea*	Beautyberry Tree	Lamiaceae	β-selinene, ar-turmerone and α-copaene	Regulate glycaemic metabolism, increase insulin, and improving microcirculation
50.	*Camellia sinensis*	green tea	Theaceae	Catechins	Antihyperglycemic
51.	*Capparis decidua*	Karira	Capparaceae	β-sitosterol	Inhibited acute elevation of blood glucose level
52.	*Capparis sepiaria*	Wild caper bush	Capparaceae	Alkaloids, glycosides, tannins, phenolics, flavonoids	Conventional hypoglycemic drugs
53.	*Capparis spinosa*	Alpine Caper Bush	Capparaceae	Docosane, nonacosane and hexadecanoic acid	*Glucose levels significantly decreases*
54.	*Caralluma adscendens*	Aak	Apocynaceae	Triterpenoids	Inhibitory activity against alpha-amylase and alpha- glucosidase.
55.	*Caralluma umbellata*	Pussur	Apocynaceae		Antihyperglycemic
56.	*Casearia esculenta*	Bairi	Flacourtiaceae		Restores glucose level
57.	*Casia fistula*	Golden Shower Tree	Fabaceae		α-amylase inhibitor
58.	*Cassia auriculata*	Avartaki or Mature Tea Tree	Caesalpiniaceae		
59.	*Cassia grandis*	Pink Shower Tree	Fabaceae		Antidiabetic potential
60.	*Catharanthus roseus*	graveyard plant	Apocynaceae		α amylase inhibitor, Reduced blood glucose levels
61.	*Cayratia trifolia*	Fox grape			
62.	*Cecropia pachystachya*	Ambay pumpwood	Urticaceae		Hypoglycemic effect
63.	*Ceiba pentandra*	Kapok Tree			α-amylase inhibition, hypoglycemic,antihyperglycemic
64.	*Centella asiatica*	gotu kola	Apiaceae		

Sl No.	Plant Species	Common name	Family	Phytochemical properties	Activity
65.	*Centratherum anthelminticum*	black/bitter cumin or kalijiri	Asteraceae		Hypoglycemic
66.	*Ceriops decandra*	Flat-leaved Spurred Mangrove	Rhizophoraceae		Controls blood glucose
67.	*Chiliadenus iphionoides*		Asteraceae		Increased insulin secretion
68.	*Chlorophytum borivilianum*	safed musli	Asparagaceae		Antidiabetic
69.	*Cinnamomum cassia and Cinnamomum japonica*	Japanese cinnamon	Lauraceae		Decreased blood glucose
70.	*Cinnamomum impressinervium*		Lauraceae		Controls Blood sugar
71.	*Cinnamomum tamala*	Indian Cassia or Indian Bay Leaf or Tej pat	Lauraceae		Hypoglycemic effect
72.	*Cinnamomum verum*	Cinnamon	Lauraceae		α-amylase inhibitor
73.	*Citrullus colocynthis*	bitter apple	Cucurbitaceae		Cucurbitaceae
74.	*Citrus sinensis*	sweet orange	Rutaceae		
75.	*Clerodendrum glandulosum* or *Clerodendrum colebrookianum*	East Indian glory bower	Lamiaceae		Inhibitors of glycemic enzyme
76.	*Clerodendrum infortunatum*	hill glory bower	Lamiaceae		Controls Blood sugar
77.	*Clerodendrum phlomidis*	Arni	Lamiaceae		Inhibitors of glycemic enzyme
78.	*Clitoria ternatea*	butterfly pea	Fabaceae		α-glucosidase, α-amylase inhibitor
79.	*Coccinia cordifolia*		Cucurbitaceae		Antidiabetic activity

Table 1. (Continued)

Sl No.	Plant Species	Common name	Family	Phytochemical properties	Activity
80.	*Coccinia grandis*	Ivy Gourd	Cucurbitaceae		Antihyperglycemic, α-glucosidase inhibitor, α-amylase inhibitor
81.	*Coccinia indica*	the ivy gourd			Inhibitors of glycemic enzyme
82.	*Cocculus hirsutus*	broom creeper	Menispermaceae		α-amylase inhibitor
83.	*Cocos nucifera*	Coconut	Arecaceae	Flavonoid, tannin, and saponin.	Potentiating the insulin effect of plasma
84.	*Coldenia procumbens*	Riceweeds	Boraginaceae		Inhibitors of glycemic enzyme
85.	*Commiphora wightii*	Indian bdellium-tree or gugal	Burseraceae		Inhibitors of glycemic enzyme
86.	*Coscinium fenestratum*	Tree turmeric or Daru Haridra	Menispermaceae		Inhibitors of glycemic enzyme
87.	*Costus igneus*	insulin plant	Costaceae		Insulin like activity
88.	*Costus pictus*	Spiral flag	Costaceae		Inhibitors of glycemic enzyme
89.	*Croton klozchianus*				Lower glucose level
90.	*Cucumis callosus*	Muskmelon	Cucurbitaceae		Controls Blood sugar
91.	*Cuminum cyminum*	spice Cumin	Apiaceae		
92.	*Curculigo orchioides*	golden eye-grass or Black Musli	Hypoxidaceae		
93.		turmeric	Zingiberaceae		
94.	*Curcuma longa* and *Curcuma domestica*	Turmeric	Zingiberaceae	Curcuminoids	Inhibition of α-glucosidase and α-amylase enzyme
95.	*Cuscuta reflexa*	Giant dodder	Convolvulaceae		
96.	*Cyamopsis tetragonoloba*	Cluster bean	Fabaceae		
97.	*Cyamopsis tetragonoloba*	Cluster bean	Fabaceae		

Sl No.	Plant Species	Common name	Family	Phytochemical properties	Activity
98.	*Cyperus kyllinga*	Whitehead spikesedge	Cyperaceae		Controls Blood sugar
99.	*Cyperus laevigatus*	Smooth flatsedge	Cyperaceae		Controls Blood sugar
100.	*Cyperus rotundus*	Papyrus sedges,	Cyperaceae		
101.	*Dendrocalamus hamiltonii*	Hamilton's bamboo	Poaceae		
102.	*Desmodium gangeticum*	salparni	Fabaceae		
103.	*Desmostachya bipinnata*	halfa grass	Poaceae		Controls Blood sugar
104.	*Dillenia indica*	Elephant Apple	Dilleniaceae		Inhibitors of glycemic enzyme
105.	*Dioscorea opposita*	Chinese yam	Dioscoreaceae		Inhibitors of glycemic enzyme
106.	*Diospyros melanoxylon*	Coromandel ebony	Ebenaceae		Inhibitors of glycemic enzyme
107.	*Diospyros peregrina*	Indian persimon,	Ebenaceae.		Inhibitors of glycemic enzyme
108.	*Diplazium esculentum*	Fiddlehead fern	Athyriaceae		
109.	*Eclipta alba*	False daisy	Asteraceae		α-glucosidase inhibitor
110.	*Elaeocarpus ganitrus*	Blueberry beads"	Elaeocarpaceae		
111.	*Elephantopus scaber*	Elephant's Foot	Asteraceae		
112.	*Embelia ribes*	False black pepper	Primulaceae		
113.	*Emblica officinalis*	Indian gooseberry	Phyllanthaceae		
114.	*Enhydra fluctuans*	Helencha or harkuch	Asteraceae		
115.	*Enicostema axillare*	Indian Whitehead	Gentianaceae		Controls Blood sugar
116.	*Erythrina indica*	Indian coral tree	Fabaceae		Inhibitors of glycemic enzyme
117.	*Erythrina variegeta*	Indian coral tree	Fabaceae		Inhibitors of glycemic enzyme
118.	*Eucalyptus citriodora*	Lemon - scented Gum	Myrtaceae		Inhibitors of glycemic enzyme
119.	*Eugenia jambolana*	Jamun	Myrtaceae		α-amylase inhibitor
120.	*Eugenia polyantha*	Indian bay-leaf	Myrtaceae		
121.	*Euphorbia caducifolia*	Leafless milk hedge	Euphorbiaceae		

Table 1. (Continued)

Sl No.	Plant Species	Common name	Family	Phytochemical properties	Activity
122.	*Euphorbia drumondii*	Caustic weed	Euphorbiaceae		Hyperglycemic
123.	*Euphorbia hirta*	Asthma Weed	Euphorbiaceae	quercetin, quercitrin, quercitol, Triterpenoid,	Decrease in blood glucose level, α-glucosidase activity
124.	*Euphorbia ligularia*	Indian spurge	Euphorbiaceae		Inhibitors of glycemic enzyme
125.	*Feronia limonia*	wood-apple	Rutaceae		Inhibitors of glycemic enzyme
126.	*Ferula assa-foetida*	Asafoetida	Apiaceae		
127.	*Ficus amplissima*	Indian Bat tree	Moraceae		Controls Blood sugar
128.	*Ficus benghalensis*	Banyan	Moraceae		Controls Blood sugar
129.	*Ficus carica*	Common fig	Moraceae		
130.	*Ficus cunia*	Drooping fig	Moraceae		α-glucosidase inhibitor
131.	*Ficus glomerata*	Cluster fig tree	Moraceae		
132.	*Ficus racemosa*	Cluster fig	Moraceae		Antihyperglycemic, hypoglycemic, α-glucosidase and α-amylase inhibitor
133.	*Ficus religiosa*	peepal tree	Moraceae		
134.	*Ficus virens*	white fig	Moraceae		
135.	*Gloriosa superba*	Gloriosa lily	Colchicaceae		Controls Blood sugar
136.	*Glycosmis pentaphylla*	Gin berry	Rutaceae		Controls Blood sugar
137.	*Glycyrrhiza glabra*	Liquorice	Fabaceae		Controls Blood sugar
138.	*Glycyrrhiza uralensis*	Chinese liquorice	Fabaceae		Controls Blood sugar
139.	*Gmelina arborea*	Beechwood	Lamiaceae		Controls Blood sugar
140.	*Grewia asiatica*	Phalsa	Malvaceae		Controls Blood sugar
141.	*Grewia hirsuta*	Nagabala	Malvaceae		Controls Blood sugar
142.	*Gymnema sylvestre*	Australian cowplant	Apocynaceae	Triterpene saponins	Stimulation in insulin secretion from the pancreas
143.	*Heinsia crinata*	Bush apple	Rubiaceae		Stimulate in insulin secretion
144.	*Helicteres isora*	Marodphali	Malvaceae		Stimulate in insulin secretion

Sl No.	Plant Species	Common name	Family	Phytochemical properties	Activity
145.	*Hemidesmus indicus*	Indian sarsaparilla	Apocynaceae		Stimulate in insulin secretion
146.	*Heritiera fomes*	Sunder	Malvaceae		Stimulate in insulin secretion
147.	*Holarrhena antidysenterica*	Kutaja	Apocynaceae		Inhibitors of glycemic enzyme
148.	*Hydnocarpus wightiana*	Chaulmoogra	Achariaceae		Inhibitors of glycemic enzyme
149.	*Ichnocarpus frutescens*	Black creeper	Apocynaceae		Inhibitors of glycemic enzyme
150.	*Imperata cylindrica*	Cogongrass	Poaceae		Stimulate in insulin secretion
151.	*Lactuca gracilis*	Lettuce	Asteraceae		Stimulate in insulin secretion
152.	*Lagenaria sicereria*	Calabash gourd	Cucurbitaceae		Stimulate in insulin secretion
153.	*Leucas aspera*	Thumbai	Lamiaceae		Controls Blood sugar
154.	*Leucas cephalotes*	Goma	Lamiaceae		Stimulate in insulin secretion
155.	*Linum usitatisumum*	Flax	Linaceae		Stimulate in insulin secretion
156.	*Luffa echinata*	Ghagarabela	Cucurbitaceae		Stimulate in insulin secretion
157.	*Mangifera indica*	Mango	Anacardiaceae		Antidiabetic, α-amylase inhibitor, antihyperlipidemic effect, hypoglycemic
158.	*Melia dubia*	Malabar Neem	Meliaceae		
159.	*Melothria maderaspatana*	Mukia Maderaspatana	Cucurbitaceae		
160.	*Mentha longifolia*	Horsemint	Lamiaceae		Inhibitors of glycemic enzyme
161.	*Mentha arvensis*	Corn Mint	Lamiaceae		Inhibitors of glycemic enzyme
162.	*Meyna laxiflora*	Muyna	Rubiaceae		Inhibitors of glycemic enzyme
163.	*Millingtonia hortensis*	Indian Cork-Tree	Bignoniaceae		Inhibitors of glycemic enzyme
164.	*Mimusops elengi*	Spanish Cherry	Sapotaceae		
165.	*Momordica charantia*	Bitter Melon	Cucurbitaceae	Charantine, charine, momordicin, momordin, cucurbitins, cucurbitacins momorcharins	Insulin secretion and glycogen synthesis
166.	*Moringa oleifera*	Drumstick tree	Moringaceae		Hypoglycemic

Table 1. (Continued)

Sl No.	Plant Species	Common name	Family	Phytochemical properties	Activity
167.	*Morus alba*	White mulberry	Moraceae		inhibition of antidiabetic, hypoglycemic, α-glucosidase and α-amylase inhibition
168.	*Mucuna gigantea*	Burny bean	Fabaceae		Stimulate in insulin secretion
169.	*Mucuna pruriens*	Velvet bean	Fabaceae		Stimulate in insulin secretion
170.	*Mukia maderaspatana*	Madras pea pumpkin	Cucurbitaceae		Stimulate in insulin secretion
171.	*Murraya koenigii*	Cucumis maderaspatanus	Rutaceae		
172.	*Murraya koenigii*	Curry Leaf Tree	Rutaceae		α amylase inhibitor, hypoglycemic effects, antihyperglycemic
173.	*Musa Sapientum*	Common banana	Musaceae		Antihyperglycemic
174.	*Musa Sapientum*				Antihyperglycemic
175.	*Nelumbo nucifera*	Sacred lotus	Nelumbonaceae		α-glucosidase, α-amylase inhibitor
176.	*Nicotiana plumbaginifolia*	Tex-mex tobacco	Solanaceae		
177.	*Nigella sativa*	black cumin	Ranunculaceae		
178.	*Nycantus arbor-tristis*	Night Blooming Jasmine	Oleaceae		Hypoglycemic
179.	*Nymphaea nouchali*	Blue lotus	Nymphaeaceae		
180.	*Nymphaea stellata*	Indian blue water lily	Nymphaeaceae		α-glucosidase inhibitor, hypoglycemic, antihyperglycemic
181.	*Ocimum sanctum*	Tulsi	Lamiaceae	Triterpenoid, eugenol, methyleugenol, and p-caryophylen	Hypoglycemic

Sl No.	Plant Species	Common name	Family	Phytochemical properties	Activity
182.	*Ocimum tenuiflorum*	holy basil	Lamiaceae		α-amylase inhibitor, hypoglycemic, antihyperglycemic
183.	*Odina wodier*	Oodi mara	Anacardiaceae		
184.	*Opuntia ficus-indica*	Prickly pear	Cactaceae		Controls Blood sugar
185.	*Oreocnide integrifolia*	Wild Rhea	Urticaceae		
186.	*Origanum vulgare*	Oregano	Lamiaceae		
187.	*Oroxylum indicum*	Indian trumpet flower	Bignoniaceae		
188.	*Oxalis corniculata*	creeping woodsorrel	Oxalidaceae		Inhibitors of glycemic enzyme
189.	*Oxalis griffithii*	Wood sorrel	Oxalidaceae		Inhibitors of glycemic enzyme
190.	*Paederia scandens*	Gandheli	Rubiaceae		
191.	*Panax ginseng*	Korean ginseng	Araliaceae	Ginsenosides-terpene glycosides, saponins, naxans, vanillic acid, and salicylates.	Improving insulin resistance, improving glucose uptake, decreasing blood glucose concentration, and protecting/regeneratingβ-cell from pancreatic islets
192.	*Pandanus fascicularis*	Fragrant screw-pine	Pandanaceae		Antihyperglycemic
193.	*Paspalum scrobiculatum*	Kodo millet	Poaceae		
194.	*Passiflora nitida*	Bell apple	Passifloraceae		
195.	*Pavonia zeylanica*	Ceylon leadwort	Plumbaginaceae		
196.	*Pergularia daemia*	Trellis-vine	Apocynaceae		Controls Blood sugar
197.	*Persea americana*	Avocado	Lauraceae		
198.	*Persea americana*				
199.	*Peucedanum praeruptorum*	Qian Hu	Apiaceae		
200.	*Phaseolus vulgaris*	Wild bean	Leguminosae		
201.	*Phoenix dactylifera*	date palm	Arecaceae		Inhibitors of glycemic enzyme

Table 1. (Continued)

Sl No.	Plant Species	Common name	Family	Phytochemical properties	Activity
202.	*Phyllanthus amarus*	Carry Me Seed	Phyllanthaceae		α-glucosidase inhibitor, hypoglycemic, α-amylase inhibitor
203.	*Phyllanthus emblica*	Indian gooseberry	Phyllanthaceae		Controls Blood sugar
204.	*Phyllanthus niruri*	gale of the wind	Euphorbiaceae		Controls Blood sugar
205.	*Phyllanthus niruri*				Controls Blood sugar
206.	*Physalis angulata*	Cutleaf groundcherry	Solanaceae		Controls Blood sugar
207.	*Physalis minima*	Bladder Cherry	Solanaceae		Controls Blood sugar
208.	*Physalis peruviana*	Cape gooseberry	Solanaceae		
209.	*Picralima nitida*	Akuamma	Apocynaceae		
210.	*Pimpinella tirupatiensis*	Saunf	Apiaceae		
211.	*Piper longum*	Indian Long Pepper	Piperaceae		
212.	*Piper longum*				Antihyperglycemic
213.	*Pisonia grandis*	Lettuce Tree	Nyctaginaceae		
214.	*Plantago ovata*	Psyllium	Plantaginaceae		
215.	*Plumbago zeylanica*	Ceylon leadwort	Plumbaginaceae		
216.	*Plumeria rubra*	Frangipani	Apocynaceae		α-amylase and α-glucosidase inhibitor
217.	*Polyalthia longifolia*	The false ashoka	Annonaceae		Antidiabetic
218.	*Polygonum hydropiper*	Marshpepper knotweed	Polygonaceae		Stimulate in insulin secretion
219.	*Pongamia pinnata*	Malapari or Karanja tree	Fabaceae		Stimulate in insulin secretion
220.	*Portulaca oleracea*	Common purslane	Portulacaceae		Stimulate in insulin secretion
221.	*Premna integrifolia*	Wind killer	Lamiaceae		Hypoglycemic
222.	*Prunus persica*	Peach	Rosaceae		

Sl No.	Plant Species	Common name	Family	Phytochemical properties	Activity
223.	*Psoralea corylifolia*	Babchi	Fabaceae		
224.	*Pterocarpus marsupium*	Piyasal	Fabaceae	Phenol and flavonoid	Lowering the glucose level, Regenerating b-cells of the pancreas islet
225.	*Pterocarpus santalinus*	Red Sandal wood	Fabaceae		
226.	*Punica granatum*	Red Sanders	Fabaceae		
227.	*Rheum emodi*	Pomegranate	Punicaceae		
228.	*Roylea cinerea*	Rhubarb	Polygonaceae		Controls Blood sugar
229.	*Rubia cordifolia*	Ashy Roylea	Lamiaceae		Controls Blood sugar
230.	*Saccharum spontaneum*	Indian madder	Rubiaceae		
231.	*Salacia chinensis*	Wild sugarcane	Poaceae		Hypoglycemic, antihyperglycaemic
232.	*Salacia oblonga*	Akan	Celastraceae		
233.	*Salacia prinoides*	Ponkoranti	Celastraceae		
234.	*Salacia reticulata*	Lolly berry	Celastraceae		Hypoglycemic, α-glucosidase inhibitor
235.	*Sesbenia aegyptiaca*	Kothala himbutu	Celastraceae		Hypoglycemic
236.	*Sida acuta*		Fabaceae		
237.	*Sida cordifolia*	Common wireweed	Malvaceae		
238.	*Solanum indicum*	Flannel weed	Malvaceae		Controls Blood sugar
239.	*Solanum trilobatum*	African egg plant	Solanaceae		Controls Blood sugar
240.	*Solanum viarum*	Red pea	Solanaceae		Controls Blood sugar
241.	*Sonchus oleraceus*	Tropical soda apple	Solanaceae		
242.	*Sphaeranthus indicus*	Common sowthistle	Asteraceae		Inhibitors of glycemic enzyme
243.	*Stereospermum suaveolens*	East Indian globe thistle	Asteraceae		Inhibitors of glycemic enzyme
244.	*Stevia rebaudiana*	Patala	Bignoniaceae		
245.	*Swertia chirayita*	Sweetleaf	Asteraceae		

Table 1. (Continued)

Sl No.	Plant Species	Common name	Family	Phytochemical properties	Activity
246.	*Syzygium cumini*	Chiretta	Gentianaceae		α-glucosidase and α-amylase inhibitor, antihyperglycemic
247.	*Syzygium densiflorum*	Java Plum	Myrtaceae		
248.	*Syzygium jambolana*	Java Plum	Myrtaceae		
249.	*Syzygium jambolanum*	Jamun	Myrtaceae		Inhibitors of glycemic enzyme
250.	*Tabernaemontana divaricate*	Jamun	Myrtaceae		Inhibitors of glycemic enzyme
251.	*Tamarindus indica*	Pinwheel	Apocynaceae		
252.	*Tamarindus indica*	tamarind	Fabaceae		α amylase inhibitor
253.	*Taxus baccata*	English yew	Taxaceae		
254.	*Tephrosia purpurea*	wild indigo	Fabaceae		Antihyperglycemic
255.	*Terminalia arjuna*	arjun tree	Combretaceae		α-amylase inhibitor
256.	*Terminalia bellirica*	baheda	Combretaceae		
257.	*Terminalia catappa*	Indian almond	Combretaceae		
258.	*Terminalia chebula*	Haritaki	Combretaceae		α-amylase inhibitor
259.	*Thespesia populnea*	Indian tulip tree	Malvaceae.		Antihyperglycemic
260.	*Tinospora cordifolia*	Amrita or Guduchi	Menispermaceae	Berberine	α-amylase inhibitors
261.	*Tinospora crispa*	Petawali	Menispermaceae	Alkaloids, flavonoid, terpenoids, Lignan, sterols	Antihyperglycemic
262.	*Tinospora sinensis*	Malabar Gulbel	Menispermaceae		Inhibition of α-glucosidase activity
263.	*Tragia involucrata*	Indian stinging nettle	Euphorbiaceae		Antihyperglycemic
264.	*Trichosanthes cucumerina*	Snake Gourd	Cucurbitaceae		
265.	*Trichosanthes dioica*	Pointed gourd	Cucurbitaceae		
266.	*Trigonella foenum-graecum*	Fenugreek	Fabaceae	Trigonelline	Regeneration of pancreatic β cells and insulin secretion

Sl No.	Plant Species	Common name	Family	Phytochemical properties	Activity
267.	*Vaccinium arctostaphylos*	European blueberry	Ericaceae		
268.	*Vernonia amygdalina*	bitter leaf	Asteraceae		
269.	*Viola odorata*	wood violet	Violaceae		
270.	*Vitex negundo Linn*	Chinese chaste tree	Lamiaceae		
271.	*Wedelia trilobata*	Yellow Creeping Daisy	Asteraceae		Inhibitors of glycemic enzyme
272.	*Withania coagulans*	Panir ke phool or Indian cheese maker	Solanaceae		Inhibitors of glycemic enzyme
273.	*Withania somnifera*	Ashwagandha	Solanaceae	alkaloids and steroidal compounds, including ergostane	Inhibitors of glycemic enzyme
274.	*Witheringia solanacea*		Solanaceae		Inhibitors of glycemic enzyme
275.	*Zaleya decandra*	Many Stamen Horse Purslane	Aizoaceae		Antidiabetic effect
276.	*Zanthoxylum armatum*	Winged Prickly Ash	Rutaceae	Tambulin, linalool, limonene and lignan	Antidiabetic effect
277.	*Zanthoxylum humile*	Winter Hardy Japanese Pepper	Rutaceae	alkaloids, coumarins, flavonoids, glycosides, saponins and terpenoids	Antidiabetic effect
278.	*Zingiber officinale*	Ginger	Zingiberaceae	Terpenoid	Lower blood glucose concentration
279.	*Ziziphus nummularia*	wild jujube or jhahrberi	Rhamnaceae	alkaloids, especially nummularine M, flavonoids, saponins, glycosides, tannins, and phenolic compounds	Stimulate in insulin secretion
280.	*Ziziphus xylopyrus*	Kath Ber	Rhamnaceae	glycosides, saponins, sterol, flavonoids, phenolic compounds, and triterpenoids	Stimulate in insulin secretion
281.	*Zizyphus mauritiana*	Indian jujube	Rhamnaceae	Vitamin C, phenolics, flavonoids, and triterpenic acids.	Stimulate in insulin secretion

Management of diabetes requires optimal medication, a suitable diet, and physical activity. The most essential step in controlling diabetes is to control the glucose level. Furthermore, diabetes can be kept under control by managing the associated consequences and modifying its risk factors.

The most common medication for diabetes is insulin, particularly in type 1 diabetes. Other treatment includes the administration of insulin, amylin, GLP-1, insulin secretagogues (repaglinide, sulfonylureas, nateglinide, etc.), biguanides, α-glucosidase inhibitors, thiazolidinediones, and dipeptidyl peptidase-4 (DPP-4) inhibitors (Subramoniam, 2016).

The main classes of contemporary pharmaceuticals used worldwide are biguanides (metformin), thiazolidinediones (glitazones), sulfonylureas, DPP-4 inhibitors, meglitinides (glinides) and α-glucosidase inhibitors (Sekhon-Loodu & Rupasinghe, 2019; Willcox et al., 2021). These are taken orally to manage blood glucose levels. In addition, insulin and insulin mimetics are two injectable drugs. However, these drugs have several undesirable side effects that lead to major medical complications during medication processing.

The metformin used in the drug prevents the synthesis of glucose molecules and increases insulin sensitivity. However, in the early stages, it has significant adverse effects such as nausea, dyspepsia, and diarrhoea. Persons with compromised heart and/or liver disease, impaired renal function, or other serious medical conditions should avoid receiving metformin treatment. Thiazolidinediones are useful in diabetes therapy because they enhance insulin sensitivity, reduce insulin resistance, while their most common side effects are weight gain and fluid retention, which can lead to peripheral edoema and heart failure. The drugs were not prescribed to people with similar conditions, such as heart failure or serious liver disease. Rosiglitazone has been associated with an increase in the risk of heart attack. Due to the increased risk of bladder cancer, pioglitazone is not accessible in several countries (Tran et al., 2020).

Nature is the main resource for most medicinal agents. Despite significant advances in synthetic drug chemistry and antibiotics, plants remain a crucial raw material for drugs that cure a variety of human diseases (Grover et al., 2002; Jain et al., 2019). In fact, the Indian medicinal plant has various antidiabetic properties that are described in Table 1 (Gaonkar & Hullatti, 2020; Maurya et al., 2021; Salehi et al., 2019).

Phytocompounds and Diabetes

Phytocompounds are well known to play a crucial role in plant sciences with the source of active pharmaceutical ingredients (Stadlbauer et al., 2016). In recent decades, the traditional medical system has become a topic of global concern. Several species of plants are considered for their therapeutic applications. The use of plants and their extracts established the foundation for current medicinal chemistry, allowing man to develop empirical drug development. In the literature, there are several species that have hypoglycemic action. Most of these plants produce bioactive substances including glycosides, alkaloids, terpenes, flavonoid, carotene, etc., which are frequently associated with an antidiabetic impact. Plant species that have potential as antidiabetics will be listed chronologically in this section (Salehi et al., 2019; Sharma et al., 2020) (Figures 1-4).

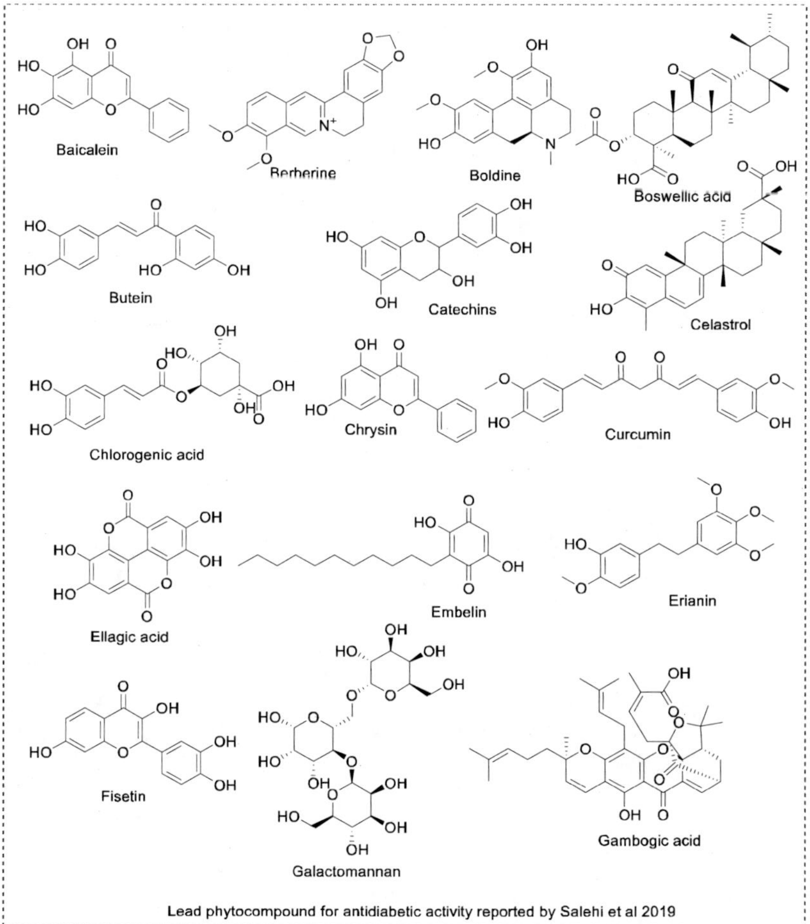

Figure 1.

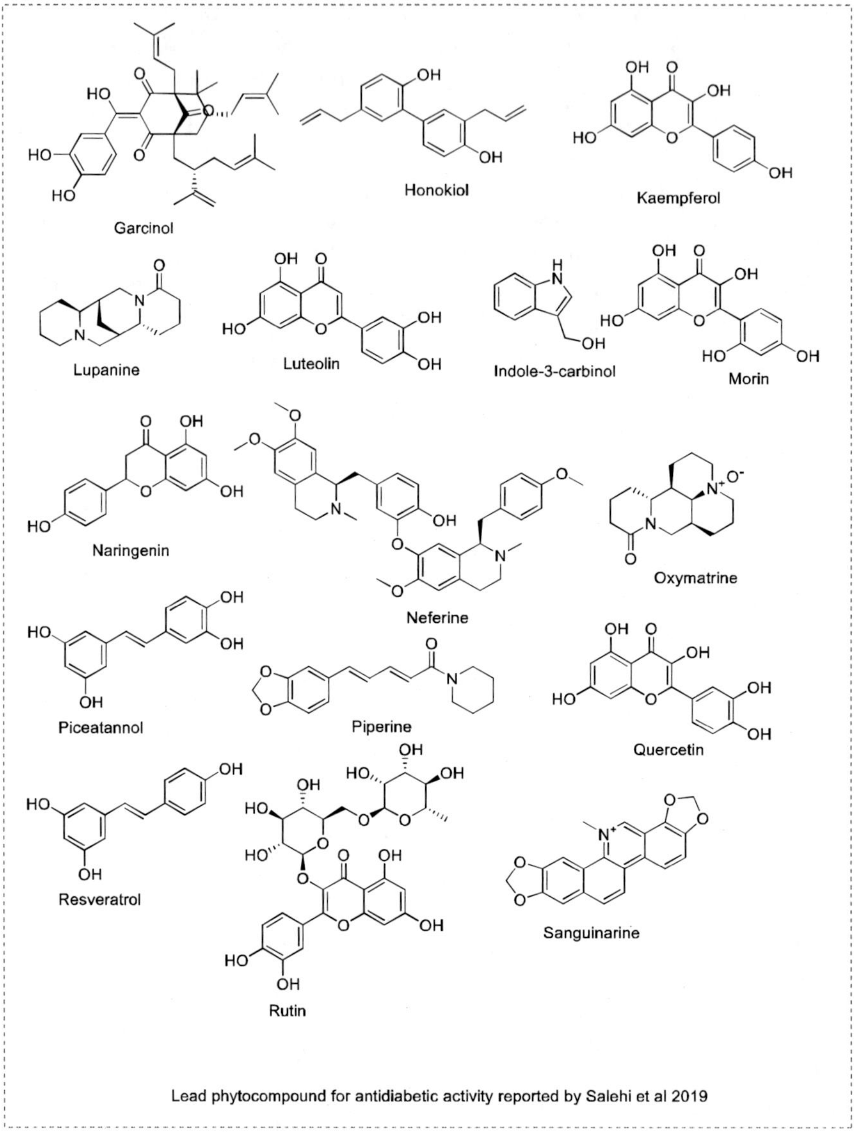
Garcinol
Honokiol
Kaempferol
Lupanine
Luteolin
Indole-3-carbinol
Morin
Naringenin
Neferine
Oxymatrine
Piceatannol
Piperine
Quercetin
Resveratrol
Rutin
Sanguinarine
Lead phytocompound for antidiabetic activity reported by Salehi et al 2019

Figure 2.

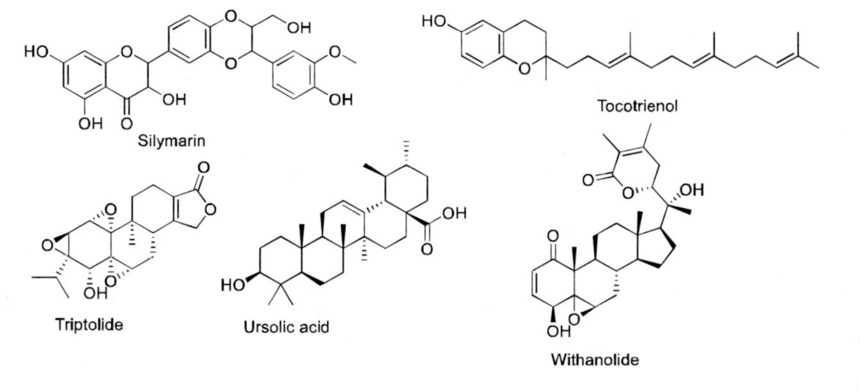

Lead phytocompound for antidiabetic activity reported by Salehi et al 2019

Figure 3.

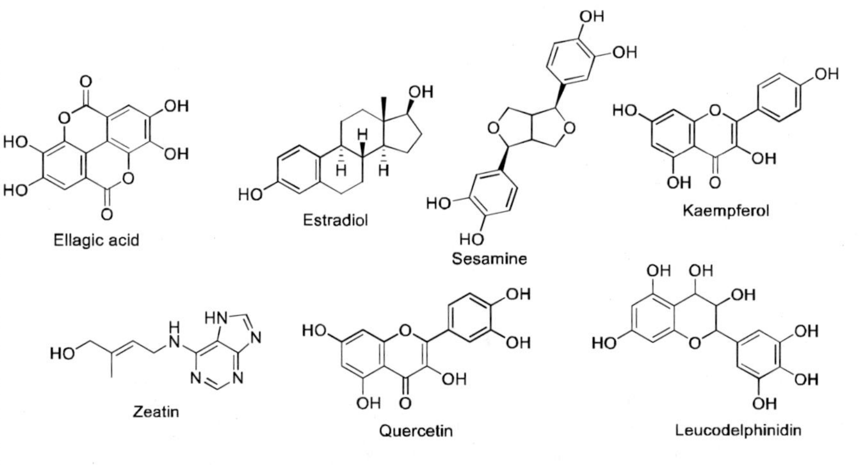

Lead phytocompound from *Phyllanthus emblica* against type 2 diabetes reported by Sharma et al 2020

Figure 4.

Figure 1-4. Leading phytocompounds for antidiabetic activities.

Conclusion

Evaluation of plant-based products that could treat diabetes mellitus due to their abundance of bioactive compounds with therapeutic potential. Using animal research, several investigators have recently reported on the antidiabetic properties of traditionally exploited Indian medicinal plants. Some more Indian medicinal plants are still to be explored, although many medicinal plants have already been evaluated for their anti-diabetic properties. Most of the medications used in the medicinal plant are said to have no side effects. Therefore, the drug developed from plants for the treatment of diabetes is an alternative option.

References

Alam, S., Sarker, M. M. R., Sultana, T. N., Chowdhury, M. N. R., Rashid, M. A., Chaity, N. I., Zhao, C., Xiao, J., Hafez, E. E., Khan, S. A. and Mohamed, I. N., 2022. Antidiabetic phytochemicals from medicinal plants: prospective candidates for the discovery and development. *Frontiers in endocrinology*, *13*.

Gaonkar, V. P. and Hullatti, K., 2020. Indian Traditional medicinal plants as a source of potent Anti-diabetic agents: A Review. *Journal of diabetes & metabolic disorders*, *19*, pp.1895-1908.

Grover, J. K., Yadav, S. and Vats, V., 2002. Medicinal plants of India with anti-diabetic potential. *Journal of ethnopharmacology*, *81*(1), pp. 81-100.

Jain, C., Khatana, S. and Vijayvergia, R., 2019. Bioactivity of secondary metabolites of various plants: a review. *Int. J. Pharm. Sci. Res*, *10*(2), pp. 494-504.

Kayarohanam, S. and Kavimani, S., 2015. Current trends of plants having antidiabetic activity: a review. *Journal of Bioanalysis & Biomedicine*, *7*(2), p. 55.

Kumar, A., Aswal, S., Semwal, R. B., Chauhan, A., Joshi, S. K. and Semwal, D. K., 2019. Role of plant-derived alkaloids against diabetes and diabetes-related complications: a mechanism-based approach. *Phytochemistry Reviews*, *18*, pp. 1277-1298.

Maurya, A., Mohan, S. and Verma, S. C., 2021. Antidiabetic potential of naturally occurring sesquiterpenes: A review. *Current Topics in Medicinal Chemistry*, *21*(10), pp. 851-862.

Patil, R., Patil, R., Ahirwar, B. and Ahirwar, D., 2011. Current status of Indian medicinal plants with antidiabetic potential: a review. *Asian Pacific Journal of Tropical Biomedicine*, *1*(2), pp. S291-S298.

Saeedi, P., Petersohn, I., Salpea, P., Malanda, B., Karuranga, S., Unwin, N., Colagiuri, S., Guariguata, L., Motala, A. A., Ogurtsova, K. and Shaw, J. E., 2019. Global and regional diabetes prevalence estimates for 2019 and projections for 2030 and 2045: Results from the International Diabetes Federation Diabetes Atlas. *Diabetes research and clinical practice*, *157*, p. 107843.

Salehi, B., Ata, A., V. Anil Kumar, N., Sharopov, F., Ramirez-Alarcon, K., Ruiz-Ortega, A., Abdulmajid Ayatollahi, S., Valere Tsouh Fokou, P., Kobarfard, F., Amiruddin Zakaria, Z. and Iriti, M., 2019. Antidiabetic potential of medicinal plants and their active components. *Biomolecules*, *9*(10), p. 551.

Sekhon-Loodu, S. and Rupasinghe, H. V., 2019. Evaluation of antioxidant, antidiabetic and antiobesity potential of selected traditional medicinal plants. *Frontiers in nutrition*, *6*, p. 53.

Sharma, P., Joshi, T., Joshi, T., Chandra, S. and Tamta, S., 2020. In silico screening of potential antidiabetic phytochemicals from Phyllanthus emblica against therapeutic targets of type 2 diabetes. *Journal of ethnopharmacology*, *248*, p. 112268.

Stadlbauer, V., Haselgrübler, R., Lanzerstorfer, P., Plochberger, B., Borgmann, D., Jacak, J., Winkler, S. M., Schröder, K., Höglinger, O. and Weghuber, J., 2016. Biomolecular characterization of putative antidiabetic herbal extracts. *PloS one*, *11*(1), p. e0148109.

Subramoniam, A., 2016. *Anti-Diabetes Mellitus Plants*. CRC Press.

Tran, N., Pham, B. and Le, L., 2020. Bioactive compounds in anti-diabetic plants: From herbal medicine to modern drug discovery. *Biology*, *9*(9), p. 252.

Willcox, M. L., Elugbaju, C., Al-Anbaki, M., Lown, M. and Graz, B., 2021. Effectiveness of medicinal plants for glycaemic control in type 2 diabetes: an overview of meta-analyses of clinical trials. *Frontiers in Pharmacology*, p. 3402.

Chapter 2

The Medicinal Herbs of Indian Origin Used to Cure Diabetes: A Review

Lakkoju Babi[1]
Nambaaru Sailaja[1]
Gundla Rambabu[2]
and Kolli Balakrishna[1,*]
[1]Department of Chemistry, GITAM (Deemed to be University), Visakhapatnam, India
[2]Department of Chemistry, GITAM (Deemed to be University), Hyderabad, India

Abstract

The term 'medicinal herbs' refers to plants with healing properties due to the ashraf of phyto chemicals. The therapeutic activities of plants were described and explained in Indian mythological history as part of Ayurveda. The Indian territory is the source of several. Due to changes in the lifestyle of modern society's lifestyle, many people today suffer from chronic diseases. Diabetes is a significant metabolic disease and it can be treated with several commercially available drugs. However, these over-the-counter medications are expensive and have several risks. Due to their low cost and less side effects, herbal medications are more attractive. The reports available on plants used as drugs to treat diabetes problems are included in the current review.

Keywords: India, medicinal plant, anti-diabetic, hyperglycemia, glucose

---

* Corresponding Author's Emails: kollibalakrishna@gmail.com and rgundla@gmail.com.

In: Antidiabetic Plants
Editor: Arpita Roy
ISBN: 979-8-88697-957-2

Introduction

The use of herbal medicines has increased dramatically in modern times and becoming increasingly popular throughout the world because they are made from natural sources and have minimal side effects. Many old-style drugs still in use are based on medicinal plants (Grover et al., 2002). Several medicinal plants have been discovered and used in traditional healthcare systems for over a million years (Scartezzini and Speroni, 2000). Worldwide, thousands of plants are used for therapeutic resolutions, according to the WHO.

India is the world's largest producer of healing herbs and is known as the 'botanical garden' (Seth and Sharma, 2004). This chapter concentrates on the herbal plants that are used in the treatment of diabetes, which causes great financial losses.

Diabates and Its Implication

Diabetes is defined as a cluster of metabolic illnesses with numerous underlying causes that is defined by persistent hyperglycemia (high blood sugar level) and altered the carbohydrates, fats and proteins metabolism as a result hitches with secretion of insulin and their action or both (W.H.O., 1999). This disease has some symptoms such as frequent urination. Diabetes causes numerous medical problems if not treated (Kitabchi, 2009).

Diabetes is classified into different types (ADA, 2019; Heise et al., 2004; Faselis et al., 2020; McIntyre et al., 2019). When insulin-producing cells in the pancreas are damaged, the pancreas cannot produce insulin, leading to type 1 diabetes which is found primarily in adults (Atkinson et al., 2014). Insulin-dependent diabetes is another name for Type 2 diabetes. In this situation, the body cannot adequately utilise the created insulin (Olokoba et al., 2012). Gestational diabetes is a type of glucose bias that manifests itself for the first time during the second or third trimester of pregnancy (Buchanan and Xiang, 2005).

Drugs and Its Negative Effects

Regardless of the availability of well-known anti-diabetic medications on the market, diabetes and its consequences remain a serious medical problem.

Table 1 lists some of the anti-diabetic medications, as well as their few side effects, physiological action, and benefits. Current diabetes medications aim to monitor and drop blood glucose levels in vessels to standard levels. However, most contemporary drugs have numerous cross-effects that can result in serious medical problems during treatment. Recent studies have shown that several newly discovered bioactive plant chemicals have greater anti-diabetic efficacy than oral hypoglycemic medications. Traditional medicine has a promising future in the treatment of diabetes due to its high clinical repetition.

Table 1. Glucose lowering agents used to treatment of diabetes and their effects (Babiker and Al Dubayee, 2017; Inzucchi et al., 2012)

Class	Compound	Physiological Action	Benefits	Side Effect/ Disadvantages
Biguanides	Metformin	Lowering Hepatic glucose production	Probability of a decrease in cardiovascular disease events	Gastrointestinal side effects
Meglitinides (glinides)	Repaglinide Nateglinide	Increases the Insulin secretion	Decreases Postprandial glucose excursions	Hyperglycemia
Thiazolidinediones	Pioglitazone Rosiglitazone	Increases Insulin sensitivity	Decrease Triacylglycerols	Weight gain
Bile acid sequestrants	Colesevelam	Decreases Hepatic glucose production	No hypoglycemia decreases	increases triacylglycerols

Natural Herbs of Indian Origin for Curing Diabetes

Medicinal plant parts are still used to treat a wide range of diseases. These are used as active therapeutic components by a wide range of civilizations. Alternative and complementary medicine is a viable option for treating illness due to its convenience, lower price and lack of side effects. Many active compounds found in medicinal plants are effective in treating a variety of diseases, including diabetes (Figure 1). In the present chapter, we discuss some Indian-originated medicinal plants and their anti-diabetic activity in this chapter.

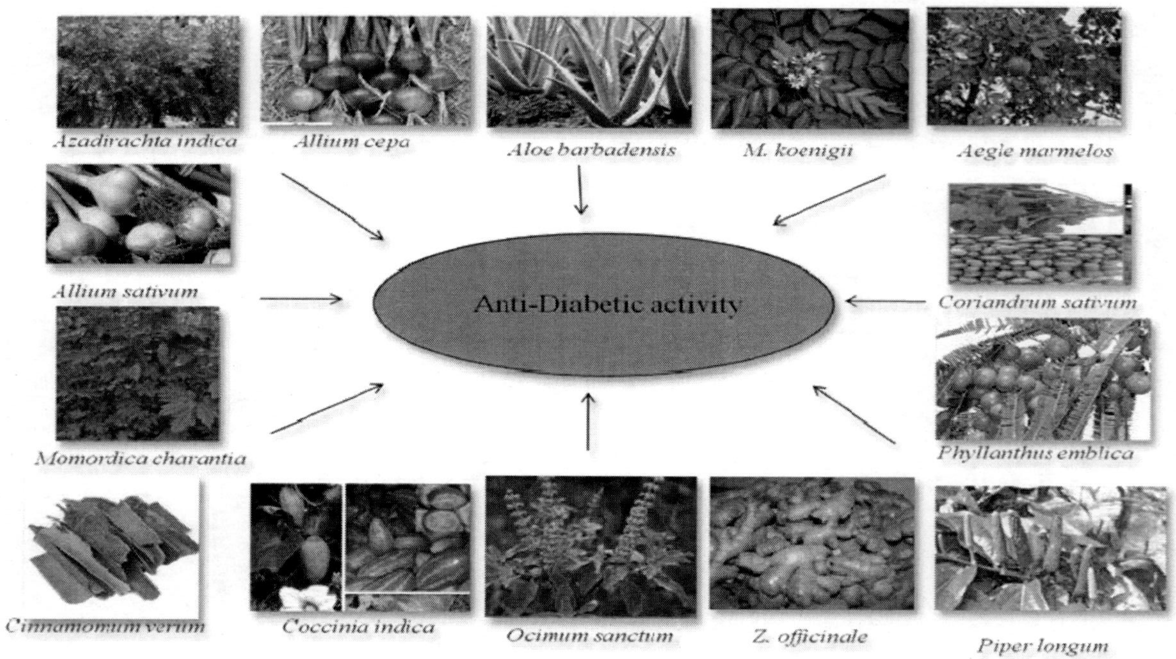
Azadirachta indica
Allium cepa
Aloe barbadensis
M. koenigii
Aegle marmelos
Allium sativum
Anti-Diabetic activity
Coriandrum sativum
Momordica charantia
Phyllanthus emblica
Cinnamomum verum
Coccinia indica
Ocimum sanctum
Z. officinale
Piper longum

Figure 1. Medicinal plants with anti-diabetic activity.

Neem (*Azadirachta Indica*)

It is a popular anti-diabetic plant with hypolipidemic, hypoglycemic, immunostimulant and hepatoprotective properties (Khosla et al., 2000). In streptozotocin-treated rats, the hydroalcoholic extracts of the neem exhibited antihyperglycemic activity because they enhanced adsorption of glucose and glycogenosis in rat hemidiaphragm (Manisha et al., 2007). Extracts of neem leaves have been observed to reduce blood glucose levels, which may be related to epinephrine that inhibits glycogenolysis and peripheral glucose utilisation (Chattopadhyay et al., 1993). The hypoglycemic activity of pure ethanolic Neem extract was compared to glimepiride in both AIDR and glucose loaded diabetic rats. In comparison to the comparable diabetic control group, *Azadirachta indica* leaf extract reduced elevated blood sugar levels (BSL) by 30.20% in AIDR (alloxan-induced diabetic rats) and by 36.91% in rats given a glucose load. This study strongly suggested that *Azadirachta indica* ethanol leaf extracts have significant anti-diabetic activity (Akter et al., 2013). In diabetic rabbits, a dose of leaf extract instigated hypoglycaemic effect 72 hours after administration, with persistence of up to 24 hours (Akhtar et al., 2011).

Onion (*Allium Cepa*)

Every country consumes plants of this genus at least once a week. The plant bulb, which contains an active ingredient known as allyl propyl disulphide, can help to prevent insulin breakdown (APDS). *Allium cepa* Linn. belongs to the Liliaceae family, which contains the onion. It can withstand harsh conditions and be stored for an extended period of time without losing biologically active compounds present within it. In diabetic rabbits, various ether insoluble and soluble fractions of dried onion powder exhibit anti-hyperglycemic activity (Mathew and Augusti, 1975). S-methyl cysteine sulphoxide was administered to AIDR and dramatically reduced blood sugar (Roman-Ramos et al., 1995; Kumari et al., 1995). S-methyl cysteine sulfoxide, a phytochemical found in onions, stimulates insulin production in the body and increases pancreatic secretion, allowing insulin to be used more effectively and interfering with dietary glucose absorption (Kumari et al., 2002).

Aloe-Vera (*Aloe Barbadensis Miller*)

Historically, various diseases have been treated using Aloe vera as a cure. This plant's main products are gel and latex. In both diabetic and normal rats, aloe gum extracts effectively improved glucose tolerance (Al-Awadi and Gumaa, 1987). *Aloe barbadensis* leaf exudates had a hypoglycaemic effect on diabetic rats that had been alloxanized, but not when given in a single dose. By promoting the production and release of insulin from pancreatic beta cells, aloe vera and its bitter component have therapeutic effects (Ajabnoor, 1990). The effects of aloe vera extract on diabetic mice and mice produced by embryonic stem cells were investigated. BSL decreased significantly after taking the everyday (Kumar et al., 2011).

Garlic (*Allium Sativum L.)*

This is a perennial herb that is grown throughout India and is originally from Asia (Singh and Kumar, 2017). Garlic is well known for having a significant amount of sulphur amino acids other than proteins, which are the source of its therapeutic activities (Ovesna et al., 2015). According to various scientific study findings, Garlic has a diverse range of biological activities, particularly antihyperglycemic, antitumour, and antibacterial activities (Batiha et al., 2020). The sulphur-containing allicin is responsible for the pungent odour. Its extract has been found to be superior to prescribed drug glipalamides in the treatment of diabetes (Eidi et al., 2006). Patients with diabetes who received the commercially available medication metformin along with garlic supplements experienced improved glycemic control (Ashraf et al., 2011). The antioxidant rank in the tissues related to blood by streptozotocin-induced diabetic rats was improved after a six-week therapy with fresh garlic homogenate (Naderi et al., 2015). The garlic ethanol extract was also shown to have anti-diabetic activity by restoring the delayed insulin response (Adinortey et al., 2019).

Indian Bael (*Aegle Marmelos*)

In traditional Indian medicine, leaf extract from Aegle marmelos was used to cure and control blood sugar. Compared to controls, the consumption of aqueous leaf extract lowers blood sugar and improves digestion in AIDR. In addition to hypoglycaemic activity, this extract has prevented the blood sugar from rising to its highest level at one hour (Karunanayake et al., 1984). According to the study, A. marmelos in vitro callus culture has the same potential for controlling diabetes as the original leaf extract. Similar anti-diabetic activity has been discovered for the methanolic extract (Arumugama et al., 2008). When administered a methanolic extract of the plant's leaves, diabetic mice had considerably lower blood glucose levels. Following a 6-day course of hypoglycemic extract treatment, there were positive results. After 12 days of extract treatment, glucose level had decreased by 54%. According to the study, the plant extract may have antioxidant properties in addition to its anti-diabetic properties (Sabu and Kuttan, 2004). Streptozotocin-induced diabetic Wistar rats received an oral dose of an aqueous extract of the A. marmelos fruit at a dose of 250 mg/kg, and their BSL significantly decreased (Kamalakkannan and Prince, 2003). And the ethanolic extract of A. marmelos controls antioxidant activity and offers an effective defense against damage from reactive oxygen species damages (Narendhirakannan, and Subramanian, 2010). A succession of phenylethyl cinnamides were extracted from A. marmelos leaves, including anhydromarmeline, glucosidase inhibitors and aegelinosides, with anhydroaegeline demonstrating high inhibitory activity.

Cinnamon Tree (*Cinnamomum Verum*)

Cinnamomum verum is a type of cinnamon. Cinnamon contains active ingredients such as cinnamic acid, which has several health advantages, as well as essential oils. In addition to anti-diabetic properties, it has a variety of therapeutic benefits, including activity against neurological disorders. According to reports, cinnamon has the ability to decrease cholesterol and blood sugar (Mang et al., 2006). Cinnamon's insulin-potentiating effect was found to be twenty times greater than that of many other spices in a comparative study (Broadhurst et al., 2000). Oral administration of purified 3 g/day of aqueous cinnamon extract effectively lowered plasma glucose levels in a double-blind trial of 79 individuals with diagnosed DM2 (Mang et al., 2006).

Ivy Gourd (*Coccinia Grandis* (L.) Voigt)

Diabetic patients received dried extracts of *Coccinia indica extracts* for six weeks. In untreated diabetics, these extracts restored the activity of the enzyme lipoprotein lipase, which had been reduced, and glucose-6-phosphate was increased (Kamble et al.). The extract of the present fruit inhibited the activity of aldose reductase by 96.6% against partially purified bovine lens aldose reductase (Kondhare and Lade, 2017). *Coccinia grandis* (L.) Voigt, a member of the Cucurbitaceae family having anti-diabetic properties. In a trial in diabetes patients, dried C. indica extract was discovered to exhibit insulin-like activities. (Kamble et al., 1998)

Holy Basil (*Ocimum Tenuiflorum L.*)

It originated in India and is broadly used in Southern Asia. The entire plant has a pleasant odour. Basil's main constituents are apigenin, linalool, and ursolic acid (Chiang et al., 2005). In rats with diabetes caused by alloxan, the aqueous extract of *Ocimum sanctum* leaves dramatically lowered BSL (Vats et al., 2002). Plasma glucose levels were reduced after 30 days of the oral administration of extract. In compared to controls, Glycogen levels decreased by 68 and 75% in the liver and skeletal muscles respectively in diabatic rats (Vats et al., 2004). A clinical trial in India found that basil leaf extract decreased fasting blood sugar by 21.0 mg/dL (Agrawal et al., 1996). The presence of many active phytochemicals in leaf power extract was found to lower plasma glucose levels (Mohana Lakshmi et al., 2012). A tetracyclic terpenoid isolated from parts of *O. sanctum* demonstrated anti-diabetic effects (Patil et al., 2011). Basil also helps reduce blood glucose levels, stimulate the nervous system, and protect against radiation (Bora et al., 2011). The *O. basilicum* extract can inhibit the activities of rat porcine pancreatic *α-amylase* and intestinal maltase, sucrase (El-Beshbishy and Bahashwan, 2012).

Indian Gooseberry (*Phyllanthus Emblica* L.)

A medicinal plant known as "Amla" is Phyllanthus emblica L., which belongs to the Euphorbiaceae family. In AIDR, the extract reduces BSL (Raphael et al., 2002). Administration of aqueous P. emblica to diabetic rats drastically poorer the fasting serum glucose levels (Ansari et al., 2014). When streptozotocin-induced diabetic rats were given the extract fraction resulted in a drastic drop in glycosylated end products with increased body weight (Rao et al., 2005). The primary biological activities of amla are accredited with its high polyphenol content, which consists primarily of tannins and flavonoids. It is well recognized that it improves glucose metabolism in addition to maintaining glucose homeostasis (Yadav et al., 2017). An impressive reduction in total lipids, as well as higher HDL cholesterol and lower LDL cholesterol levels, was observed in a trial in diabetic volunteers treated with a dose of 3 g/day of P. emblica powder (Akhtar et al., 2011).

Black Plum (*Syzygium Cumini* (L.) Skeels or Jamun

It has been used to delicacy diabetes in India for many years and a member of the Myrtaceae family. Cholesterol, postprandial glucose, blood glucose, and free fatty acid levels were all lower in diabatic rats (Prince et al., 2004). The tribes in India consume stem bark decoction to treat the said disease (Chhetri et al., 2005). *S. cumini* extracts have also been shown to inhibit –glucosidase (Shinde et al., 2008). The existence of inorganic constituents in *S. cumini* seeds has also been investigated for hypoglycemic and hypolipidemic activity (Ravi et al., 2005). In diabetic animals, glucokinase and phosphofructokinase, two liver enzymes involved in glucose metabolism, had significantly lower enzyme activities (Grover et al., 2000). In diabetic Wistar rats, oral intake of aqueous and ethanolic extracts of *S. cumini* bark for three weeks showed in significant droppage glucose in blood (Tripathi, and Kohli, 2014). *S. cumini* is well recognized for its normoglycemia properties and reduces blood glucose levels by enhancing oral glucose tolerance (Pandey and Khan, 2002; Ravi et al., 2004). According to research, *S. cumini* is an effective glucosidases inhibitor. Only murine liver glucosidases were inhibited by methanolic extract of *S. cumini* (Bhat et al., 2011). Administration of *S. cumini* seed extract (aqueous) for three weeks, it has a modulatory impact on the inflammatory and hyperglycemic circumstances seen in diabetes and has a defensive effect in opposition to the pathophysiological manifestations of diabetes in its early stages (Bitencourt et al., 2015). In rats with type 2 diabetic rats, administration of *S. cumini* seed extract (aqueous) exhibited significant insulin sensitisation and β-cell protective effects (Sharma et al., 2017).

Ginger (*Zingiber officinale Roscoe*)

It belongs to the Zingiberaceae family and is more often referred to as ginger. It has a wide range of medicinal applications. Ginger has been shown in studies to have anti-diabetic, hypoglycemic, anti-oxidant, hypolipidemic and hypocholesterolemic properties (Rani et al., 2012). Powdered ginger supplementation for three months improved antioxidant status and glycaemic index in type 2 diabetic patients (Shidfar et al., 2015). Gingerol, a key ingredient in Z. officinale, increased insulin secretion and facilitated glucose uptake in skeletal muscles in diabetic mice (Samad et al., 2017). Other studies have shown that ginger can control tissue glycogen content in diabetic rats (Abdulrazaq et al., 2012). It was also discovered that the fresh ginger solution inhibited alpha-amylase and alpha-glucosidase activities (Akinyemi et al., 2014). Furthermore, ginger powder can lower blood glucose levels (Mohd Sahardi, and Makpol, 2019).

Conclusion

Diabetes is a significant economic burden on patients. Uninhibited diabetes also causes severe constant complications such as kidney failure. Many traditional medicines have come to light as a result of the negative effects of modern therapies. Furthermore, natural mine which is available in the form of plant can now be combined with standard drugs. Each type of mine contains energetic components that can change blood sugar levels and manage diabetes hurdle. The isolation, purification, and identification of bioactive substances in plants will be the focus of future research. This review hopes to provide the necessary information for the management of diabetes.

References

Abdulrazaq, N. B., Cho, M. M., Win, N. N., Zaman, R. and Rahman, M. T., 2012. Beneficial effects of ginger (Zingiber officinale) on carbohydrate metabolism in streptozotocin-induced diabetic rats. *British Journal of Nutrition*, *108*(7), pp.1194-1201.

Adinortey, M. B., Agbeko, R., Boison, D., Ekloh, W., Kuatsienu, L.E., Biney, E. E., Affum, O.O., Kwarteng, J. and Nyarko, A.K., 2019. Phytomedicines used for diabetes mellitus in Ghana: A systematic search and review of preclinical and clinical evidence. *Evidence-Based Complementary and Alternative Medicine*, *2019*.

Agrawal, P., Rai, V. and Singh, R.B., 1996. Randomized placebo-controlled, single blind trial of holy basil leaves in patients with noninsulin-dependent diabetes mellitus. *International journal of clinical pharmacology and therapeutics*, *34*(9), pp.406-409.

Ajabnoor, M. A., 1990. Effect of aloes on blood glucose levels in normal and alloxan diabetic mice. *Journal of ethnopharmacology*, *28*(2), pp.215-220.

Akhtar, M. S., Ramzan, A., Ali, A. and Ahmad, M., 2011. Effect of Amla fruit (Emblica officinalis Gaertn.) on blood glucose and lipid profile of normal subjects and type 2 diabetic patients. *International journal of food sciences and nutrition*, *62*(6), pp.609-616.

Akhtar, N., Khan, B.A., Majid, A., Khan, H. M., Mahmood, T. and Saeed, T., 2011. Pharmaceutical and biopharmaceutical evaluation of extracts from different plant parts of indigenous origin for their hypoglycemic responses in rabbits. *Acta Poloniae Pharmaceutica*, *68*(6), pp.919-925.

Akinyemi, A. J., Ademiluyi, A. O. and Oboh, G., 2014. Inhibition of angiotensin-1-converting enzyme activity by two varieties of ginger (Zingiber officinale) in rats fed a high cholesterol diet. *Journal of medicinal food*, *17*(3), pp.317-323.

Akter, R., Mahabub-Uz-Zaman, M., Rahman, M. S., Khatun, M. A., Abdullah, A. M., Ahmed, N .U. and Islam, F., 2013. Comparative studies on antidiabetic effect with phytochemical screening of Azadirachta indicia and Andrographis paniculata. *IOSR Journal of Pharmacy and Biological Sciences*, *5*(2), pp.122-128.

Al-Awadi, F. M. and Gumaa, K. A., 1987. Studies on the activity of individual plants of an antidiabetic plant mixture. *Acta diabetologia latina*, *24*, pp.37-41.

American Diabetes Association, 2019. 2. Classification and diagnosis of diabetes: standards of medical care in diabetes—2019. *Diabetes care*, *42*(Supplement_1), pp.S13-S28.

Ansari, A., Shahriar, M.S. Z., Hassan, M. M., Das, S. R., Rokeya, B., Haque, M. A., Haque, M.E., Biswas, N. and Sarkar, T., 2014. Emblica officinalis improves glycemic status and oxidative stress in STZ induced type 2 diabetic model rats. *Asian Pacific journal of tropical medicine*, *7*(1), pp.21-25.

Arumugam, S., Kavimani, S., Kadalmani, B., Ahmed, A. B. A., Akbarsha, M. A. and Rao, M. V., 2008. Antidiabetic activity of leaf and callus extracts of Aegle marmelos in rabbit. *Sci. Asia*, *34*(3), pp.317-321.

Ashraf, R., Khan, R. A. and Ashraf, I., 2011. Garlic (Allium sativum) supplementation with standard antidiabetic agent provides better diabetic control in type 2 diabetes patients. *Pak. J. Pharm. Sci.*, *24*(4), pp.565-570.

Atkinson, M.A., Eisenbarth, G.S. and Michels, A.W., 2014. Type 1 diabetes. *The Lancet*, *383*(9911), pp.69-82.

Babiker, A. and Al Dubayee, M., 2017. Anti-diabetic medications: How to make a choice?. *Sudanese Journal of Paediatrics*, *17*(2), p.11.

Bhat, M., Zinjarde, S.S., Bhargava, S.Y., Kumar, A.R. and Joshi, B.N., 2011. Antidiabetic Indian plants: a good source of potent amylase inhibitors. *Evidence-Based Complementary and Alternative Medicine*, *2011*.

Bitencourt, P. E. R., De Bona, K. S., Cargnelutti, L. O., Bonfanti, G., Pigatto, A., Boligon, A., Athayde, M.L., Pierezan, F., Zanette, R.A. and Moretto, M.B., 2015. Syzygium cumini seed extract ameliorates adenosine deaminase activity and biochemical parameters but does not alter insulin sensitivity and pancreas architecture in a short-term model of diabetes. *Journal of Complementary and Integrative Medicine*, *12*(3), pp.187-193.

Bora, K. S., Arora, S. and Shri, R., 2011. Role of Ocimum basilicum L. in prevention of ischemia and reperfusion-induced cerebral damage, and motor dysfunctions in mice brain. *Journal of ethnopharmacology*, *137*(3), pp.1360-1365.

Broadhurst, C. L., Polansky, M. M. and Anderson, R. A., 2000. Insulin-like biological activity of culinary and medicinal plant aqueous extracts in vitro. *Journal of agricultural and food chemistry*, *48*(3), pp.849-852.

Buchanan, T. A. and Xiang, A. H., 2005. Gestational diabetes mellitus. *The Journal of clinical investigation*, *115*(3), pp.485-491.

Chattopadhyay, R. R., Chattopadhyay, R. N. and Maitra, S. K., 1993. Effect of Azadirachta indica leaf extract on hepatic glycogen in rats. *Indian Journal of Pharmacology*, *25*(3), p.174.

Chhetri, D. R., Parajuli, P. and Subba, G. C., 2005. Antidiabetic plants used by Sikkim and Darjeeling Himalayan tribes, India. *Journal of Ethnopharmacology*, *99*(2), pp.199-202.

Chiang, L. C., Ng, L. T., Cheng, P. W., Chiang, W. and Lin, C. C., 2005. Antiviral activities of extracts and selected pure constituents of Ocimum basilicum. *Clinical and Experimental Pharmacology and Physiology*, *32*(10), pp.811-816.

Eidi, A., Eidi, M. and Esmaeili, E., 2006. Antidiabetic effect of garlic (Allium sativum L.) in normal and streptozotocin-induced diabetic rats. *Phytomedicine*, *13*(9-10), pp.624-629.

El-Beshbishy, H. A. and Bahashwan, S. A., 2012. Hypoglycemic effect of basil (Ocimum basilicum) aqueous extract is mediated through inhibition of α-glucosidase and α-amylase activities: An in vitro study. *Toxicology and Industrial Health*, *28*(1), pp.42-50.

El-Saber Batiha, G., Magdy Beshbishy, A., G. Wasef, L., Elewa, Y.H., A. Al-Sagan, A., Abd El-Hack, M.E., Taha, A.E., M. Abd-Elhakim, Y. and Prasad Devkota, H., 2020. *Chemical constituents and pharmacological activities of garlic (*Allium sativum L.): A review. *Nutrients*, *12*(3), p.872.

Faselis, C., Katsimardou, A., Imprialos, K., Deligkaris, P., Kallistratos, M. and Dimitriadis, K., 2020. Microvascular complications of type 2 diabetes mellitus. *Current vascular pharmacology*, *18*(2), pp.117-124.

Grover, J. K., Vats, V. and Rathi, S. S., 2000. Anti-hyperglycemic effect of Eugenia jambolana and Tinospora cordifolia in experimental diabetes and their effects on key metabolic enzymes involved in carbohydrate metabolism. *Journal of Ethnopharmacology*, *73*(3), pp.461-470.

Grover, J. K., Yadav, S. and Vats, V., 2002. Medicinal plants of India with anti-diabetic potential. *Journal of ethnopharmacology*, *81*(1), pp.81-100.

Heise, T., Nosek, L., Rønn, B. B., Endahl, L., Heinemann, L., Kapitza, C. and Draeger, E., 2004. Lower within-subject variability of insulin detemir in comparison to NPH insulin and insulin glargine in people with type 1 diabetes. *Diabetes*, *53*(6), pp.1614-1620.

Inzucchi, S. E., Bergenstal, R. M., Buse, J. B., Diamant, M., Ferrannini, E., Nauck, M., Peters, A. L., Tsapas, A., Wender, R. and Matthews, D.R., 2012. Management of hyperglycemia in type 2 diabetes: a patient-centered approach: position statement of the American Diabetes Association (ADA) and the European Association for the Study of Diabetes (EASD). *Diabetes care*, *35*(6), pp.1364-1379.

Kamalakkannan, N. and Prince, P. S. M., 2003. Hypoglycaemic effect of water extracts of Aegle marmelos fruits in streptozotocin diabetic rats. *Journal of ethnopharmacology*, *87*(2-3), pp.207-210.

Kamble, S. M., Kamlakar, P. L., Vaidya, S. and Bambole, V.D., 1998. Influence of Coccinia indica on certain enzymes in glycolytic and lipolytic pathway in human diabetes. *Indian journal of medical sciences*, *52*(4), pp.143-146.

Karunanayake, E. H., Welihinda, J., Sirimanne, S. R. and Adorai, G. S., 1984. Oral hypoglycaemic activity of some medicinal plants of Sri Lanka. *Journal of ethnopharmacology*, *11*(2), pp.223-231.

Kitabchi, A. E., Umpierrez, G. E., Miles, J. M. and Fisher, J. N., 2009. Hyperglycemic crises in adult patients with diabetes. *Diabetes care*, *32*(7), pp.1335-1343.

Kitabchi, A. E., Umpierrez, G. E., Miles, J.M. and Fisher, J. N., 2009. Hyperglycemic crises in adult patients with diabetes. *Diabetes care*, *32*(7), pp.1335-1343.

Kumar, R., Sharma, B., Tomar, N. R., Roy, P., Gupta, A. K. and Kumar, A., 2011. In vivo evalution of hypoglycemic activity of Aloe spp. and identification of its mode of action on GLUT-4 gene expression in vitro. *Applied biochemistry and biotechnology*, *164*, pp.1246-1256.

Kumari, K. and Augusti, K. T., 2002. *Antidiabetic and antioxidant effects of S-methyl cysteine sulfoxide isolated from onions (Allium cepa Linn) as compared to standard drugs in alloxan diabetic rats.*

Kumari, K., Mathew, B. C. and Augusti, K. T., 1995. Antidiabetic and hypolipidemic effects of S-methyl cysteine sulfoxide isolated from Allium cepa Linn. *Indian journal of biochemistry & biophysics*, *32*(1), pp.49-54.

Lakshmi, M. S., Rani, S. K. and Reddy, U. K., 2012. A review on diabetes mellitus and the herbal plants used for its treatment. *Asian J. Pharm. Clin. Re.s*, *5*(4), pp.15-21.

Mang, B., Wolters, M., Schmitt, B., Kelb, K., Lichtinghagen, R., Stichtenoth, D.O. and Hahn, A., 2006. Effects of a cinnamon extract on plasma glucose, HbA1c, and serum lipids in diabetes mellitus type 2. *European journal of clinical investigation*, *36*(5), pp.340-344.

Martínez, N., Rodríguez, Y., Salguero, O., Requena, D., Triana, L. and Pérez-Ybarra, L., 2014. A study of hypoglycemic effects of Azadirachta indica (Neem) in human blood cells. *Emirates Journal of Food and Agriculture*, pp.623-629.

Mathew, P. T. and Augusti, K. T., 1975. Hypoglycaemic effects of onion, Allium cepa Linn. on diabetes mellitus-a preliminary report. *Indian Journal of physiology and pharmacology*, *19*(4), pp.213-217.

McIntyre, H. D., Catalano, P., Zhang, C., Desoye, G., Mathiesen, E.R. and Damm, P., 2019. Gestational diabetes mellitus. *Nature reviews Disease primers*, *5*(1), p.47.

Modak, M., Dixit, P., Londhe, J., Ghaskadbi, S. and Devasagayam, T.P.A., 2007. Indian herbs and herbal drugs used for the treatment of diabetes. *Journal of clinical biochemistry and nutrition*, *40*(3), pp.163-173.

Mohd Sahardi, N. F. N. and Makpol, S., 2019. Ginger (Zingiber officinale Roscoe) in the prevention of ageing and degenerative diseases: review of current evidence. *Evidence-Based Complementary and Alternative Medicine*, *2019*.

Naderi, R., Mohaddes, G., Mohammadi, M., Alihemmati, A., Badalzadeh, R., Ghaznavi, R., Ghyasi, R. and Mohammadi, S., 2015. Preventive effects of garlic (Allium sativum) on oxidative stress and histopathology of cardiac tissue in streptozotocin-induced diabetic rats. *Acta physiologica hungarica*, *102*(4), pp.380-390.

Narendhirakannan, R. T. and Subramanian, S., 2010. Biochemical evaluation of the protective effect of Aegle marmelos (L.), Corr. leaf extract on tissue antioxidant defense system and histological changes of pancreatic β-cells in streptozotocin-induced diabetic rats. *Drug and chemical toxicology*, *33*(2), pp.120-130.

Olokoba, A. B., Obateru, O. A. and Olokoba, L. B., 2012. Type 2 diabetes mellitus: a review of current trends. *Oman medical journal*, *27*(4), p.269.

Ovesná, J., Mitrová, K. and Kučera, L., 2015. Garlic (A. sativum L.) alliinase gene family polymorphism reflects bolting types and cysteine sulphoxides content. *BMC genetics*, *16*, pp.1-10.

Pandey, M. and Khan, A., 2002. *Hypoglycaemic effect of defatted seeds and water soluble fibre from the seeds of Syzygium cumini (Linn.) skeels in alloxan diabetic rats.*

Patil, R., Patil, R., Ahirwar, B. and Ahirwar, D., 2011. Isolation and characterization of anti-diabetic component (bioactivity—guided fractionation) from Ocimum sanctum L.(Lamiaceae) aerial part. *Asian Pacific journal of tropical medicine*, *4*(4), pp.278-282.

Prince, P. S. M., Kamalakkannan, N. and Menon, V. P., 2004. Antidiabetic and antihyperlipidaemic effect of alcoholic Syzigium cumini seeds in alloxan induced diabetic albino rats. *Journal of ethnopharmacology*, *91*(2-3), pp.209-213.

Rani, M. P., Krishna, M. S., Padmakumari, K. P., Raghu, K. G. and Sundaresan, A., 2012. Zingiber officinale extract exhibits antidiabetic potential via modulating glucose uptake, protein glycation and inhibiting adipocyte differentiation: an in vitro study. *Journal of the Science of Food and Agriculture*, *92*(9), pp.1948-1955.

Rao, T. P., Sakaguchi, N., Juneja, L. R., Wada, E. and Yokozawa, T., 2005. Amla (Emblica officinalis Gaertn.) extracts reduce oxidative stress in streptozotocin-induced diabetic rats. *Journal of medicinal food*, *8*(3), pp.362-368.

Raphael, K. R., Sabu, M. C. and Kuttan, R., 2002. *Hypoglycemic effect of methanol extract of Phyllanthus amarus Schum & Thonn on alloxan induced diabetes mellitus in rats and its relation with antioxidant potential.*

Ravi, K., Rajasekaran, S. and Subramanian, S., 2005. Antihyperlipidemic effect of Eugenia jambolana seed kernel on streptozotocin-induced diabetes in rats. *Food and Chemical Toxicology*, *43*(9), pp.1433-1439.

Ravi, K., Sekar, D. S. and Subramanian, S., 2004. Hypoglycemic activity of inorganic constitutents in Eugenia jambolana seed on streptozotocin-induced diabetes in rats. *Biological Trace Element Research*, *99*, pp.145-155.

Roman-Ramos, R., Flores-Saenz, J. L. and Alarcon-Aguilar, F. J., 1995. Anti-hyperglycemic effect of some edible plants. *Journal of Ethnopharmacology*, *48*(1), pp.25-32.

Sabu, M. C. and Kuttan, R., 2004. Antidiabetic activity of Aegle marmelos and its relationship with its antioxidant properties. *Indian Journal of physiology and pharmacology*, *48*(1), pp.81-88.

Samad, M. B., Mohsin, M., Bin, N. A., Razu, B. A., Hossain, M. T., Mahzabeen, S., Unnoor, N., Muna, I. A., Akhter, F., Kabir, A. U. and Hannan, J. M. A., 2017. [6]-Gingerol, from Zingiber officinale, potentiates GLP-1 mediated glucose-stimulated insulin secretion pathway in pancreatic β-cells and increases RAB8/RAB10-regulated membrane presentation of GLUT4 transporters in skeletal muscle to improve hyperglycemia in Leprdb/db type 2 diabetic mice. *BMC complementary and alternative medicine*, *17*(1), pp.1-13.

Scartezzini, P. and Speroni, E., 2000. Review on some plants of Indian traditional medicine with antioxidant activity. *Journal of ethnopharmacology*, *71*(1-2), pp.23-43.

Seth, S.D. and Sharma, B., 2004. Medicinal plants in India. *Indian Journal of Medical Research*, *120*(1), p.9.

Sharma, S., Pathak, S., Gupta, G., Sharma, S. K., Singh, L., Sharma, R. K., Mishra, A. and Dua, K., 2017. Pharmacological evaluation of aqueous extract of syzigium cumini for its antihyperglycemic and antidyslipidemic properties in diabetic rats fed a high cholesterol diet—Role of PPARγ and PPARα. *Biomedicine & Pharmacotherapy*, *89*, pp.447-453.

Shidfar, F., Rajab, A., Rahideh, T., Khandouzi, N., Hosseini, S. and Shidfar, S., 2015. The effect of ginger (Zingiber officinale) on glycemic markers in patients with type 2 diabetes. *Journal of complementary and integrative medicine*, *12*(2), pp.165-170.

Shinde, J., Taldone, T., Barletta, M., Kunaparaju, N., Hu, B., Kumar, S., Placido, J. and Zito, S.W., 2008. α-Glucosidase inhibitory activity of Syzygium cumini (Linn.) Skeels seed kernel in vitro and in Goto–Kakizaki (GK) rats. *Carbohydrate research*, *343*(7), pp.1278-1281.

Singh, V. and Kumar, R., 2017. Study of phytochemical analysis and antioxidant activity of Allium sativum of Bundelkhand region. *International Journal of Life-Sciences Scientific Research*, *3*(6), pp.1451-1458.

Tripathi, A. K. and Kohli, S., 2014. Pharmacognostical standardization and antidiabetic activity of Syzygium cumini (Linn.) barks (Myrtaceae) on streptozotocin-induced diabetic rats. *Journal of Complementary and Integrative Medicine*, *11*(2), pp.71-81.

Vats, V., Grover, J. K. and Rathi, S. S., 2002. Evaluation of anti-hyperglycemic and hypoglycemic effect of Trigonella foenum-graecum Linn, Ocimum sanctum Linn and Pterocarpus marsupium Linn in normal and alloxanized diabetic rats. *Journal of ethnopharmacology*, *79*(1), pp.95-100.

Vats, V., Yadav, S. P. and Grover, J. K., 2004. Ethanolic extract of Ocimum sanctum leaves partially attenuates streptozotocin-induced alterations in glycogen content and carbohydrate metabolism in rats. *Journal of ethnopharmacology*, *90*(1), pp.155-160.

World Health Organization, 1999. *Definition, diagnosis and classification of diabetes mellitus and its complications: report of a WHO consultation. Part 1, Diagnosis and classification of diabetes mellitus* (No. WHO/NCD/NCS/99.2). World health organization.

Yadav, S. S., Singh, M. K., Singh, P. K. and Kumar, V., 2017. Traditional knowledge to clinical trials: A review on therapeutic actions of Emblica officinalis. *Biomedicine & Pharmacotherapy*, *93*, pp.1292-1302.

Chapter 3

Antidiabetic Plants from an African Region

Mohsina Patwekar* and Faheem Patwekar

Luqman College of Pharmacy, Gulbarga, Karnataka, India

Abstract

In Africa, diabetes mellitus is one of the main health problems. Most of those who are affected cannot afford typical oral synthetic anti diabetic medication that are available to address the condition since they are expensive. It is interesting that the continent is rich in medicinal plants that have been researched by us for their traditional use in the treatment of diabetes mellitus. In this review article, many of these investigations are methodically collated, but there is no repository of data on these plants that may serve as a guide between January 2000 and July 2013 are methodically collated in this review article, with a closer look at certain important plants from the continent's subregions. The most researched plants are those of the Asteraceae and Lamiaceae families, and West Africa has the highest number of these species.

Keywords: diabetes mellitus, antidiabetic plant, North Africa, East Africa, West Africa, South Africa

---

* Corresponding Author's Email: mohsina.patwekar@gmail.com.

In: Antidiabetic Plants
Editor: Arpita Roy
ISBN: 979-8-88697-957-2

Introduction

DM is a diverse collection of metabolic illnesses caused by a problem with insulin secretion and action that results in persistent hyperglycemia (Malviya et al., 2010) and protein, lipid and carbohydrate metabolism (Maritim AC et al., 2003). Because there is not enough medication available to treat diabetes mellitus, especially in underdeveloped African and Asian nations, the condition is considered a risk to public health. The lack of effective management and therapy for diabetes mellitus may be the cause of the increasing prevalence of morbidity and death associated with it (Dailey, 2011). Worldwide, there are about 366 million diabetics, according to the International Diabetic Federation (DF) (International Diabetes Federation, 2014), and by 2030, there may be 552 million. More than 14 million Africans are said to have diabetes, with Nigeria and South Africa having the highest incidence rates. Poor socioeconomic conditions make it practically impossible to appropriately monitor and manage DM in Africa. Nigeria and Côte d'lvoire held the top two spots in terms of the number of DM cases recorded in West Africa. South Africa (2.0 million diabetics) is at the top of the list in Southern Africa, followed by the Democratic Republic of the Congo (737000 diabetics). With 720730 diabetics, Kenya ranked sixth in Africa and first in the Eastern area, while Cameroon (517860 diabetic) had the highest Number in the middle of the continent. No country in the top ten list of African countries with DM was found in North Africa that had the fewest diabetics among African subregions (International Diabetes Federation (Brussels), 2012). In Africa, medicinal plants are a common component of traditional medicine, which is widely practised. Traditional medicine is widely known throughout Africa and is even regulated in some nations, such as Ghana, where it is integrated into primary healthcare.

Various methods, including contemporary synthetic anti-diabetic medicine and lifestyle changes, are currently employed to control DM. This comprises glycoside inhibitors (acarbose), sulfonyl urea (glibenclamide), and biguanide (metformin). However, the serious side effects of these synthetic oral hypoglycemic drugs have a recognisable profile. These include liver, and heart failure, hypoglycemia, nausea, diarrhoea, and gastrointestinal pain (Michael et al., 2013) in common thyme,, German thyme,, garden thyme and Just thyme are all names for the thyme vulgarises plant species, from the western Mediterranean to Southern Italy there are plant species that are unique to Southern Europe. It is a complete green subshrub with a bushy appearance and a woody base, heights of 15-30cm (6-12in) and widths of 40-16 in. It has small highly aromatic, grey-green leaves and clusters of purple or pink flowers in the early summer. In addition to being fairly expensive and out of reach for most Africans. Researchers are motivated to validate the traditional uses of a variety of antidiabetic African medicinal plants as a potential alternative treatment by conducting scientific studies due to these restrictions and the exponential rise in the prevalence of DM. This is in part due to the fact that the health care delivery system in African nations places high priority on the use of natural products and herbs (Cragg et al., 2013). According to the World Health Organisation (WHO), 80% of the population in several African nations relies mainly on herbal remedies and traditional treatments in general (Calixto, 2000). This is due to both the perceived efficiency of plant -based medicines and the accessibility of these medicinal plants, which make up around 25% of all higher plants in the world and exceed 5 400 medicinal plants, which make known medicinal applications (Van et al., 2008). DM is currently one of the illnesses that is treated most frequently using conventional drugs made from several African subregions, including West Africa (Adebayo, 2009). East (Keter et al., Moshi et al. 2002, Rutebemberwa et al., 2013), North (Rachid et al., 2012, Eddouks et al., 2002, Afolayan, 2010), Southern (Mahop et al., 2007, Din et al., 2011), and Central Africa (Makri et al., 2007); in this article, we had to perform a thorough analysis of all African antidiabetic medicinal plants that had been studied scientifically, and the findings of those studies had been published between January 2000 and July 2013. The government organisation, the scientific community, and a map of Africa showing the countries regions are in this review. Data collected on these plants involved their common and scientific name families (Tables 1-4). The medicinal plants discussed in this review are as follows.

Table 1. Antidiabetic plants in the African region

Sr no	North Africa	East Africa	South	West
1	*Ocimum basilicum L.*	*Aspilia pluriseta Schweinf*	*Agava Americana*	*Aloe perryi baker*
2	*Pinax ginsing*	*Cathaedulis Vahl.*	*Bridelila micrantha*	*Bridelila ferrguinea benth*
3	*Thymus vulgaries*	*Ficus syconorus L.*	*Bryophyllum pinnatum Lam.*	*Chrysophyllum cainito L.*
4	*Zingiber Officinale Roscoe*	*Pappea capensis Eckl. And Zeyh*	*Catharantusroseus L. G. Don*	*Detarium microcarpum Guill. And perr*
5	*Ziziphusspina-christi L.*	*Strychnos henningsi Gilg*	*Eucleaundulata Thunb. Var. Myrtina*	*Ficus asperifolia L*

Methodology

Searching Medline, Google Scholar, Science Direct and PubMed for medicinal plants of African origin that have been explored and investigated for their antidiabetic therapeutic potentials in vivo resulted in the collection of pertinent literature. Some papers were located by looking up citations from other works by going directly to the journals' websites. They were analysed on the geographical area where they originated. The literature taken into account covered the time period from January 2000 to July 2013. An antihyperglycemia, antihyperglycemia, medicinal plant, an anti-diabetic and Africa keyword search was conducted. Another combination of keywords, such as plant, hypoglycemia, and Africa, was used to find further data. 256 studies that reported in vivo activity as opposed to invitro activity were chosen and published in this study, which yielded a total of 313 papers. After the search, the plants were organised and displayed according to where they were found.

Antidiabetic Plants in the North Africa Regions

Ocimum basilicum L.

Family: Lamiaceae

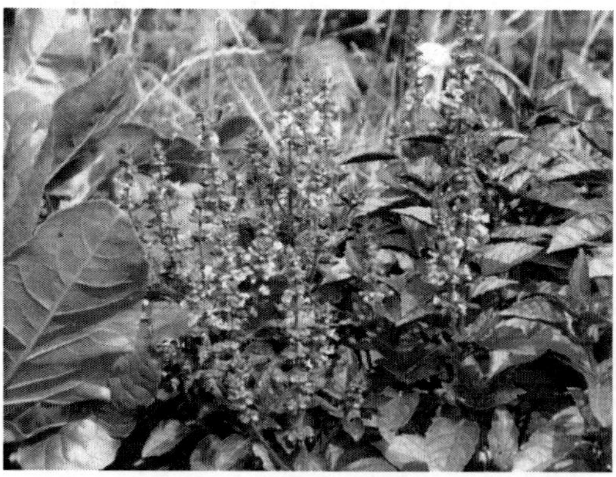

Figure 1. *Ocimum basilicum* L.

Ocimum basilicum L. (Figure 1), a member of the Lamiaceae family, is used primarily in cooking and has a strong aroma and flavour. Although it is indigenous to Asia, Africa, Central America, and South America, it is widely framed around the world, particularly in the Mediterranean region. It is tall, glossy, green plants with Lance -shaped, scented leaves that can grow to Hight around 90cm. Based on the variation in composition, basil is known to have between 50 and 150 species (Makri O et al., 2007). Basil is referred to as the "lord of herbs" because of its amazing aroma.

Pinax ginseng

Family: Araliaceous

You have certainly heard the term "ginseng" mentioned particularly in connection with natural remedies and dietary supplements. However, ginseng is truly present in a variety of species around the world. *Pinax ginseng* (Figure 2), also known as Korean ginseng and commonly referred to as panax ginseng by Mayer, is *Pinax quinquefolium*, also known as American ginseng because it is a plant that occurs naturally in both Canada and the USA. *Pinax japonicus, sometimes* called Japanese ginseng, is an additional (Kiefer D. S et al. 2003).

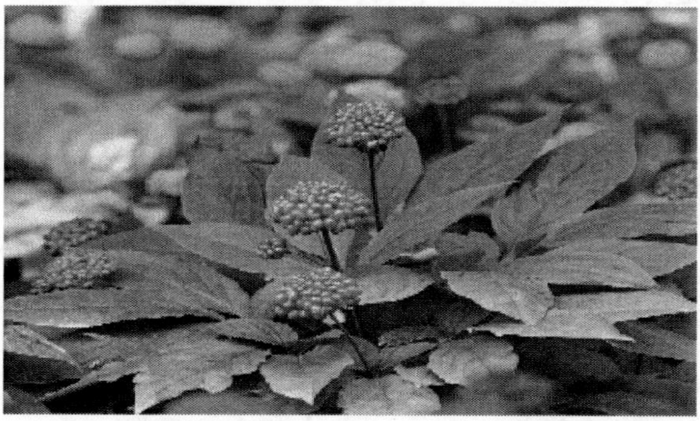

Figure 2. *Pinax ginseng*.

Thymus vulgaris

Family: Lamiaceae

German thyme (Figure 3), common thyme,, garden thyme and just thyme are all names for the Thymus vulgaris plant species, which is endemic to southern Europe from the western Mediterranean to southern Italy. It is an evergreen woody subshrub that reaches height of 15-30cm (6-12 in) and a width of 40-16 in. It has grey green leaves, small, and highly aromatic, and bunch of pink or purple flowers in the early summer (Kuete (2017), Patwekar et al. 2022).

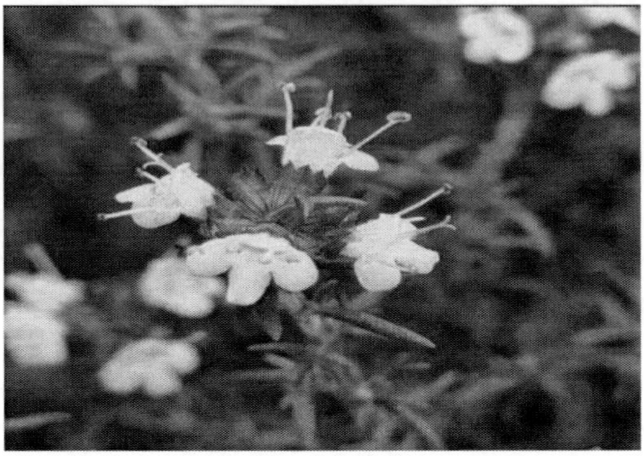

Figure 3. *Thymus vulgaris*.

Zingiber Officinale Roscoe

Family: Zingiberaceae

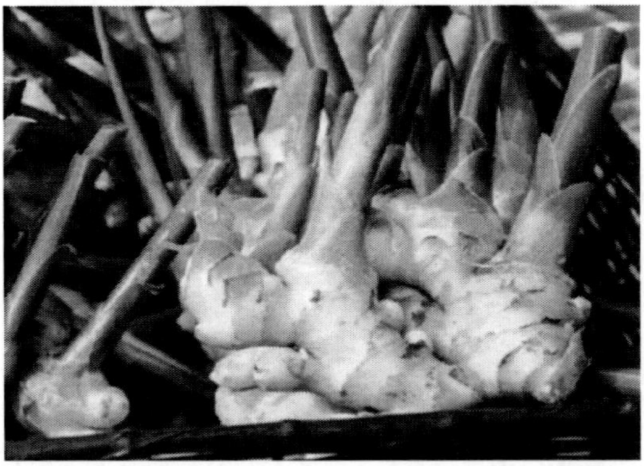

Figure 4. *Zingiber officinale Roscoe*.

Ginger (Figure 4), African ginger, and black ginger are all popular names for officinale Roscoe. It is a member of the Zingiberaceae family. Ginger is a perennial with up to foot -long, grass-like leaves. Most commonly found in Asia, Mexico, Jamaica, Africa, Hawaii, and India (Njeru et al., 2020; Faheem et al., 2021). *Z. officinale* Roscoe has been widely used as an antimalarial agent in West African nations.

Ziziphusspina -christi L.

Family: Rhamnaceae

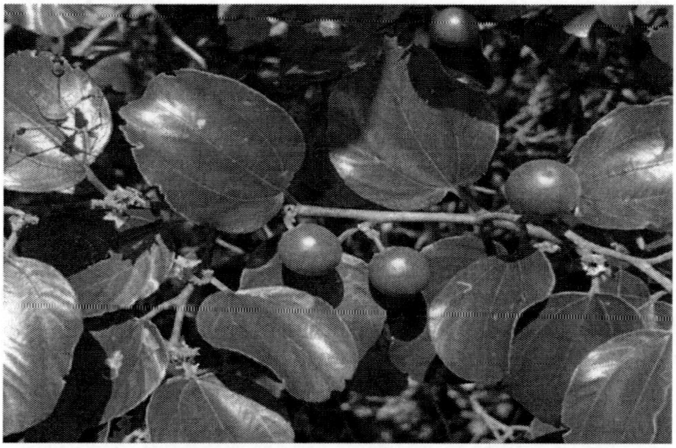

Figure 5. *Ziziphusspina -christi* L.

Table 2. Antidiabetic medicinal plants from North Africa

Scientific Name	Common name	Family	Part used	Type of effect	Country	Reference
Ocimum basilicum L	Sweet basil	Lamiaceae	Leaf	Antihyperglycemic and antihyperlipidemic	Morocco/ Egypt	(Mohsina et al., 2022, Zeggwagh et al., 2007)
Pinax ginsing	Korean ginsing	Araliaceae	Root	Antihyperglycemic Antioxidative and insulin no tropic	Egypt	(Dawidar et al., 2010)
Thymus Vulgaries	Thyme	Lamiaceae	Oil	Antihyperglycemic and Anti hypoglycemic	Egypt	(Eseyin, 2007)
Zingiber Officinale Roscoe	Ginger	Zingiberaceae	Rhizome	Antihyperglycemic and antihyperlipidemic	Egypt	(Abdel-Zahera et al., 2005)
Ziziphusspina -christi L.	Christ's Thorn Jujube	Rhamnaceae	Leaf	Antihyperglycemic and insulin no tropic	Egypt	(Michel et al., 2011)

Ziziphusspina -christi (Figure 5), also known as Christ's thorn jujube, is an evergreen plant or tree that is indigenous to southern and western Asia, as to well as northern and tropical Africa. It is indigenous to certain tropical nations, as well as the Levant, East Africa, and Mesopotamia. Fruit and leaves were employed in traditional Egyptian cuisine and rituals (Mahmoodi et al., 2021).

Antidiabetic Plants in East Africa

Aspilia pluriseta Schweinf

Family: Asteraceae

In Kenya (Cowling et al., 2005), as well as in central, southern and also east Africa (Tits et al., 1991), *A. pluriseta* (Figure 6) is a widely used herb. With little to no scientific support, *A. pluriseta* is traditionally used to manage and treat stomach ailments, cough, wound, burn wounds, pimple, nose, eye, ear infection, kwashiorkor disorders, and diabetes mellitus.

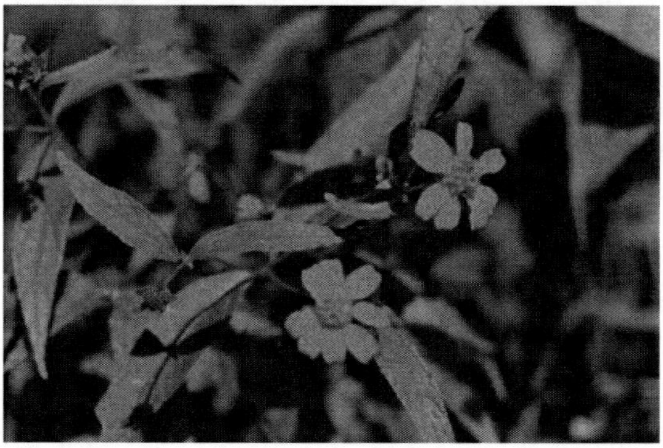

Figure 6. *Aspilia pluriseta Schweinf.*

Cathaedulis Vahl

Family: Celastraceae

Native to parts of East Africa and the Arabian Peninsula, *Catha edulis* (Vahl) Endl (Figure 7). It is also known as Khat and is frequently chewed as a natural stimulant in customs and practises there (Graziani et al., 2008). For several decades, Catha edulis was historically controlled in the region for use in rituals, ceremonies, and medicine (Gebisssa, 2004). Due to emigration from the Horn of Africa in the early 1990s, *Catha edulis* spread to Europe, North America, and Australia (Boye et al., 1992).

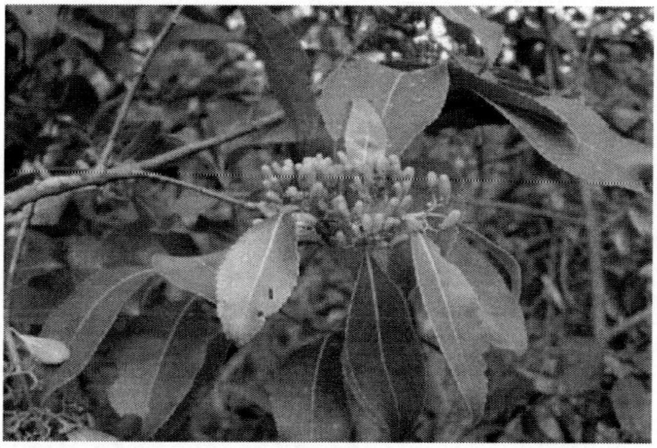

Figure 7. *Cathaedulis Vahl.*

Ficus syconorus L.

Family: Moraeceae

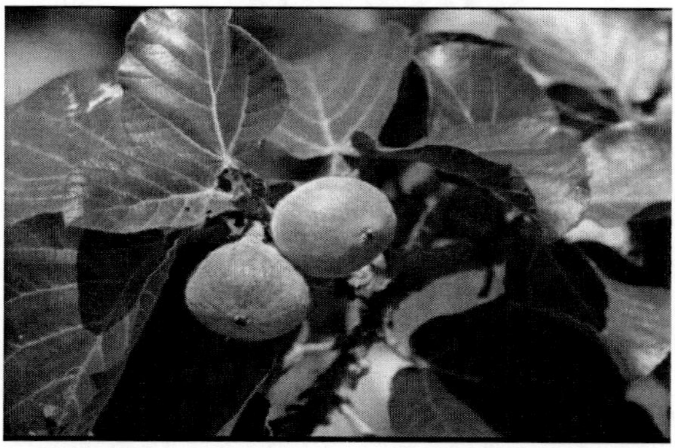

Figure 8. *Ficus syconorus* L.

Semi -deciduous *Ficus sycomorus* subsp (Figure 8). Sycomorus trees can grow up to 35 metres tall. Young branches have long greenish-yellow hairs covering the bark; older branches and steam, however, have pale brown to yellowish- brown hairs that flake in papery strips. The diameter of the main trunk might occasionally exceed 2 metres. Simple, up to 170mm -150mm, oval to elliptical, lobed base; rounded leaf tip; elevated veins on lower surface; rough to the touch; leave on new growth. Stipules that protect the growing tip. On immature leaves, the 20-30 mm long leaf stalks are hairy; however, older leaves become glabrous (Faheem et al., 2020, Mohsina et al., 2022).

Pappeacapensis Eckl. and Zeyh

Family: Sapindaceae

Pappea capesis Eckl and zeyh (Figure 9), the only species of genus pappea (Sapindaceae), is a small to medium-sized tree with a dense crowd that can be found in various subtropical thickets (Lemmens et al., 2012) on termite mounds and among rocks. The bark is smooth and varies in size color from light grey to brownish, with those from a drier location being smaller than those from a wetter condition. The tree, which is located in Africa, is most frequently found in wide open spaces, by river, on termite mounds and among rocks.

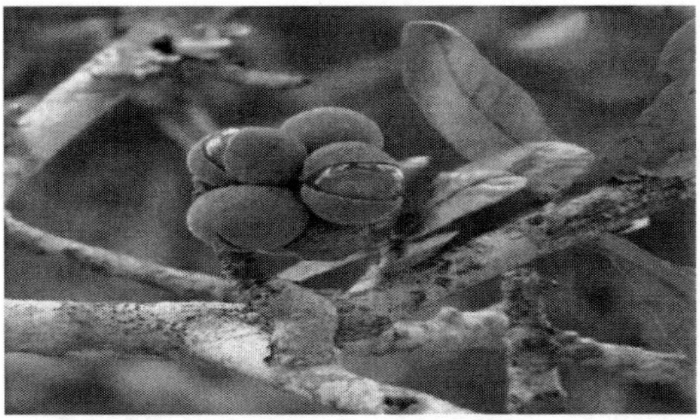

Figure 9. *Pappea capesis* Eckl and Zehy.

Strychnoshenningsi Gilg.

Family: Longaniaceae

Strychnos honningsii (Figure 10) is a small, densely branched tree or shrub that can reach height of up to 20 metres. It is topically grown between 2 and 12 metres tall.

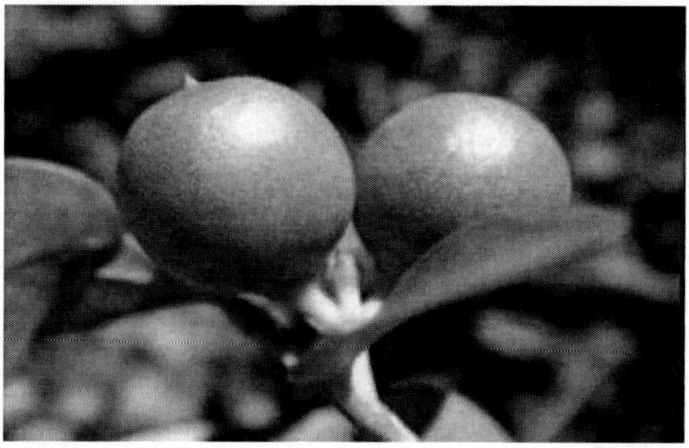

Figure 10. *Strychnos honningsi* Gilg.

Table 3. Antidiabetic medicinal plants from East Africa

Scientific name	Common name	Family	Part used	Type of effect	Country	Reference
Aspilia pluriseta Schweinf	Dwarfaspilia	Asteraceae	Root	Antihyperglycemic	Kenya	(Cowling et al., 1991)
Cathaedulis Vahl	Bushman's tea	Celastraceae	Root	Antihyperglycemic	Kenya	(Boye et al., 1992)
Ficus syconorus L.	Fig-mulberry	Moraecea	Steam bark	Antihyperglycemic	Kenya	((Faheem et al., 2020, Mohsina et al., 2022))
Pappeacapensis Eckl And Zeyh	Jacket plum	Sapindaceae	Leaf/ steam bark	Antihyperglycemic	Kenya	(Lemmens et al. 2012)
Strychnoshenningsi Gilg	Red bitter berry	Longaniaceae	Leaf	Antihyperglycemic	Kenya	(Quazi A et al., 2022)

The plant is taken wild for use in local medicine; some of the compounds in the plants are extracted for use in commerce. The bole can be of 40 to 50 cm. The plant is a good ornamental option due to its attractive shadow, lustrous foliage, and fragrant blossoms (Quazi et al., 2022).

Antidiabetic medicinal plants from South Africa

Agava americana

Family: Agavaceae

Agava americana (Figure 11), despite being known as the century plant, has a 10-to-30-year life span of only 10 to 30 years. Its grey-green leaves are 0.9 to 1.5 m (3-5ft) long with a pink margin and a heavy spike at the tip that can be pierced deeply. Its spread is approximately 1.8-3 m (6-10 ft). The plant sends a tall branching stalk that can grow up to 8 to 9 metres tall as it near the end of its life and is covered in yellow blooms (Hulle et al., 2015).

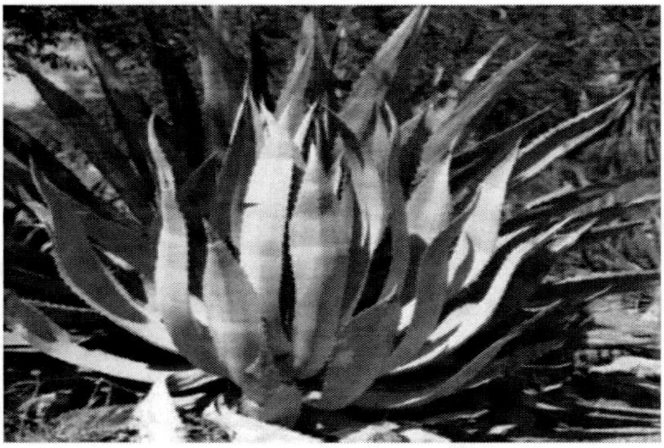

Figure 11. *Agava americana*.

Bridelia micrantha

Family: Phyllanthaceae

The small to medium -sized *Bridelia micrantha* (Hochst.) Bail (Figure 12). The tree, also known as mitzeerie or coastal golden leaf, is a member of the phyllanthaceae (formerly Euphorbiaceae) family. *B. micrantha* is a small to medium -sized monoecious evergreen or deciduous tree with a rounded crown and a short, frequently twisted bole up to 100 cm in diameter (Mburu et al., 2016), various species of Bridelia are used as anti-bacterial, ant anemic, anthelmintic, anticonvulsants, antidiabetic antidiarrheal, antimalarial, antinociceptive anti-inflammatory, hypoglycemic antiviral, and for abdominal pain, sexual diseases, gynecological and cardiovascular in traditional medicine around the world. Therefore, it is not surprising that tropical Africa uses *the* bark, leaves, and roots extensively for herbal medicine (Okeleye et al., 2011).

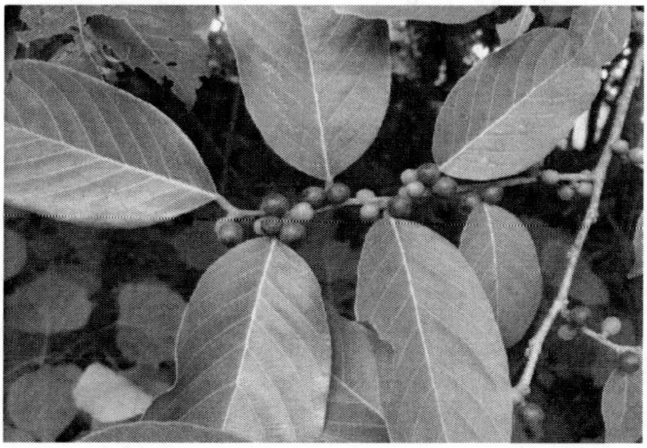

Figure 12. *Bridelia micrantha.*

Bryophyllum pinnatum Lam

Family: Life Plant

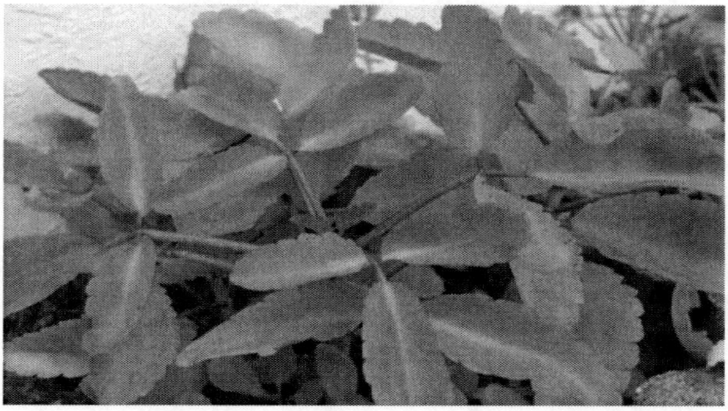

Figure 13. *Bryophyllum pinnatum* Lam.

The leaves of the oval, thick, fleshy, curved, or serrated margin species leaves are frequently crimson in colour (Figure 13). The leaves are pinnately affected at the top and simple at the base of the steam. They are 10-30 cm (4-12 in) long and have up to three to five pairs of meaty limb lobes. The propensity of the leaves to hatch bulbils is extraordinary. Adventitious buds, which create roots, stalks, and leaves, begin to develop at their edge, in between the teeth. The plantlets root as they hit the ground and grow into larger plants. The section *Bryophyllum* exhibits this characteristic quite frequently. The persistent calyx and corolla contain follicles (10-15mm in diameter) that are the fruits (Kamboj and Saluja, 2009).

Catharanthus roseus

Family: Phyllanthaceae

The tropical hardy plant *Catharanthus roseus* (Figure 14) is used as a potted ornamental plant for its pink or white blossoms. The common name for it is Madagascar periwinkle. It is a small perennial herbaceous evergreen species that is indigenous to the island of Madagascar. The plant has excellent heat tolerance, can reach a height of one to two feet, has glossy, dark green leaves that are one to two inches long and still bloom in hot weather. Horticulture has created variation with hues purple "eye" in the centre 'eye'. Due to the plant's alkaloids, medicine greatly benefits from it. More than 200 alkaloids are used as medications to treat various disorders (Gajalakshmi et al., 2013).

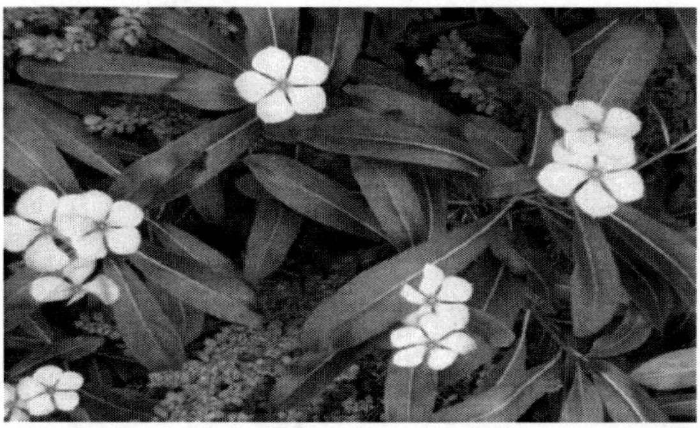

Figure 14. *Catharanthus roseus*.

Euclea undulata Thunb. Var. Myrtina

Family: Crassulaceae

Uncurved Euclea in South Africa, the Shrub Thunb. Var. Myrtina (Figure 15) is widely distributed. Diabetes is treated with the roots by conventional healers. Epicatechin and amyrin-30-(5-hydroxy) ferulic acid, two secondary metabolites that can be used to treat diabetes, have been established in plant roots, according to the research. Epicatechin decreases blood glucose levels, while amyrin -30 –(5hydroxy) ferulic acid inhibits -glucoside (Deutschländer et al., 2011).

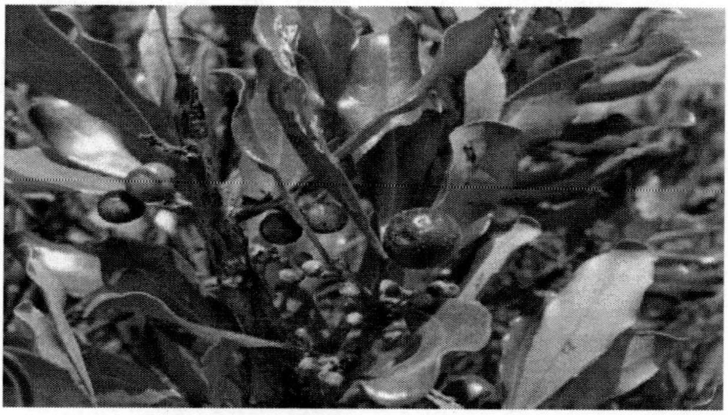

Figure 15. *Euclea undulata* Thunb. Var. Myrtina.

Table 4. Antidiabetic medicinal plants from South Africa

Scientific name	Common name	Family	Part used	Type of effect	Country	Reference
Agava Americana	American aloe	Agavaceae	Leaves	Antihyperglycemic	South Africa	(Hulle et al., (2015)
Bridelila micrantha	Mitzeerie/ coastal golden leaf	Phyllanthaceae	Leaf	Antihyperglycemic	South Africa	(Kamboj and Saluja 2009)
Bryophyllum pinnatum Lam.	Life plant	Crassulaceae	Leaf	Antihyperglycemic	South Africa	(Kamboj and Saluja 2009)
Catharanthus roseus L. G. Don	Madagascar Periwinkle	Apocynaceae	Leaf	Antihyperglycemic and hypoglycemia	South Africa	(Gajalakshmi, et al., 2013)
Euclea undulata Thunb. var. myrtina	Fire fighter's blessing	Ebenaceae	Root	Antihyperglycemic	South Africa	(Deutschländer, et al., 2011)

Aloe perryi

Family: Asphodelaceae

In the Arabian Peninsula, *Aloe perryi* (Figure 16) is the most widely cultivated aloe species and constipation and eye infection are treated with conventional treatment and current promising antitumorigenesis and scientific data (Ibegbulem and Chikezie, 2013) recently examined the chemical makeup of the methanolic extract of *A. perryi* and *A. vera* and demonstrate that the both chemical compositions are abundant anthrones, chromes, Anthraquinones and flavonoids, with *A. perryi* having higher concentrations of all this substance. Furthermore, the same authors have demonstrated that the methanolic extract of *Arabian perryi* and *Arabian vera* has strong antioxidant and free radical scavenging properties and also the ability to inhibit the glucosidase enzyme, suggesting that it may have hypoglycemic and antidiabetic effects.

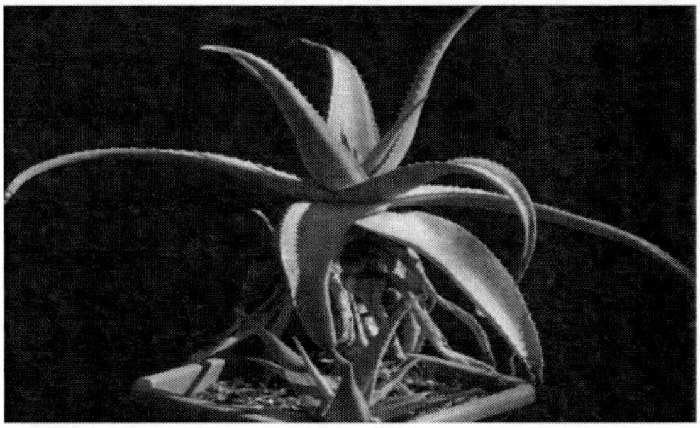

Figure 16. *Aloe perryi*.

Bridelia ferrguinea Benth

Family: Euphorbiaceae

A shrub or a tiny, nonlactiferous, sour tree, *Bridelia ferruguinea* (Figure 17) grows up to 15 m tall. The plant girth increases to 1.5 metres and its twisted bole branches downward. *Bridelia ferruguinea* has a dark grey, slash, thin steam bark, rough, and cracked It is distinguished by having long, thin branches that occasionally (typically when young) have short spines attached. The leaves are small to medium sized, simple petiolate with stipules, alternating, spiral, or distichous arrangement, and have somewhat wavey edges. It has an apex and an entirely acute or acuminate border on its broadly elliptic lamina. Male and female flowers generally coexist in each flower cluster. The female is sub-sessile, while the male flower is pedicellate and yellowish green (Mahomoodally et al., 2021).

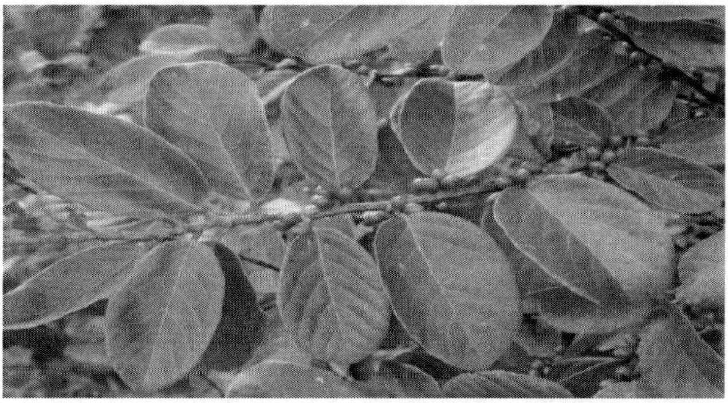

Figure 17. *Bridelia ferrguinea* benth.

Chrysophyllum cainito L.

Family: Anacardiaceae

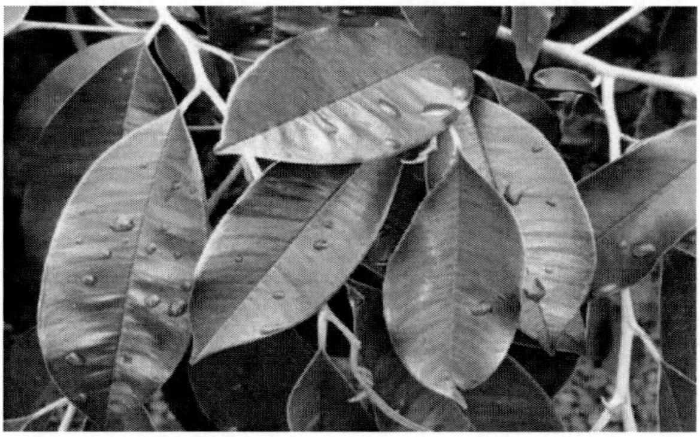

Figure 18. *Chrysophyllum cainito* L.

Chrysophyllum cainito L. (Figure 18) is a tropical fruit tree. Sometimes known as the 'star apple' has been demonstrated to have a variety of biological purposes such as anti-inflammatory, antihypertensive antioxidant, wound-healing, antidiabetic activity, antibacterial, and wound healing are just a few of the scientifically proven benefits of *C. cainito.* Traditional uses of the stem bark decoction include tonic, stimulant antidiarrheal, and anti-diabetic properties. Although many countries have used the fruit, leaves and stem of the *C. cainito* plant as alternative treatments for diabetic patients, there is little pharmacological support for therapeutic use (Luo et al., 2002).

Detarium microcarpum Guill and Perr

Family: Caesalpiniaceae

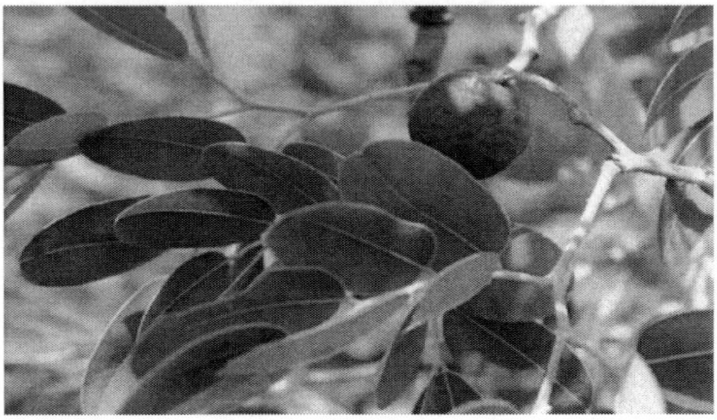

Figure 19. *Datarium microcarpum* Guill and perr).

Detarium microcarpum Guill (Figure 19) and perr have been utilised for decades to treat variety of diseases in countless societies in Africa. The Kalbi tribe of North East Nigeria has reportedly used steam and root bark as a treatment for newborn illnesses such as 'Gedigedi' or "Tando" (Hausa), stomach problems, wounds, and other conditions. As a vegetable and condiment, seeds and leaves are consumed. The pulp of the fruit is utilized to treat skin diseases in Burkina Faso. The leaves, bark and roots of D. microcarpum have also been used medicinally as astringents and diuretic. The various sections have been linked to anti -rheumatic and antiplasmodial properties (Mariod et al., 2009).

Ficus asperifolia

Family: Moraeceae

The *Ficus asperifolia* (Figure 20), sometimes known as 'sand paper', is a terrestrial or epiphytic tree of the size of a tiny to average -sized terrestrial or epiphytic tree that can grow to a height of 29 meters. *F. asperifolia* is widely distributed, gigantic and spirally shown; its limbs are mostly oval or elliptical shape, and its roots are often and magnificent. It is one of the several high-medicine herbs with wide range of applications, including analgesic, anti-cancer, diuretic, and pain relief during the maturation cycle. It is used to treat

in addition, Senegal, Uganda and South Africa are affected. It can be found in all Nigerian states (Nkafamiya et al., 2010).

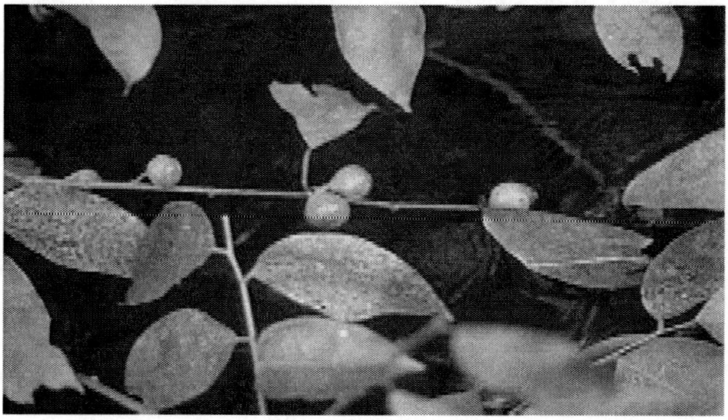

Figure 20. *Ficus asperifolia.*

Conclusion

Africa has a wealth of antidiabetic plant resources, but it is difficult to pinpoint the best reported activity. This review article systematically complies with all antidiabetic plant studies done in African plant between numerous of these medicinal plants, the antidiabetic properties have been confirmed by scientific research, but there is no repository of data on these plants that could serve as a guide for future studies done in African plant between January 2000 and July 2013 while also taking a closer look at a few plants have been studied the most, while the Asteraceae and Lamiaceae group of plants have been studied the most, while West Africa has the most plants have been studied. Unfortunately, only a few studies reported partial characterization of the bioactive principle and mechanism of action, despite the fact that many cases reported promising results. The government, pharmaceutical industry and scientific community are urged to look into some of these plants for potential future study, if possible, commercialisation.

Acknowledgments

Authors would like to offer her special thanks to Luqman College of pharmacy for allowing her to carry out this work. I am particularly grateful for the assistance, and coordination support provided by Ustad Almas.

References

Abdel-Zaher, A. O., Salim, S. Y., Assaf, M. H. and Abdel-Hady, R. H., 2005. Antidiabetic activity and toxicity of Zizyphus spina-christi leaves. *Journal of ethnopharmacology*, *101*(1-3), pp. 129-138.

Afolayan, A. J. and Sunmonu, T. O., 2010. In vivo studies on antidiabetic plants used in South African herbal medicine. *Journal of clinical biochemistry and nutrition*, *47*(2), pp. 98-106.

Boye, G. L., Sarpong, K. and Mensah, E. A. eds., 1992. *Ghana Herbal Pharmacopoeia*. Advent Press.

Calixto, J. B., 2000. Efficacy, safety, quality control, marketing and regulatory guidelines for herbal medicines (phytotherapeutic agents). *Brazilian Journal of medical and Biological research*, *33*, pp. 179-189.

Cos, P., Hermans, N., De Bruyne, T., Apers, S., Sindambiwe, J. B., Witvrouw, M., De Clercq, E., Berghe, D. V., Pieters, L. and Vlietinck, A. J., 2002. Antiviral activity of Rwandan medicinal plants against human immunodeficiency virus type-1 (HIV-1). *Phytomedicine*, *9*(1), pp. 62-68.

Cowling, R. M., Procheş, Ş., Vlok, J. H. J. and Van Staden, J., 2005. On the origin of southern African subtropical thicket vegetation. *South African Journal of Botany*, *71*(1), pp. 1-23.

Cragg, G. M. and Newman, D. J., 2013. Natural products: a continuing source of novel drug leads. *Biochimica et Biophysica Acta (BBA)-General Subjects*, *1830*(6), pp. 3670-3695.

Dailey, G., 2011. Overall mortality in diabetes mellitus: where do we stand today?. *Diabetes technology & therapeutics*, *13*(S1), pp. S-65.

Dawidar, A. M., Abdel-Mogib, M., Abou-Elzahab, M. M., Berghot, M. A., Mahfouz, M., El-Ghorab, A. H. and Hussien, K. H., 2010. Effect of photo-oxygenation on biological activities of some commercial Egyptian essential oils. *Revista latinoamericana de química*, *38*(3), pp. 168-179.

Deutschländer, M. S., Lall, N., Van de Venter, M. and Hussein, A. A., 2011. Hypoglycemic evaluation of a new triterpene and other compounds isolated from Euclea undulata Thunb. var. myrtina (Ebenaceae) root bark. *Journal of Ethnopharmacology*, *133*(3), pp. 1091-1095.

Din, N., Dibong, S. D., Mpondo, E. M., Priso, R. J., Kwin, N. F. and Ngoye, A., 2011. Inventory and identification of plants used in the treatment of diabetes in Douala Town (Cameroon). *European Journal of Medicinal Plants*, *1*(3), pp. 60-73.

Eddouks, M., Maghrani, M., Lemhadri, A., Ouahidi, M. L. and Jouad, H., 2002. Ethnopharmacological survey of medicinal plants used for the treatment of diabetes mellitus, hypertension and cardiac diseases in the south-east region of Morocco (Tafilalet). *Journal of ethnopharmacology*, *82*(2-3), pp. 97-103.

Eseyin, O. A., 2007. Hypoglycemic Effect of the Seed Extract of Telfairia occidentalis in Rat'Olorunfemi A. Eseyin, "Patrick Ebong," Arit Ekpo," Arnold Igboasoiyi and" Emmanuel Oforah" Faculty of Pharmacy, University of Uyo, Nigeria "Department of Biochemistry, University of Calabar, Nigeria" Department of Biochemistry,

University of Uyo, Nigeria. *Pakistan Journal of Biological Sciences*, *10*(3), pp. 498-501.

Faheem, I. P., Gopalakrishana, B., Mohsina, F. P. and Ahmad, N., 2020. Antidiabetic activity OF FICUS dalhousiae miq leaves ethanolic extract ON streptozotocin induced diabtes IN wistar albino rats. *World Journal of Pharmaceutical Research*, *10*(1), p. 1258.

Faheem, I. P., Gopalakrishna, B., Mohsina, F. P. and Priya, S., 2021. Antioxidant activity of leaves and bark extracts of Crataeva magna plant. *World Journal of Biology Pharmacy and Health Sciences*, *5*(1), pp. 001-008.

Faheem, I. P., Gopalakrishna, B., Mohsina, F. P. and Priya, S., 2021. Antidiabetic potential of ethanolic leaf extract of Crataeva magna in streptozotocin-induced diabetic model. *Innovations in Pharmaceuticals and Pharmacotherapy*, *9*, pp. 1-7.

Gajalakshmi, S., Vijayalakshmi, S. and Devi, R. V., 2013. Pharmacological activities of Catharanthus roseus: a perspective review. *International Journal of Pharma and Bio Sciences*, *4*(2), pp. 431-439.

Gbolade, A.A., 2009. Inventory of antidiabetic plants in selected districts of Lagos State, Nigeria. *Journal of ethnopharmacology*, *121*(1), pp. 135-139.

Hulle, A., Kadole, P. and Katkar, P., 2015. Agave Americana leaf fibers. *Fibers*, *3*(1), pp. 64-75.

Ibegbulem, C. O. and Chikezie, P. C., 2013. Hypoglycemic properties of ethanolic extracts of Gongronema latifolium, Aloe perryi, Viscum album and Allium sativum administered to alloxan-induced diabetic albino rats (Rattus norvegicus). *Pharmacognosy Communications*, *3*(2), p. 12.

International Diabetes Federation (Brussels). *Diabetes at a glance, 2012,* Africa (AFR). Available at https://www.idf.org/sites/default/files/IDF_AFR_5E_Update_FactSheet_0.pdf. Accessed February 13, 2013.

International Diabetes Federation (IDF) *Diabetes Atlas. 7th edition.* Brussels, Belgium: Int Diabetes Federation; 2014.

Kamboj, A. and Saluja, A., 2009. Bryophyllum pinnatum (Lam.) Kurz.: phytochemical and pharmacological profile: a review. *Pharmacognosy Reviews*, *3*(6), p. 364.

Keter, L. K. and Mutiso, P. C., 2012. Ethnobotanical studies of medicinal plants used by Traditional Health Practitioners in the management of diabetes in Lower Eastern Province, Kenya. *Journal of Ethnopharmacology*, *139*(1), pp. 74-80.

Kiefer, D. S. and Pantuso, T., 2003. Panax ginseng. *American family physician*, *68*(8), pp. 1539-1542.

Kuete, V., 2017. Thymus vulgaris. *Medicinal spices and vegetables from Africa*, pp. 599-609.

Lemmens, R. H. M. J., Louppe, D. and Oteng-Amoako, A. A., 2012. Plant Resources of Tropical Africa 7 (2). Timbers 2. *PROTA Foundation*. CTA, Wageningen, Netherlands.

Luo, X. D., Basile, M. J. and Kennelly, E. J., 2002. Polyphenolic antioxidants from the fruits of Chrysophyllum cainito L. (star apple). *Journal of Agricultural and food chemistry*, *50*(6), pp. 1379-1382.

Mahmoodi, A. R., Mesdaghi, M., Amirkhani, M. and Kargari, E., 2021. *An Investigation on Some Ecological Characteristics of Ziziphus spina chirsti (L.) in Southern Iran.*

Mahomoodally, M. F., Jugreet, S., Sinan, K. I., Zengin, G., Ak, G., Ceylan, R., Jekő, J., Cziáky, Z., Angelini, P., Angeles Flores, G. and Venanzoni, R., 2021. Pharmacological potential and chemical characterization of Bridelia ferruginea benth.—a native tropical african medicinal plant. *Antibiotics*, *10*(2), p. 223.

Mahop, T. M. and Mayet, M., 2007. Enroute to biopiracy? Ethnobotanical research on antidiabetic medicinal plants in the Eastern Cape Province, South Africa. *African Journal of Biotechnology*, *6*(25), pp. 2945-2952.

Makri, O. and Kintzios, S., 2008. Ocimum sp.(basil): Botany, cultivation, pharmaceutical properties, and biotechnology. *Journal of herbs, spices & medicinal plants*, *13*(3), pp. 123-150.

Mariod, A., Mirghani, M., Abdul, A. and Abdelwahab, S., 2009. Detarium microcarpum Guill and Perr fruit proximate chemical analysis and sensory characteristics of concentrated juice and jam. *African Journal of Biotechnology*, *8*(17).

Maritim, A. C., Sanders, A. and Watkins Iii, J. B., 2003. Diabetes, oxidative stress, and antioxidants: a review. *Journal of biochemical and molecular toxicology*, *17*(1), pp. 24-38.

Mburu, C., Kareru, P. G., Kipyegon, C., Madivoli, E. S., Maina, E. G., Kairigo, P. K., Kimani, P. K. and Marikah, D. M., 2016. Phytochemical screening of crude extracts of Bridelia micrantha. *European Journal of Medicinal Plants*, *16*(1), pp. 1-7.

Kane, M. P., Abu-Baker, A. and Busch, R. S., 2005. The utility of oral diabetes medications in type 2 diabetes of the young. *Current Diabetes Reviews*, *1*(1), pp. 83-92.

Michel, C. G., Nesseem, D. I. and Ismail, M. F., 2011. Anti-diabetic activity and stability study of the formulated leaf extract of Zizyphus spina-christi (L.) Willd with the influence of seasonal variation. *Journal of ethnopharmacology*, *133*(1), pp. 53-62.

Mohsina, F. P., Quazi, A., Faheem, I. P., Almas, U. and Rohin, S., Ethnopharmacology, Phytochemistry, Traditional Uses, Pharmacology and Chemistry of Crataeva magna and Ficus dalhousie.

Mohsina, F. P., Quazi, A., Faheem, I. P., Anuradha, M., Mukim, M. and Patil, A., 2022. Botanical, Ethnopharmacological, phytochemical & pharmacological standards of plant Ichnocarpus frutescens. *Research & Review: Drugs and Drugs Development*, *4*(1), pp. 1-12.

Moshi, M. J. and Mbwambo, Z. H., 2002. Experience of Tanzanian traditional healers in the management of non-insulin dependent diabetes mellitus. *Pharmaceutical Biology*, *40*(7), pp. 552-560.

Malviya, N., Jain, S. and Malviya, S. A. P. N. A., 2010. Antidiabetic potential of medicinal plants. *Acta pol pharm*, *67*(2), pp.113-118.

Njeru, S. N. and Muema, J. M., 2020. Antimicrobial activity, phytochemical characterization and gas chromatography-mass spectrometry analysis of Aspilia pluriseta Schweinf. extracts. *Heliyon*, *6*(10), p. e05195.

Nkafamiya, I. I., Osemeahon, S. A., Modibbo, U. U. and Aminu, A., 2010. Nutritional status of non-conventional leafy vegetables, Ficus asperifolia and Ficus sycomorus. *African Journal of Food Science*, *4*(3), pp. 104-108.

Okeleye, B. I., Bessong, P. O. and Ndip, R. N., 2011. Preliminary phytochemical screening and in vitro anti-Helicobacter pylori activity of extracts of the stem bark of Bridelia micrantha (Hochst., Baill., Euphorbiaceae). *Molecules*, *16*(8), pp. 6193-6205.

Patwekar, M., Patwekar, F., Mezni, A., Sanaullah, S., Fatema, S. R., Almas, U., Ahmad, I., Tirth, V. and Mallick, J., 2022. Assessment of antioxidative and alpha-amylase potential of polyherbal extract. *Evidence-based Complementary and Alternative Medicine, 2022*.

Quazi, A., Mohsina, F. P., Faheem, I. P. and Priya, S., 2022. Silico ADMET analysis, molecular docking and in vivo anti diabetic activity of polyherbal tea bag formulation in streptozotocin-nicotinamide induced diabetic rats. *International Journal of Health Sciences*, *6*, pp. 343-372.

Rachid, A., Rabah, D., Farid, L., Zohra, S. F., Houcine, B. and Nacéra, B., 2012. Ethnopharmacological survey of medicinal plants used in the traditional treatment of diabetes mellitus in the North Western and South Western Algeria. *Journal of medicinal plants research*, *6*(10), pp. 2041-2050.

Rutebemberwa, E., Lubega, M., Katureebe, S. K., Oundo, A., Kiweewa, F. and Mukanga, D., 2013. Use of traditional medicine for the treatment of diabetes in Eastern Uganda: a qualitative exploration of reasons for choice. *BMC international health and human rights*, *13*, pp. 1-7.

Tits, M., Damas, J., Quetin-Leclercq, J. and Angenot, L., 1991. From ethnobotanical uses of Strychnos henningsii to antiinflammatories, analgesics and antispasmodics. *Journal of ethnopharmacology*, *34*(2-3), pp. 261-267.

Van Wyk, B. E., De Wet, H. and Van Heerden, F. R., 2008. An ethnobotanical survey of medicinal plants in the southeastern Karoo, South Africa. *South African Journal of Botany*, *74*(4), pp. 696-704.

Watt, J. M. and Breyer-Brandwijk, M. G., 1962. The Medicinal and Poisonous Plants of Southern and Eastern Africa being an Account of their Medicinal and other Uses, Chemical Composition, Pharmacological Effects and Toxicology in Man and Animal. *The Medicinal and Poisonous Plants of Southern and Eastern Africa being an Account of their Medicinal and other Uses, Chemical Composition, Pharmacological Effects and Toxicology in Man and Animal.*, (Edn 2).

Zeggwagh, N. A., Sulpice, T. and Eddouks, M., 2007. Anti-hyperglycaemic and hypolipidemic effects of Ocimum basilicum aqueous extract in diabetic rats. *American journal of Pharmacology and toxicology*, *2*(3), pp. 123-129.

Chapter 4

Plant-Based Compounds in Diabetic Management

Chathurangani D. A. U.[1]
Dinusha N. Udukala[1,*]
and Medha J. Gunaratna[2]
[1]Institute of Chemistry Ceylon, College of Chemical Sciences, Rajagiriya, Sri Lanka
[2]Department of Chemistry, Faculty of Science, University of Kelaniya, Kelaniya, Sri Lanka

Abstract

Diabetes mellitus (DM) is one of the most common medical problems in the world, regardless of age, gender and income of the individuals. Therefore, control or mitigation of DM is highly demanded. Among the currently available therapeutics against DM, the use of α-amylase and α-glucosidase inhibitors plays a vital role. These inhibitors assist in preventing the fast breakdown of sugars and consequently manage blood sugar levels by inhibiting glycosidase activity. Herbal medications are often accepted due to their therapeutic relevance and because they are recognised to have fewer side effects. In nature, there are numerous sources of compounds having α-amylase and α-glucosidase inhibitory actions. In this chapter, 115 compounds isolated from plants that exhibit α-amylase and α-glucosidase inhibitory activities are summarised. Compounds with higher inhibitory activities could be clinically developed as natural nutraceuticals to treat DM.

Keywords: diabetes, management, plants, compounds

---

* Corresponding Author's Email: dinusha@ichemc.edu.lk.

In: Antidiabetic Plants
Editor: Arpita Roy
ISBN: 979-8-88697-957-2

Introduction

Diabetic mellitus (DM) is one of the most common chronic diseases that affect humans. It is caused by an absolute or relative deficiency of insulin and/or reduced insulin action that leads to hyperglycemia and / or abnormalities in the metabolism of carbohydrates, fats, and protein metabolism (Patil et al., 2011). DM is associated with a higher production of free radicals and oxidative stress in the body due topersistent high blood glucose levels. Over time, this causes several complications, such as retinopathy, cardiovascular disease, diabetic foot, neuropathy, and nephropathy. DM is a non-communicable disease that ranked among the top five global morbidities (Alam et al., 2022). It is a major health issue that has an increasing incidence rate and results in numerous deaths around the world. According to the International Diabetes Federation, 537 million adults (20-79 years) had diabetes in 2021; by2045, that number is projected to increase to 783 million. Furthermore, in 2021, this organisation reported 6.7 million deaths from diabetes-related complications (Kambale et al., 2022). Therefore, researchers are frantically working to discover effective therapeutics to treat DM and its side effects. Among them, herbal medications are often accepted because of their therapeutic relevance and because they are recognised to have fewer side effects (Modak et al., 2007). The application of herbal treatments for the control of DM has also been endorsed by the World Health Organisation (WHO) (Bailey and Clifford J. Day, 1989). Although numerous novel compounds have been isolated and identified from plants that possess antidiabetic actions, further research is still needed to find more effective therapeutics. Therefore, this chapter provides a detailed review of plant-based compounds that can be used to treat DM in humans.

There are two major types of DM classified as type 1 and type 2 which are also called insulin-dependent diabetes mellitus (IDDM) and noninsulin-dependent diabetes mellitus (NIDDM), respectively (Zulcafli et al., 2020). IDDM occurs due to deficient insulin production in the body that is mainly caused by the damage to pancreatic islet beta cells. Patients with IDDM are more likely to develop ketoacidosis and require daily insulin administration to keep blood glucose levels under control. IDDM affects children and adolescents (Salehi et al., 2019). NIDDM is the most widespread type of diabetes that usually manifests in maturity and primarily affects obese adults over the age of 40 (Meuleneire 2008). Patients with NIDDM have hyperglycemia as a result of pathophysiological abnormalities that affect insulin secretion and resistance. NIDDM has a higher genetic association compared to IDDM (Ozougwu 2013) and denotes a disorder with altered metabolism of fat and carbohydrates.. The risk factors for the development of NIDDM are ethnicity, a family history of the disease, a history of gestational diabetes, older age, overweight and obesity, an unhealthy diet, inactivity, and smoking (Salehi et al., 2019). DM often has relationships with hypertension, hyperlipidemia, hyperinsulinemia, and atherosclerosis. Both types of DM exhibit common signs, such as elevated blood sugar levels, unusual thirst, severe hunger, frequent urination, acute weakness, impaired vision, etc. (Khan et al., 2012).

Role of α-Amylase and α-Glucosidase Enzymes

The two key enzymes involved in starch digestion within the body are α-amylase and α-glucosidase (Figure 1). Therefore, inhibiting these enzymes is a fundamental approach in the treatment of NIDDM (Rasouli et al., 2020).

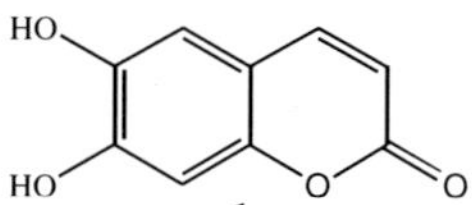

1

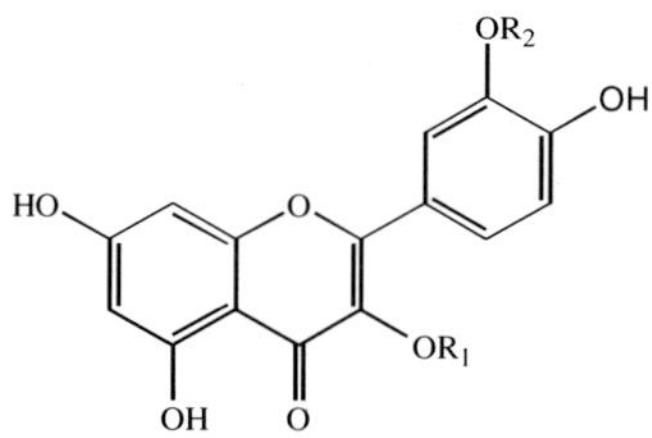

2. 47. R_1, R_2 = H
3. R_1 = H, R_2 = CH_3
5. R_1 = β-D-Glc*p*, R_2 = H
6. R_1 = β-D-Glc*p*, R_2 = CH_3
9. R_1 = (6”-acetyl)-β-D-Glc*p*, R_2 = H
16. R_1 = (6”-α-L-Rha*p*)-β-D-Glc*p*, R_2 = H

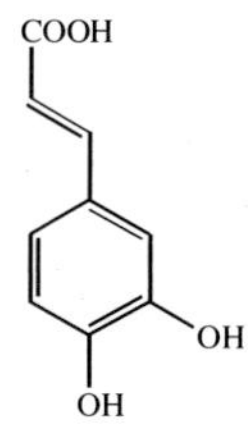

4, 24

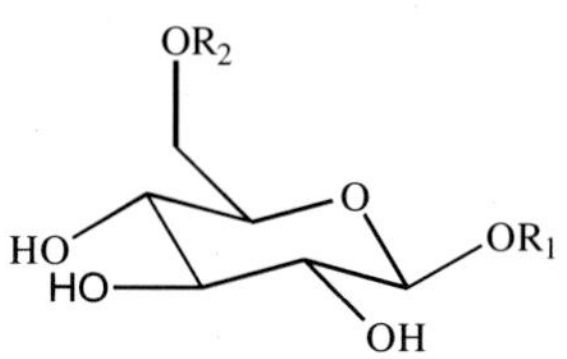

11. R_1 = protocatechuoyl, R_2 = H
13. R_1 = H, R_2 = protocatechuoyl
14. R_1 = vanilloyl, R_2 = H
15. R_1 = H, R_2 = vanilloyl

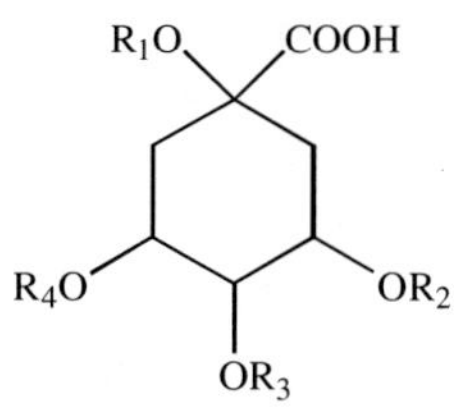

7. R_1, R_3 = H, R_2, R_4 = caffeoyl
8. R_1, R_2 = H, R_3, R_4 = caffeoyl
10. R_2, R_3 = H, R_1, R_4 = caffeoyl
12. R_1, R_3, R_4 = H, R_2 = caffeoyl

Figure 1. (Continued)

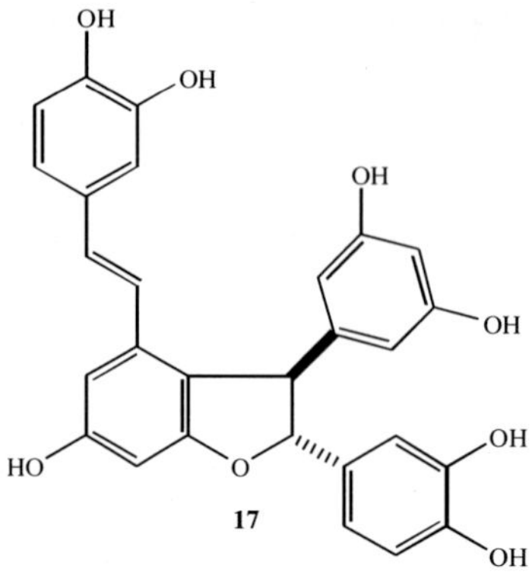

17

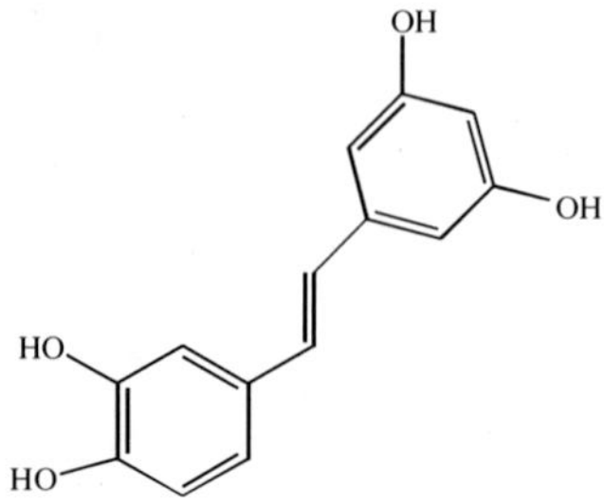

18

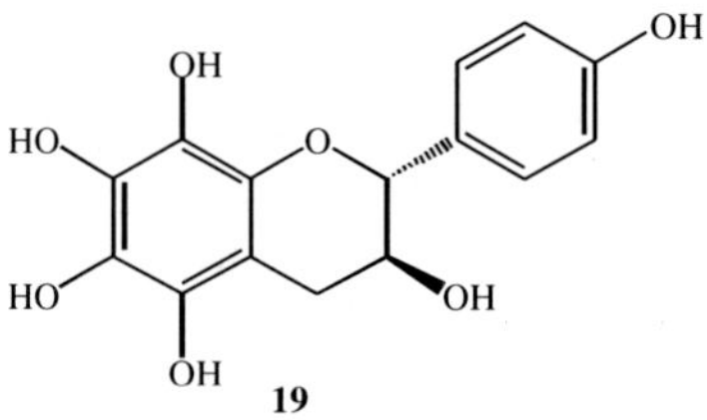

19

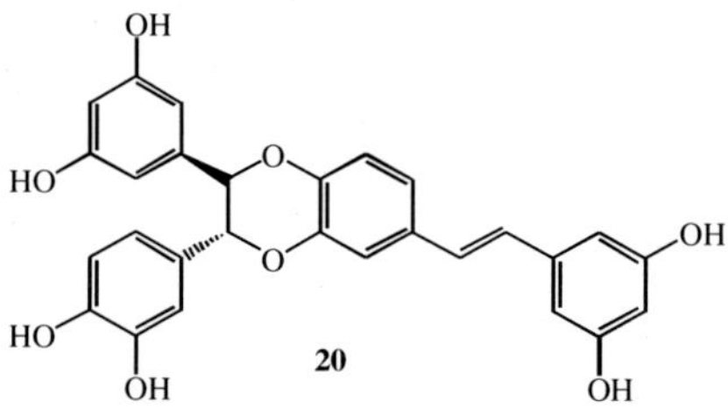

20

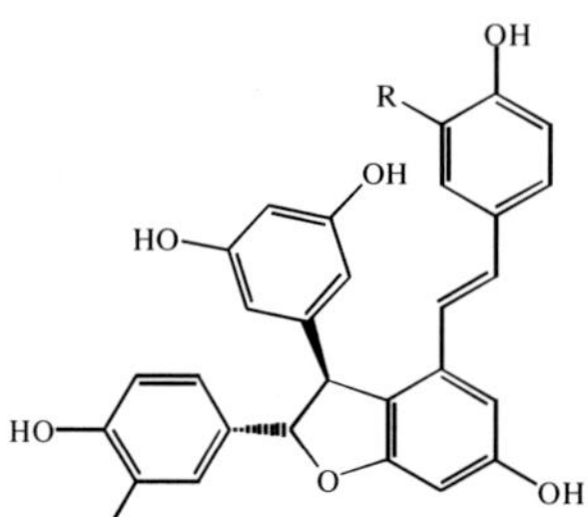

21. R= OH
22. R= H

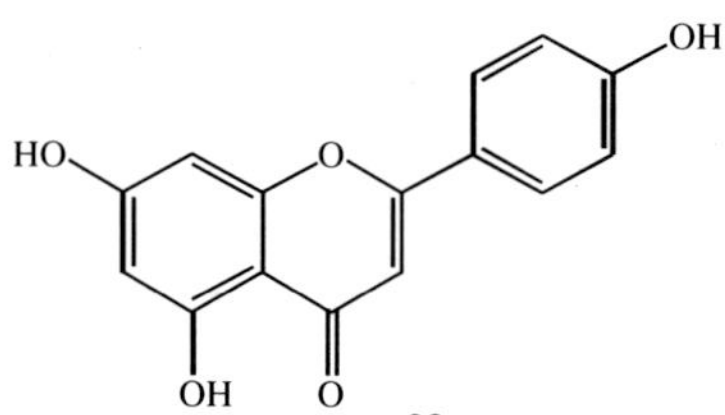

23

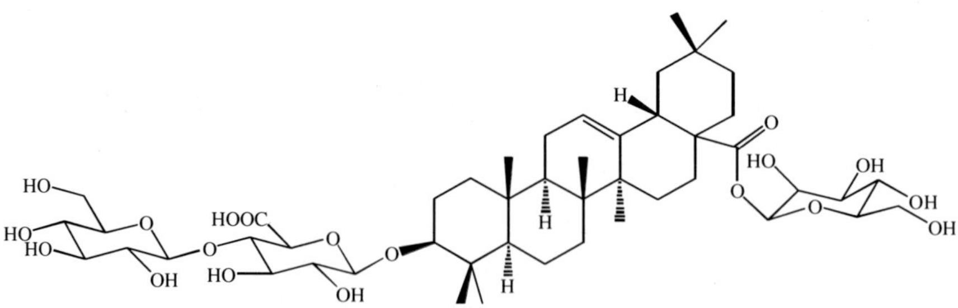

25

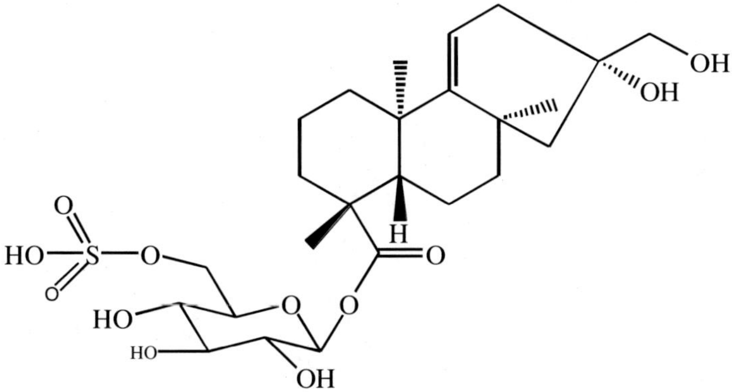

26

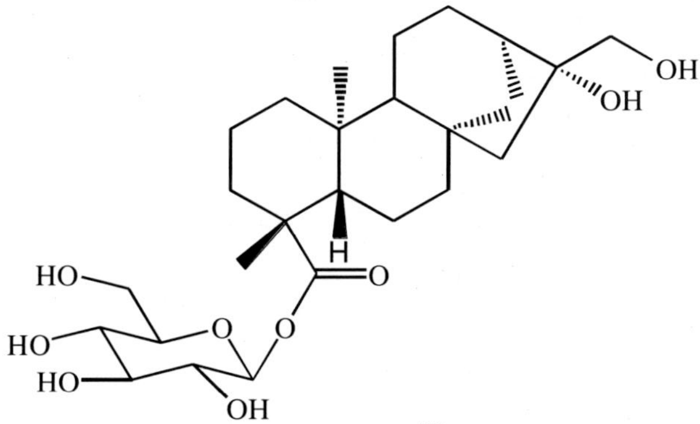

27. $\Delta^{9,11}$

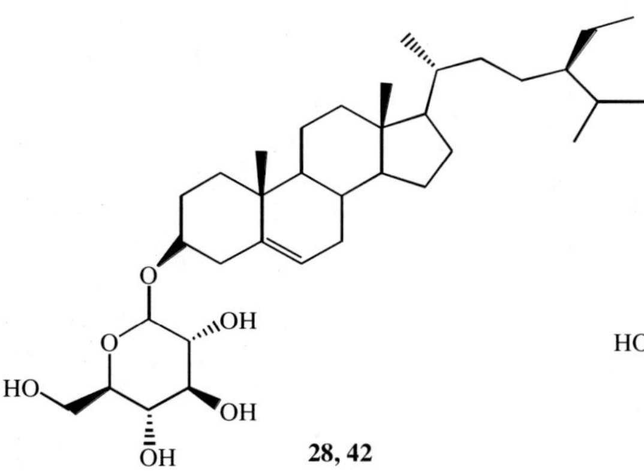

28, 42

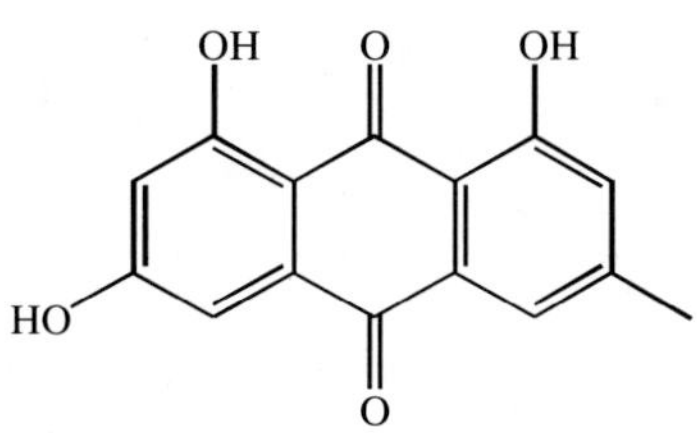

29

Figure 1. (Continued)

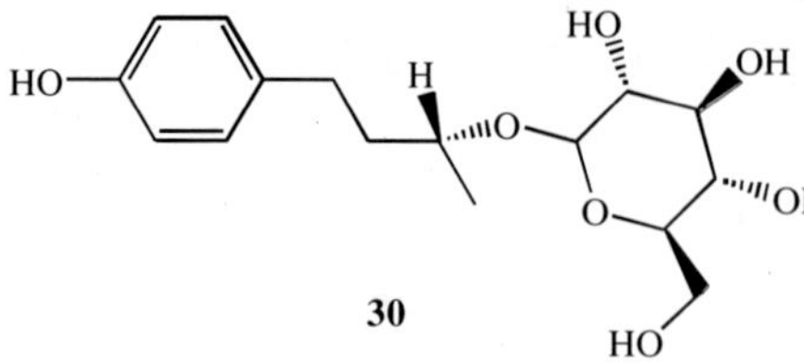

30

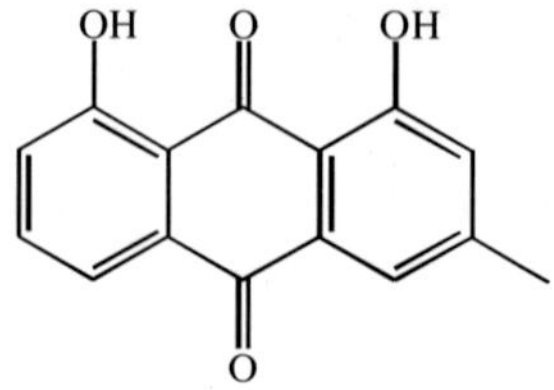

31

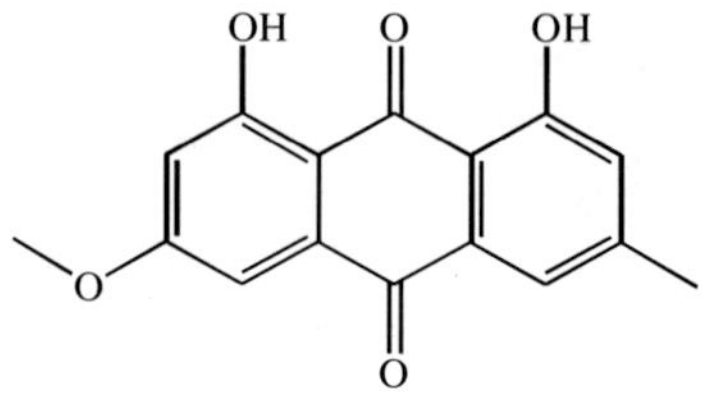

32

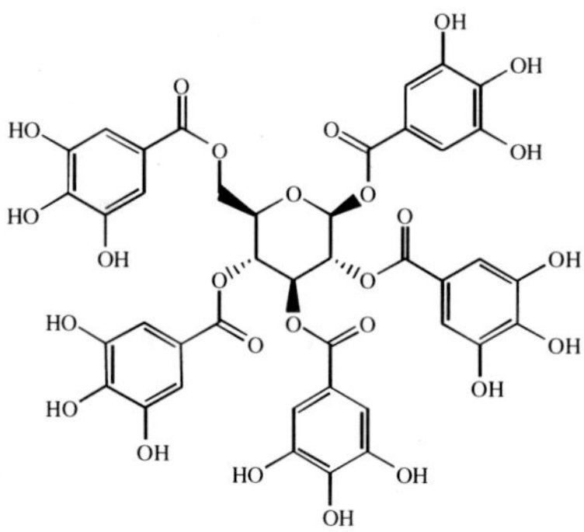

33, 71

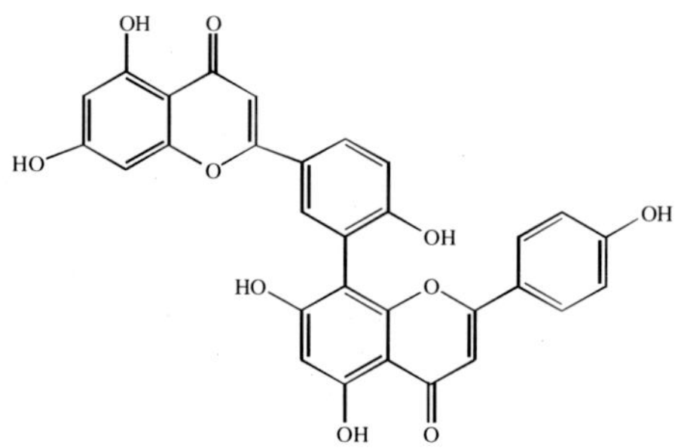

34

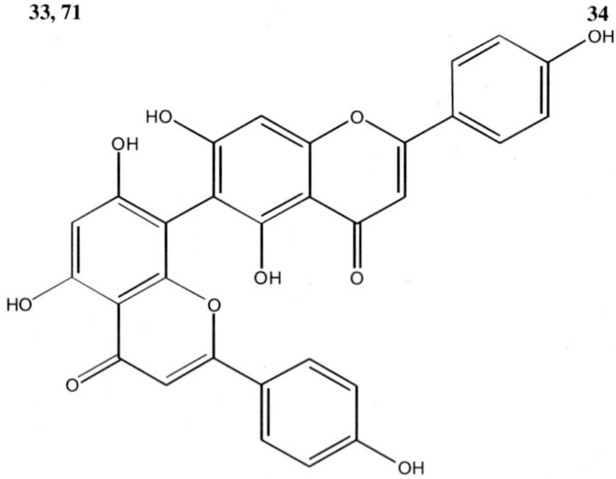

35

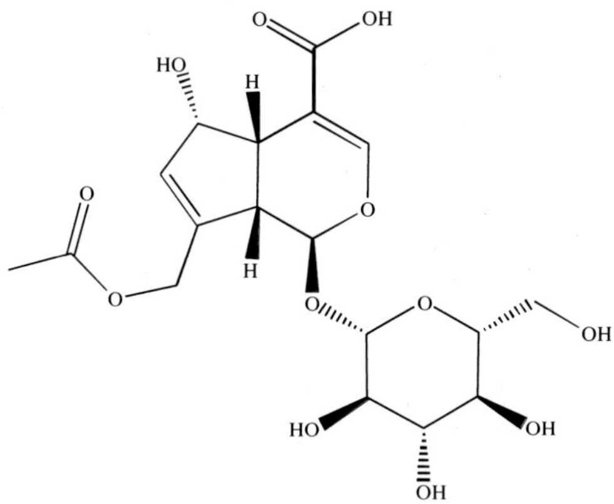

36

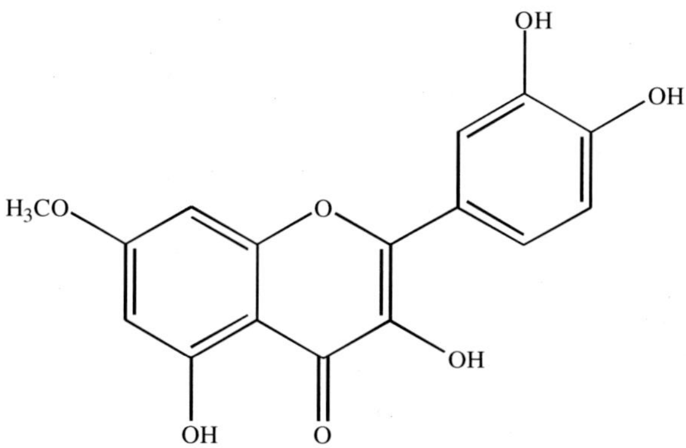

37

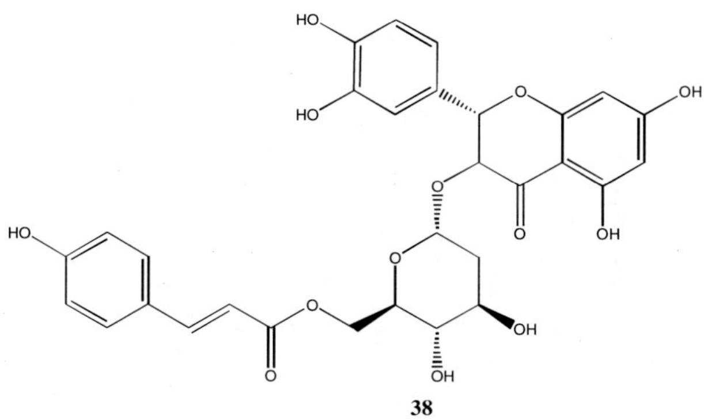

38

Figure 1. (Continued)

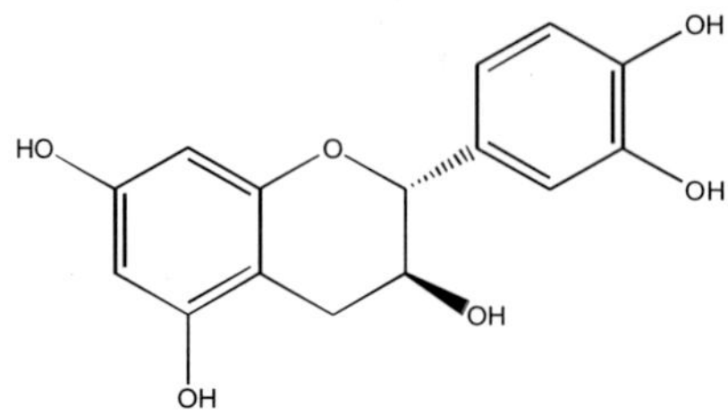

39

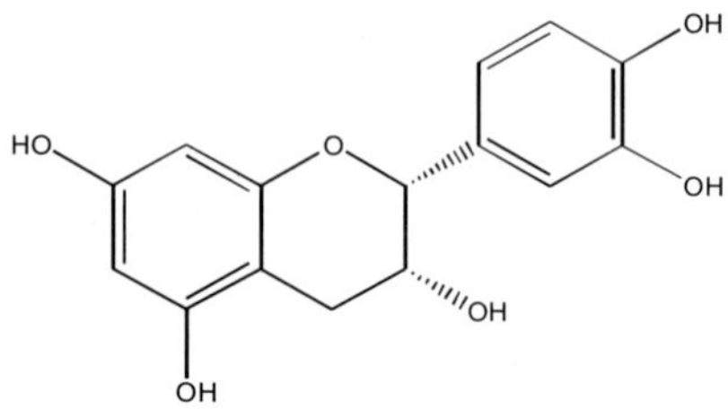

40

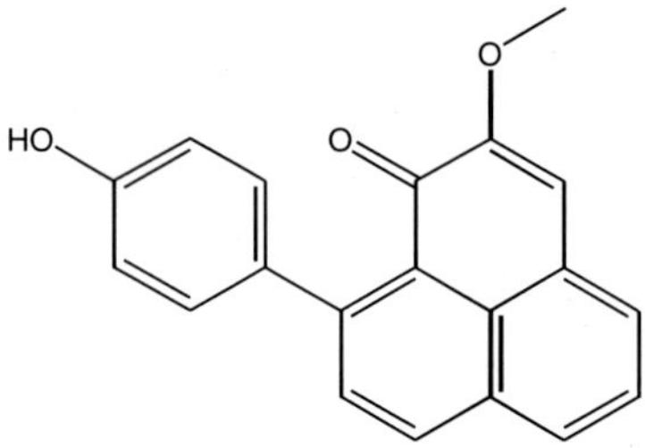

41

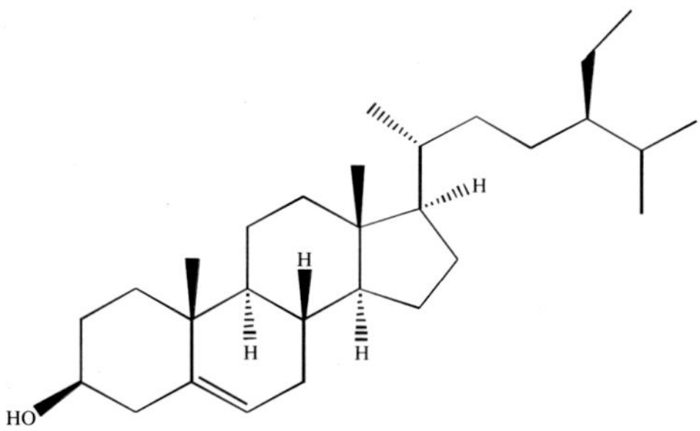

43

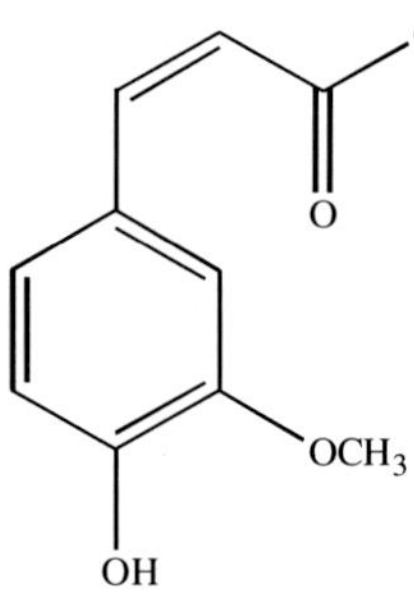

44

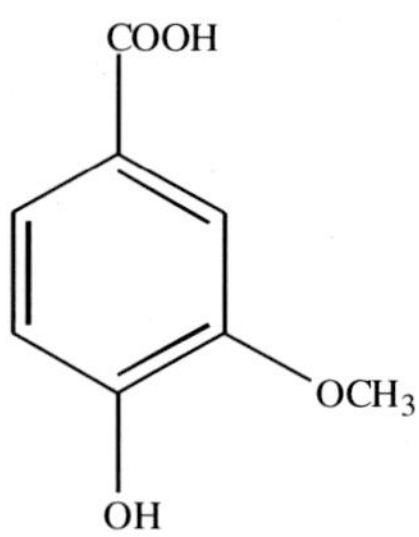

45

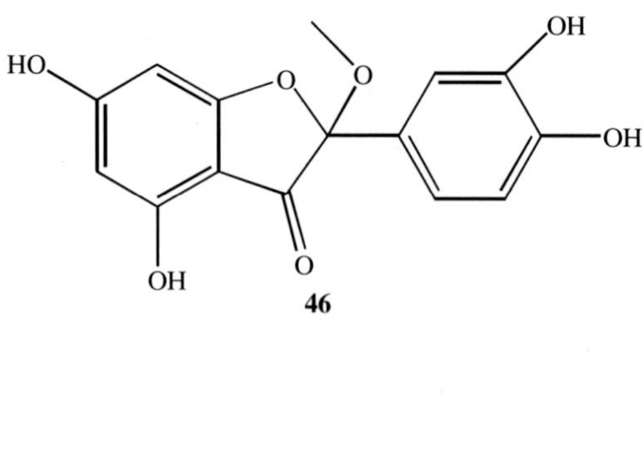

46

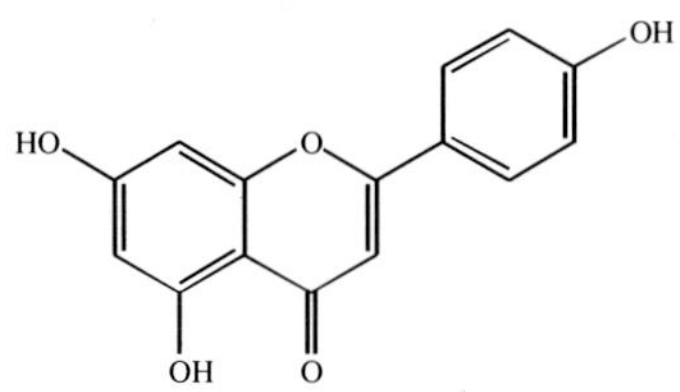

48, 57

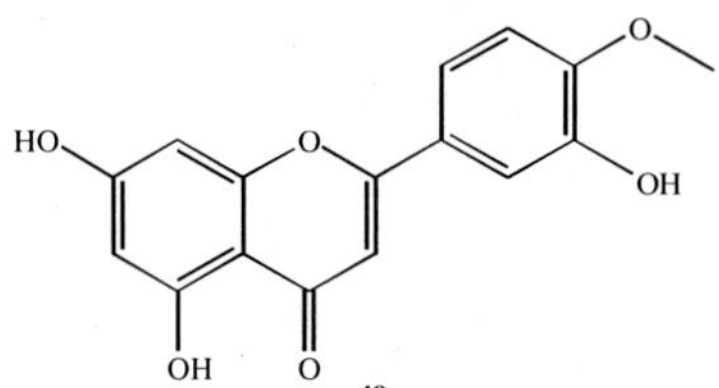

49

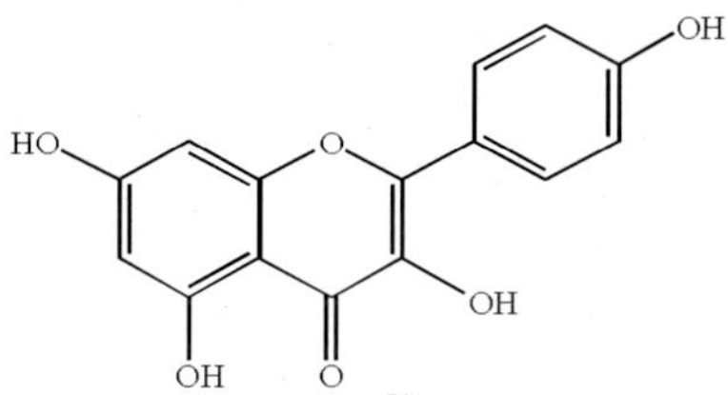

50

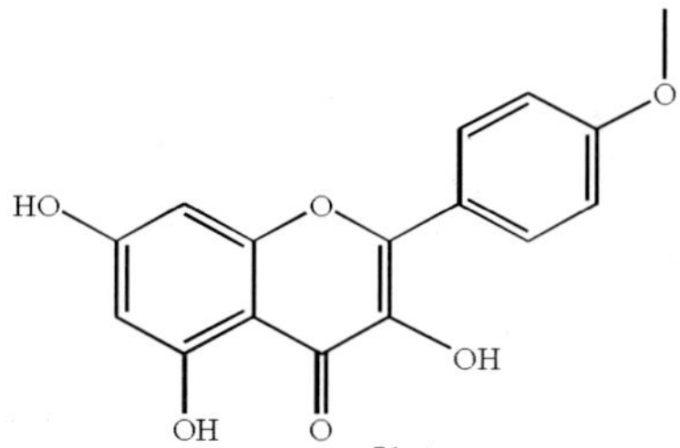

51

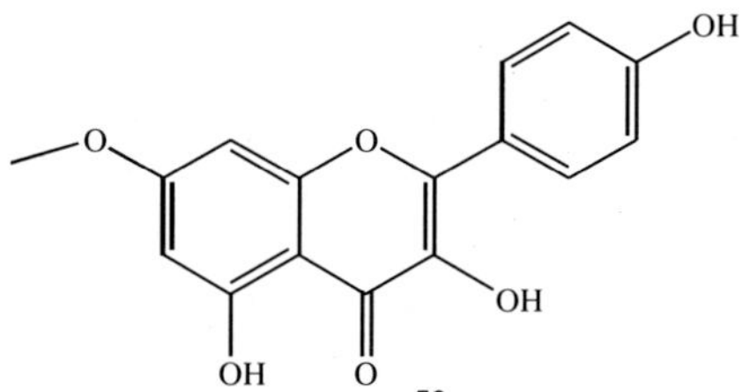

52

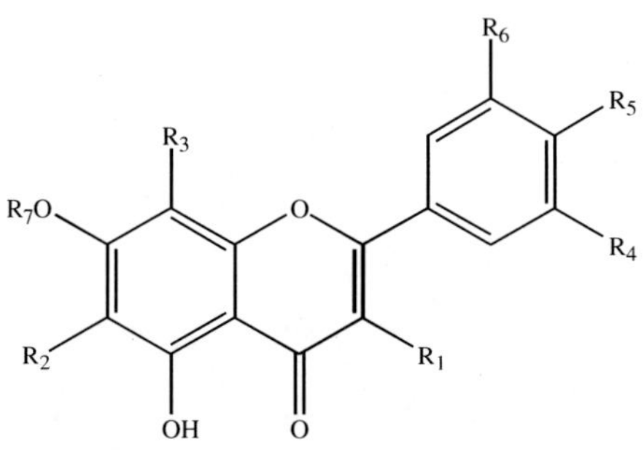

54. R_1 = OMe, R_2 = Br, R_3 = Br, R_4 = Br, R_5 = OH, R_6 = Br, R_7 = Me
55. R_1 = OMe, R_2 = Br, R_3 = Br, R_4 = OH, R_5 = OMe, R_6 = Br, R_7 = Me
56. R_1 = H, R_2 = H, R_3 = H, R_4 = OH, R_5 = OH, R_6 = H, R_7 = H
58. R_1 = H, R_2 = OMe, R_3 = OMe, R_4 = OH, R_5 = OMe, R_6 = H, R_7 = Me
59. R_1 = OH, R_2 = H, R_3 = H, R_4 = OH, R_5 = OMe, R_6 = OH, R_7 = H
60. R_1 = OH, R_2 = H, R_3 = H, R_4 = H, R_5 = OH, R_6 = H, R_7 = Me
61. R_1 = OMe, R_2 = H, R_3 = H, R_4 = OH, R_5 = OMe, R_6 = H, R_7 = Me
62. R_1 = OMe, R_2 = H, R_3 = Br, R_4 = H, R_5 = OH, R_6 = H, R_7 = Me
63. R_1 = OH, R_2 = H, R_3 = H, R_4 = OMe, R_5 = OH, R_6 = OMe, R_7 = Me

Figure 1. (Continued)

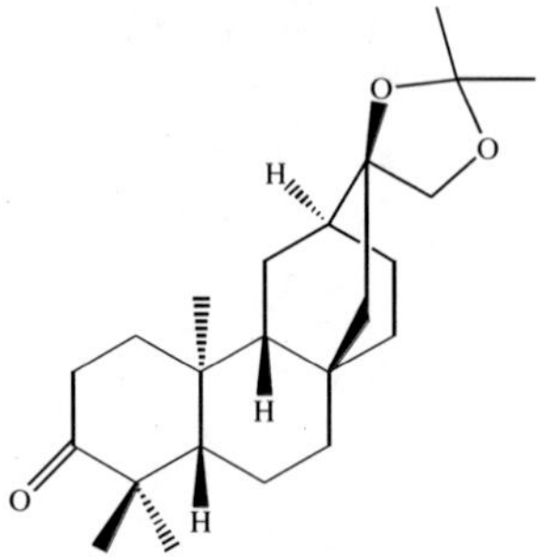

64

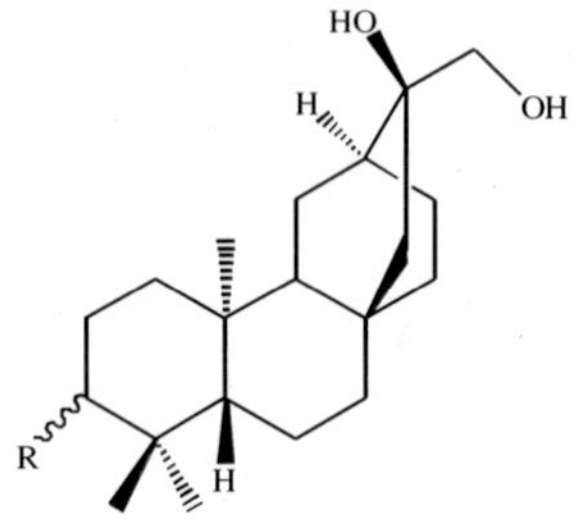

65

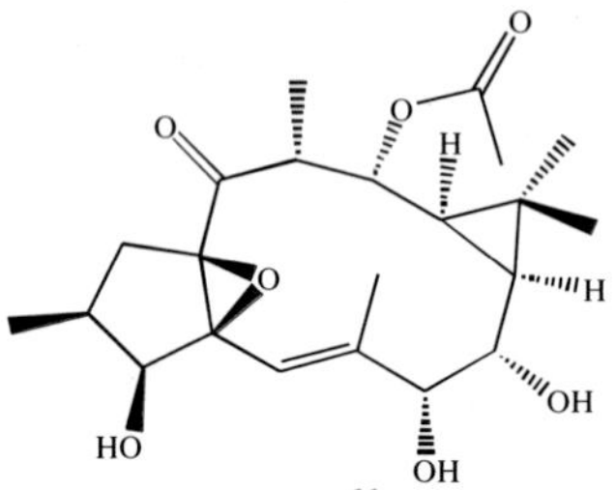

66

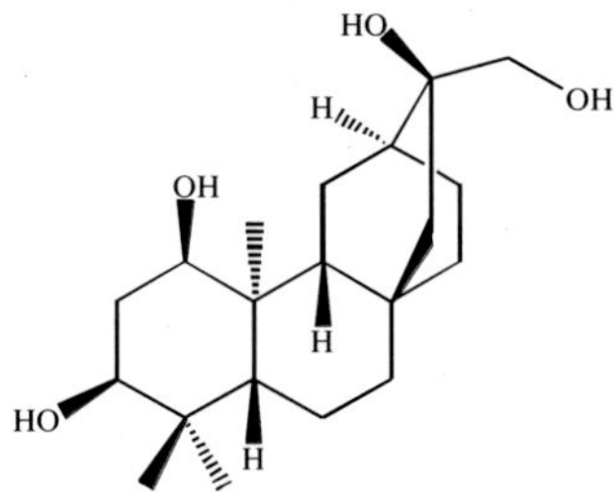

67

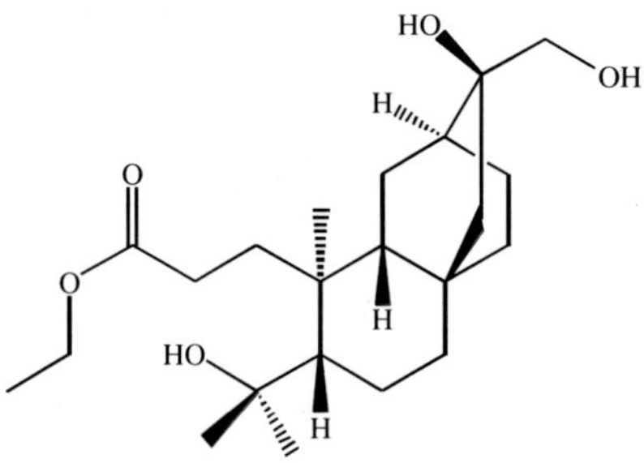

68

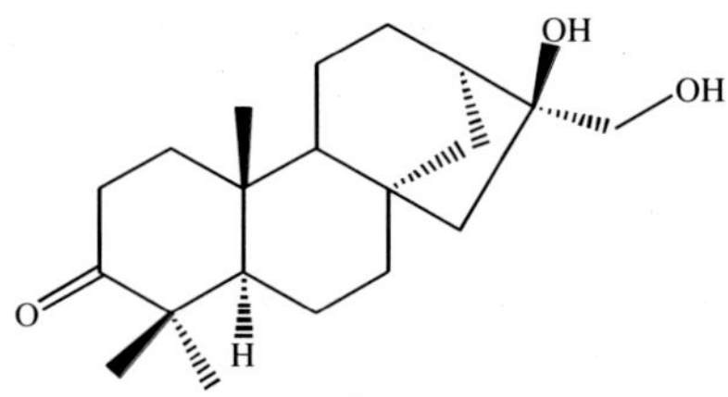

69

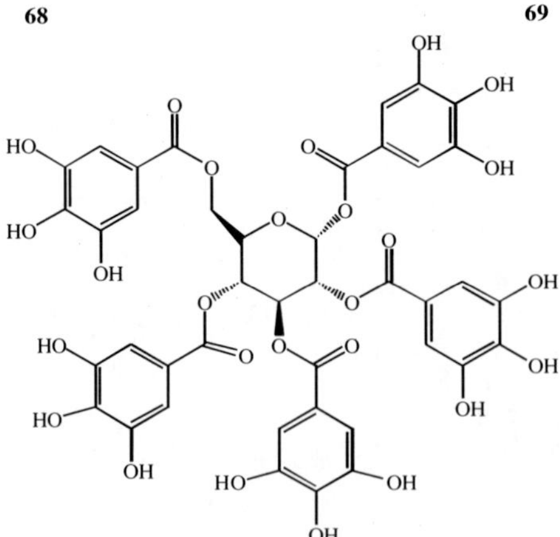

70

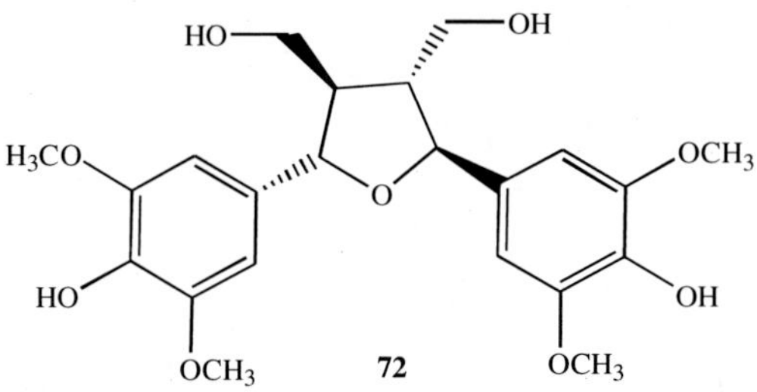

72

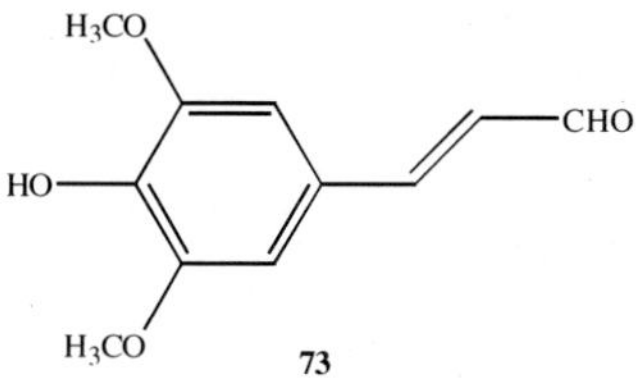

73

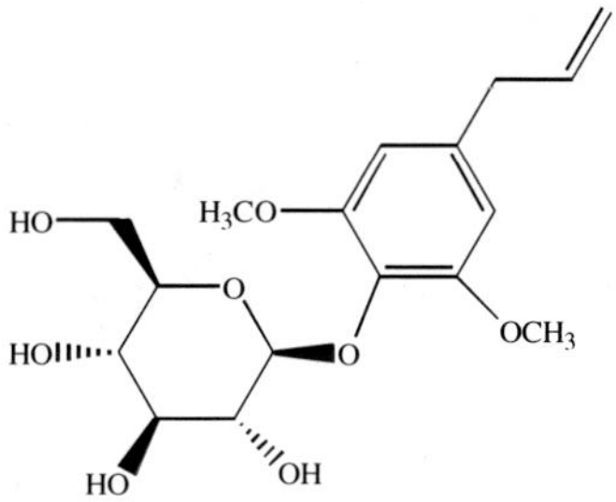

74

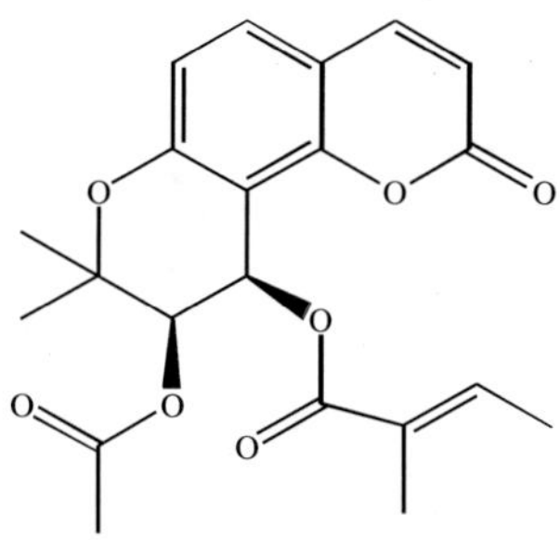

75

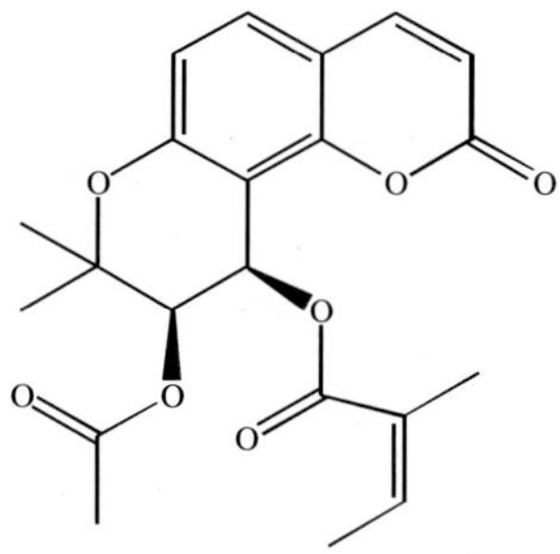

76

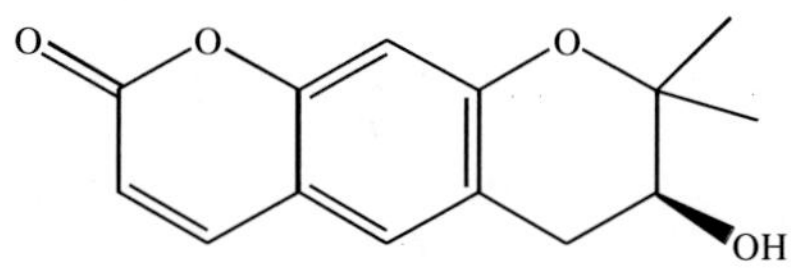

77

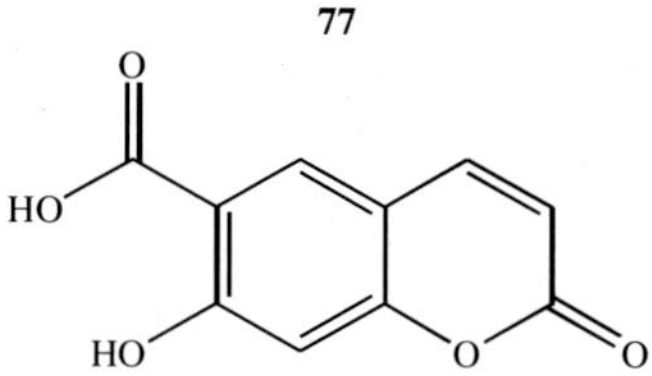

82

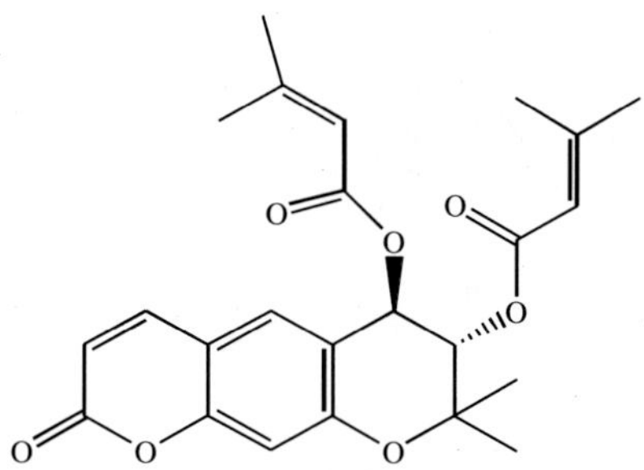

80

Figure 1. (Continued)

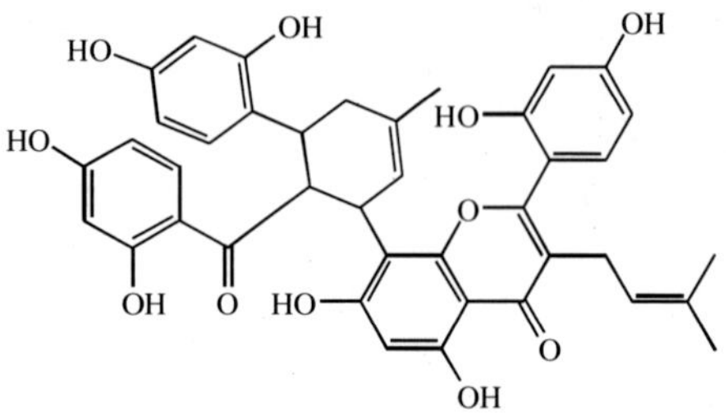

89

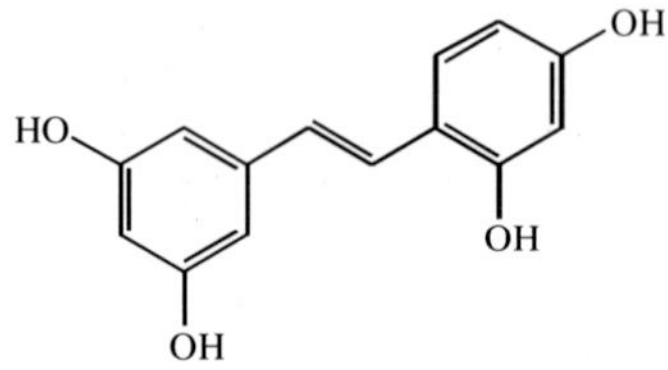

90

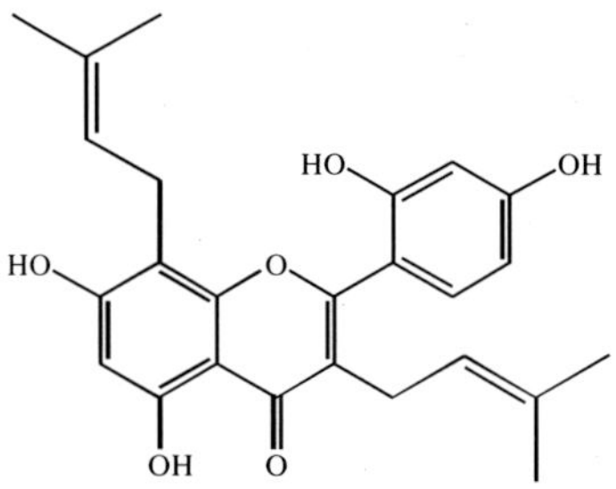

91

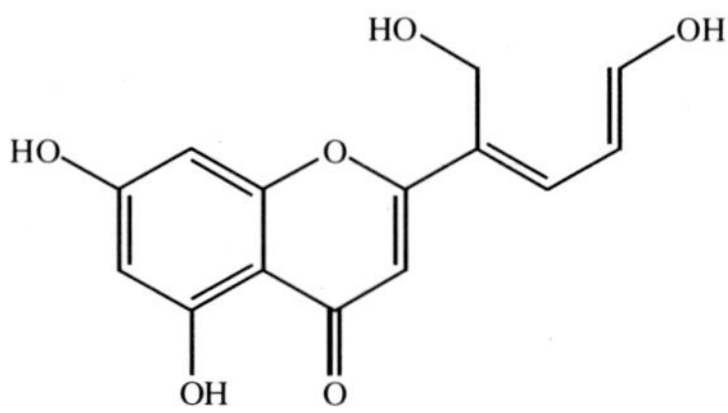

92

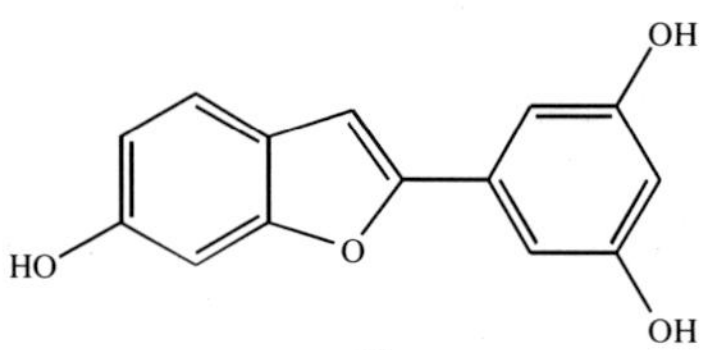

93

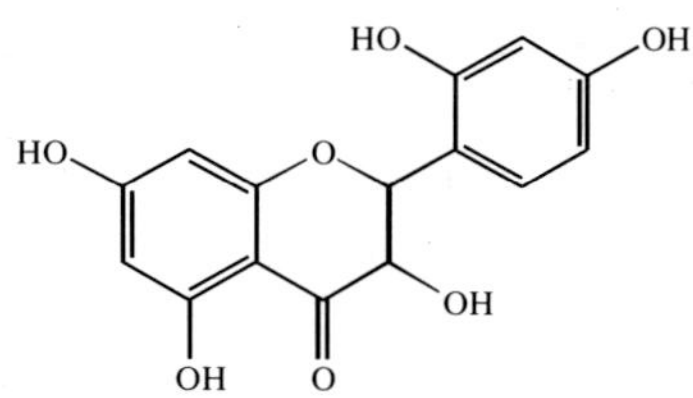

94

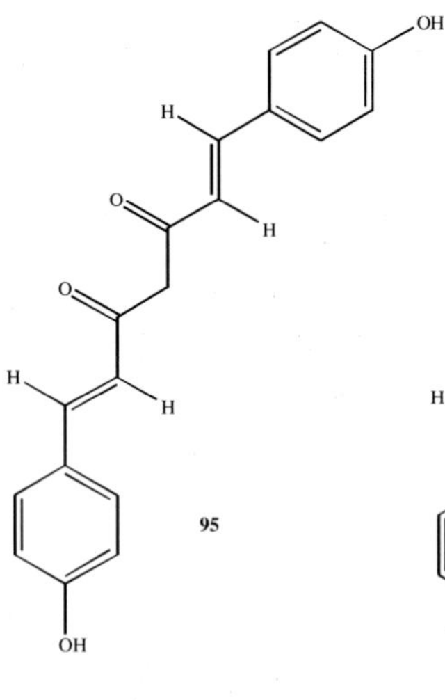

95

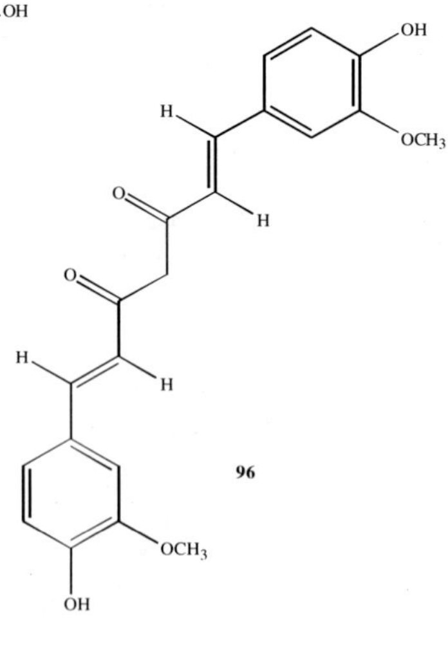

96

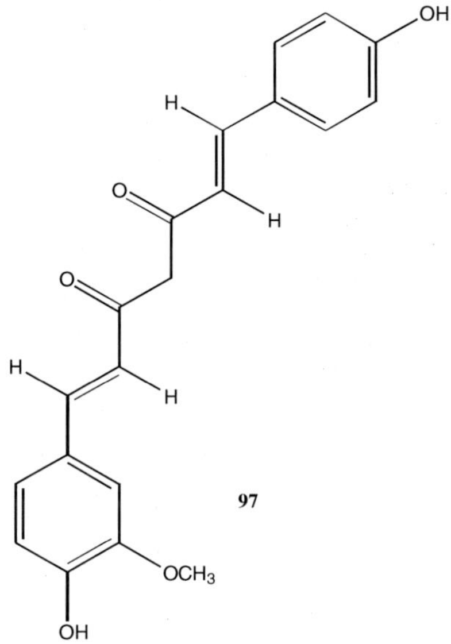

97

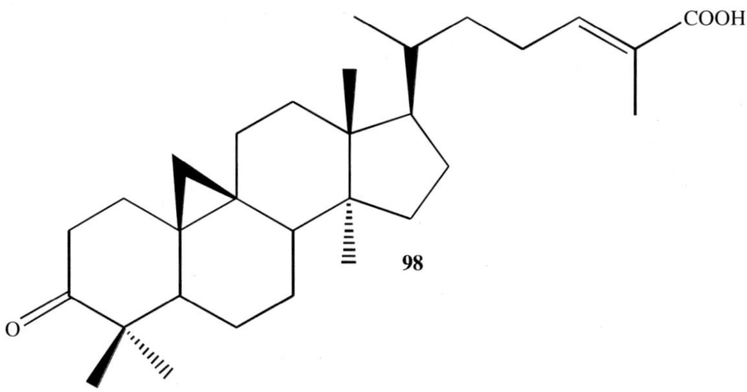

98

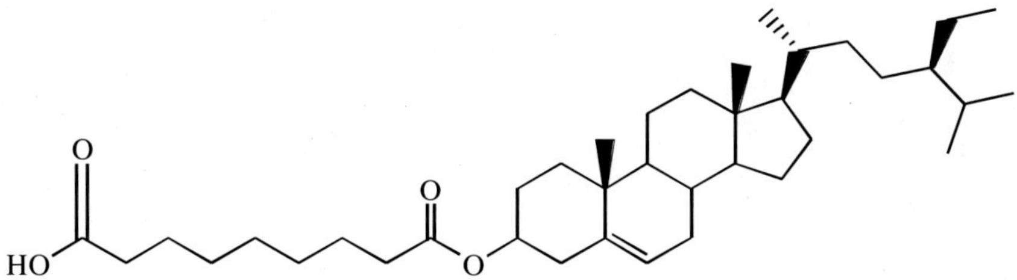

99

Figure 1. (Continued)

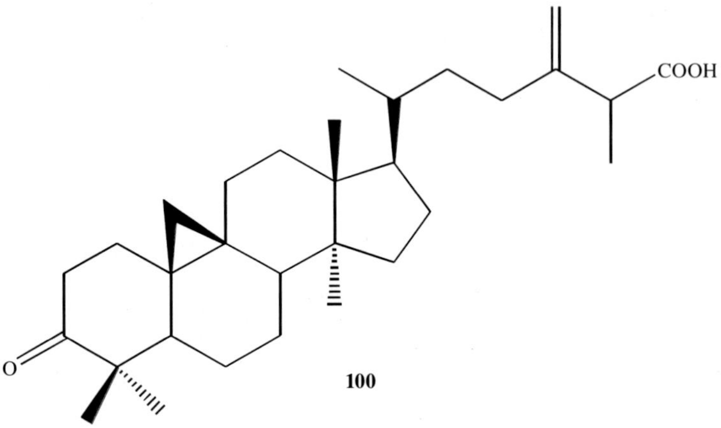

100

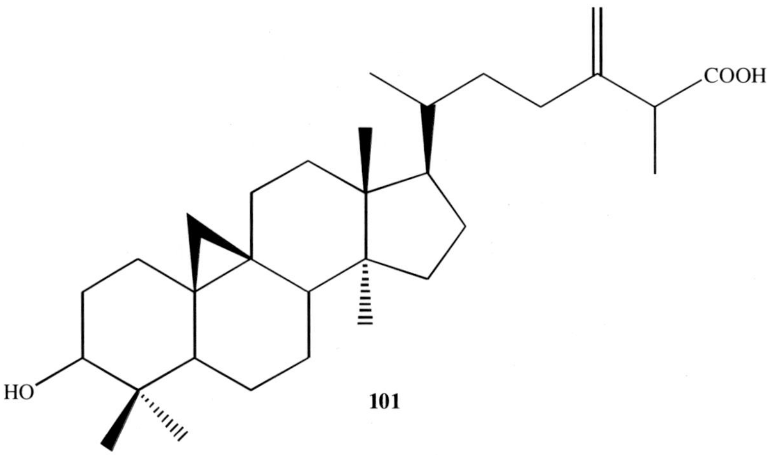

101

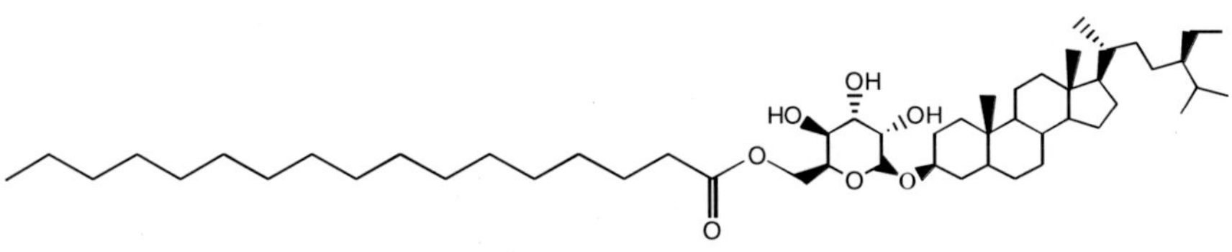

102

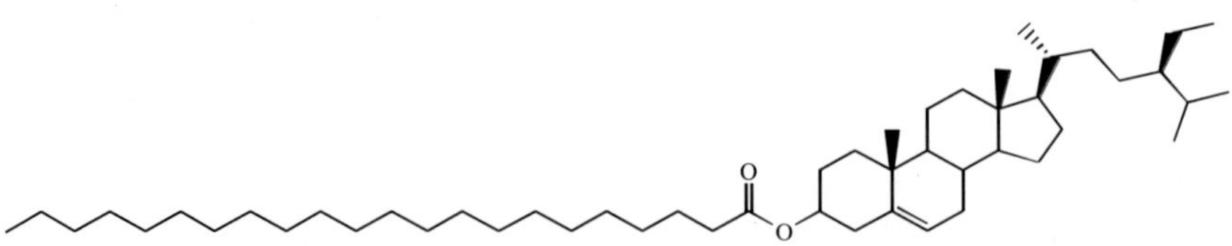

103

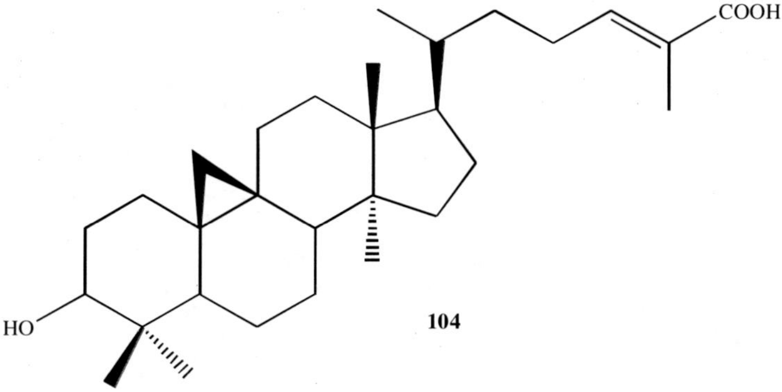

104

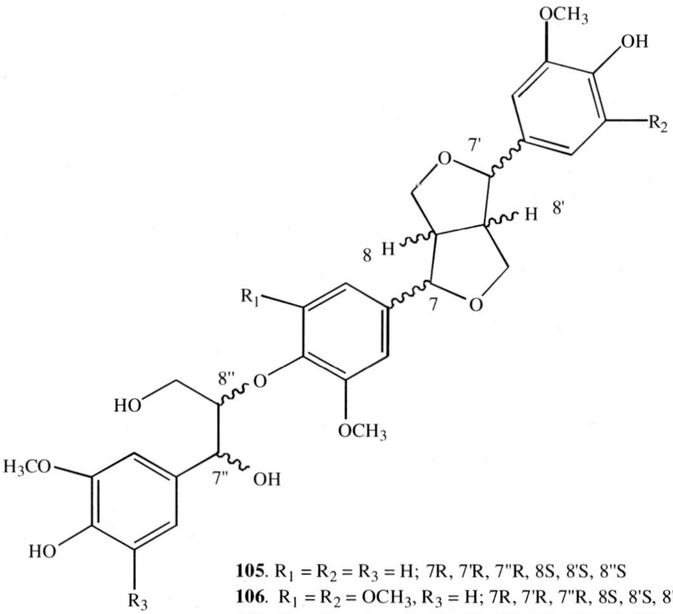

105. $R_1 = R_2 = R_3 = H$; 7R, 7'R, 7''R, 8S, 8'S, 8''S
106. $R_1 = R_2 = OCH_3$, $R_3 = H$; 7R, 7'R, 7''R, 8S, 8'S, 8''S
107. $R_1 = R_2 = R_3 = OCH_3$; 7S, 7'S, 7''S, 8R, 8'S, 8''S

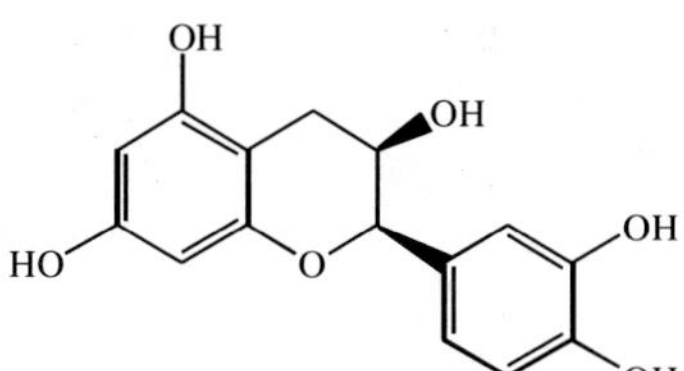

108

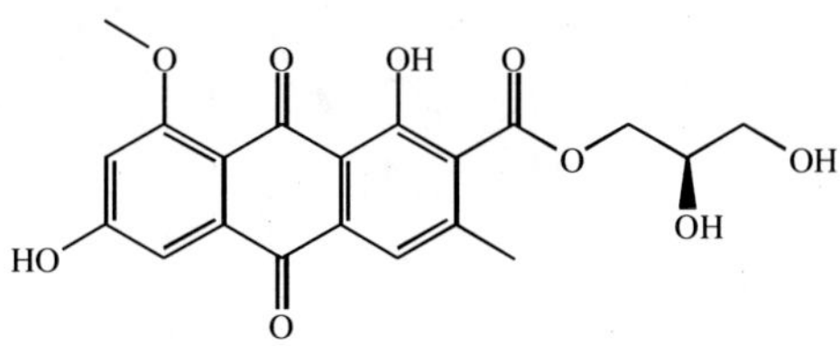

109

Figure 1. (Continued)

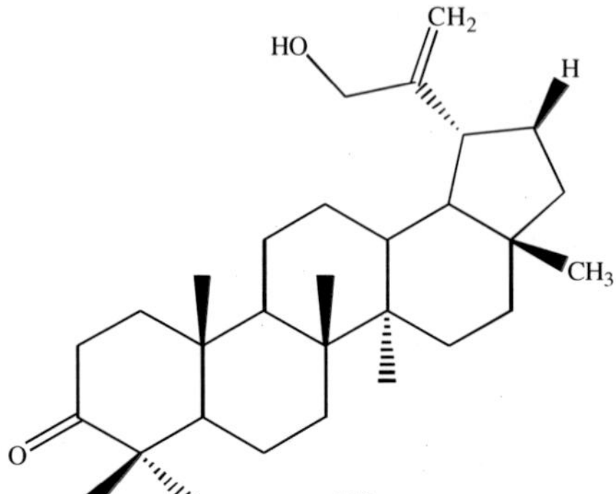

110

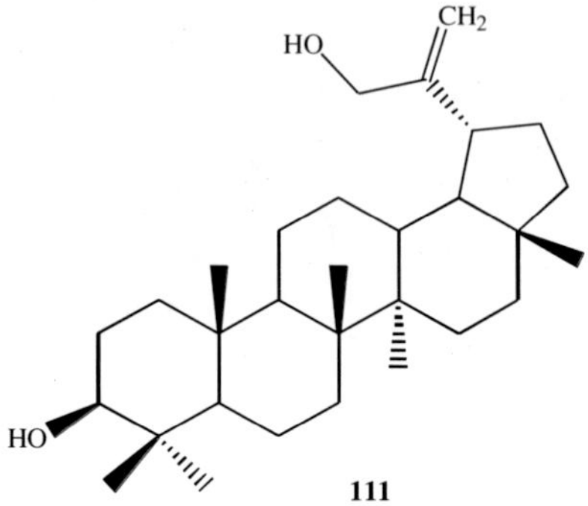

111

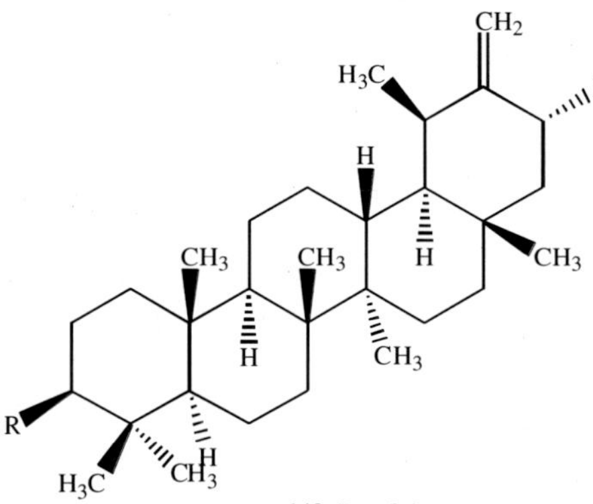

112. R = OAc
113. R = OH

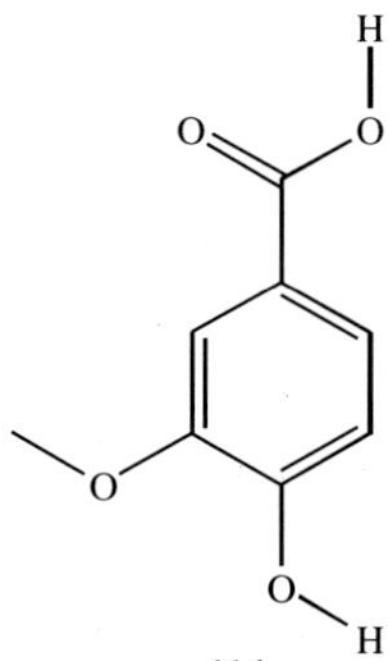

114

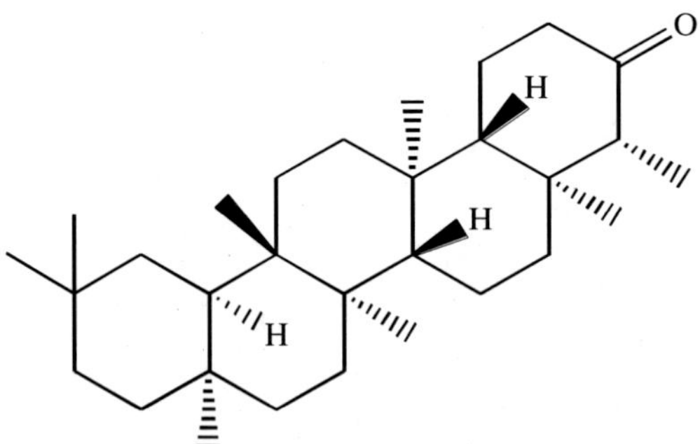

115

Figure 1. Isolated bioactive α-amylase and α-glucosidase inhibitory compounds.

Alpha-amylase (1,4-α-D-glucan-glucanohydrolase, EC 3.2. 1.3) catalyses the hydrolysis of 1,4-D-glucan linkages in starch, maltodextrins and maltooligosaccharides. This enzyme is found in fungi, bacteria, plants, animals, and humans (Svensson, 1988). In animals, α-amylase is produced primarily in the salivary glands, pancreas, and small intestine. In humans, multiple steps are involved in starch digestion. The initial partial digestion of polymeric substrates into shorter oligomers is caused by salivary amylase (Truscheit et al., 1981). Therefore, inhibiting α-amylase, which is involved in starch and glycogen, is suggested to be a strategy to treat carbohydrate intake, such as diabetes and obesity (Rasouli et al., 2017).

Alpha-glucosidase (EC 3.2.1.20) is a carbohydrate hydrolytic enzyme that can be found in tissues of humans, animals, plants, and microbes (Kumar et al., 2011). The luminal surface of enterocytes contains α-glucosidase, which is secreted into the small intestine (Yihai Wang et al., 2013). Maltose and sucrose are hydrolysed into glucose and fructose by the enzyme α-glucosidase. Hence, inhibiting α-glucosidase activity prevents postprandial hyperglycemia and increased blood sugar levels (Kim, Rioux and Turgeon 2014).

As a result of consuming carbohydrates such as starch that break down into smaller molecules, hydrolysing enzymes like α-amylase and α-glucosidase causes an accumulation of free glucose in the blood (Jhong et al., 2015). The main issue in DM is hyperglycemia, a condition in which there is a high concentration of glucose molecules in the blood. Therefore, the treatment of hyperglycemia is associated with the decrease or modulation of glucose production from the digestion of complex carbohydrates and/or its absorption from the small intestine (Rasouli et al., 2020).

Medicinal Plants as Antidiabetic Agent

Natural products, especially those of plant origin, are crucial to maintaining the health of both individuals and society. A variety of medicinal plants offer a rich source of bioactive compounds that have potent pharmacological effects. They are the key source for discovering lead candidates and are crucial for future drug development initiatives (Salehi et al., 2019). Plant-based preparations are the dominant player among all accessible medicines, especially in rural areas (Singab et al., 2014), due to their easy accessibility, affordability, and minimum negative side effects. Furthermore, many of the pharmaceuticals currently on the market have been prepared directly or indirectly from plants, which have long been a major source of medication

(Arumugam, Manjula and Paari 2013). Therefore, the use of medicinal plants in the treatment of disorders such as DM is recommended, as these plants contain a variety of pharmacoactive constituents, including flavonoids, terpenoids, saponins, carotenoids, alkaloids, glycosides, etc. (Afrisham et al., 2015).

Several studies have been conducted to investigate the potential role of medicinal plants as α-glucosidase and α-amylase inhibitors. Numerous plants have been shown to inhibit α-glucosidase and α-amylase in the treatment of NIDDM. In the literature, antidiabetic activities of about 800 plant species have been reported (Arumugam, Manjula and Paari 2013). Numerous interesting pharmacophores have been isolated and their structures have been identified as a result of research on novel bioactive chemicals derived from plants (de Sales et al., 2012).

Biochemical Methods to Identify Antidiabetic Agents

The α-amylase and α-glucosidase inhibitory assays have been conducted using spectrophotometric methods to identify plant-based α-amylase and α-glucosidase inhibitors.

In the α-amylase inhibitory assay, potato starch has been commonly used as a substrate. Maltose released from starch during its enzymatic hydrolysis is reacted with 3,5-dinitrosalicylic acid (DNS) to produce 3-amino-5-nitrosalicylic acid (ANSA) and maltonic acid. The ANSA produced has been monitored at 540 nm using a microplate spectrophotometer. Acarbose has been used as a standard for the α-amylase inhibitory assay (Gök et al., 2020), (Dehghan, Salehi, and Amiri, 2018).

The α-glucosidase inhibition has been evaluated using p-nitrophenyl-α-D-glucopyranoside (p-NPG) as a substrate, and the subsequent release of p-nitrophenol is measured using a microplate spectrophotometer at 405 nm. Acarbose, quercetin, genistein, and deoxynojirimycin have been used as standards for the α-glucosidase inhibitory assay of -glucosidase (Yuwei Wang et al., 2021), (Gök et al., 2020).

Table 1. Isolated compounds with α-amylase and α-glucosidase inhibitory activity of -amylase and -glucosidase

Compound reference No	Plant name	Plant part used	Compound name	Activity	IC$_{50}$ Value (μM)		Reference article
					Compound	Reference	
1.	*Calendula officinalis*	Leaves	Aesculetin	α-Amylase inhibitor	5.72	14.78 (Acarbose)	(Olennikov and Kashchenko 2014)
2.			Quercetin		5.92		
3.			Isorhamnetin		8.79		
4.			Caffeic acid		14.04		
5.			isoquercetin		15.45 μg/mL	9.54 μg/mL (Acarbose)	
6.			isorhamnetin-3-*O*-*β*-D-glucopyranoside		23.41 μg/mL		
7.			3,5-di-*O*-caffeoylquinic acid		25.63 μg/mL		
8.			4,5-di-*O*-caffeoylquinic acid		26.65 μg/mL		
9.			quercetin-3-*O*-(6''-acetyl)-*β*-D-glucopyranoside		32.70 μg/mL		
10.			1,5-di-*O*-caffeoylquinic acid		37.15 μg/mL		
11.	*Calendula officinalis*	Leaves	1'-*O*-protocatechuoyl-*β*-D-glucopyranose	α-Amylase inhibitor	62.46 μg/mL	9.54 μg/mL (Acarbose)	(Olennikov and Kashchenko 2014)
12.			3-*O*-caffeoylquinic acid		65.42 μg/mL		
13.			6'-*O*-protocatechuoyl-*β*-D-glucopyranose		66.52 μg/mL		
14.			1'-*O*-vanilloyl-*β*-d-glucopyranose		73.69 μg/mL		
15.			6'-*O*-vanilloyl-*β*-D-glucopyranose		79.18 μg/mL		
16.			Rutin		89.85 μg/mL		
17.	*Callistemon rigidus*	Stem bark	Scirpusin B	α-Amylase inhibitor	90.5	45.4 (Acarbose)	(Kobayashi et al., 2006)
18.			Piceatannol		457.0		

Table 1. (Continued)

Compound reference No	Plant name	Plant part used	Compound name	Activity	IC$_{50}$ Value (µM)		Reference article
19.	*Cyperus rotundus*	Rhizomes	(2RS,3SR)-3,40,5,6,7,8-hexahydroxyflavane	α-Amylase inhibitor	24.2 ± 1.1	776.1 ± 36.7 (Acarbose)	(H. H. T. Tran et al., 2014)
20.			Cassigarol E	α-Amylase inhibitor	21.7 ± 1.4		
				α-Glucosidase inhibitor	210.5 ± 17.3	2060 ± 97.5 (Acarbose)	
21.	*Cyperus rotundus*	Rhizomes	Scirpusin B	α-Glucosidase inhibitor	94.3 ± 6.8 µg/mL	2060 ± 97.5 µg/mL (Acarbose)	(H. H. T. Tran et al., 2014)
22.			Scirpusin A		168.1 ± 12.5 µg/mL		
23.	*Wedelia trilobata*	Leaves	5,7,4'-trihydroxyflavone	α-Glucosidase inhibitor	27.54 ± 1.12 µg/mL	450.56 ± 2.31 µg/mL (Acarbose)	(Luyen et al., 2019)
24.			3,4-dihydroxy-cinnamic acid	α-Amylase inhibitor	181.97 ± 2.62 µg/mL	6.78 ± 0.32 µg/mL (Acarbose)	
				α-Glucosidase inhibitor	173.78 ± 2.37 µg/mL	450.56 ± 2.31 µg/mL (Acarbose)	
25.			3-*O*-[β-D-glucopyranosyl(1-4)-β-D-glucoronopyranosyl] oleanolic acid 28-*O*-β-D-glucopyranosyl ester	α-Amylase inhibitor	52.08 ± 0.56 µg/mL	6.78 ± 0.32 µg/mL (Acarbose)	
				α-Glucosidase inhibitor	190.40 ± 2.01 µg/mL	450.56 ± 2.31 µg/mL (Acarbose)	
26.			Wedtriloside B	α-Amylase inhibitor	87.10 ± 1.89 µg/mL	6.78 ± 0.32 µg/mL (Acarbose)	
27.			Wedtriloside A	α-Amylase inhibitor	112.20 ± 2.87 µg/mL	6.78 ± 0.32 µg/mL (Acarbose)	(Luyen et al., 2019)
28.	*Rheum turkestanicum*	Root	Daucosterol	α-Amylase inhibitor	46.4 ± 1.5	47.4 ± 1.1 (Acarbose)	(Dehghan, Salehi, and Amiri 2018)
				α-Glucosidase inhibitor	17.0 ± 1.0	16.4 ± 0.9 (Acarbose)	

Compound reference No	Plant name	Plant part used	Compound name	Activity	IC_{50} Value (µM)		Reference article
29.			Emodin	α-Amylase inhibitor	184.7 ± 4.0	47.4 ± 1.1 (Acarbose)	
				α-Glucosidase inhibitor	42.5 ± 1.4	16.4 ± 0.9 (Acarbose)	
30.			Rhododendrin	α-Amylase inhibitor	107.5 ± 3.6	47.4 ± 1.1 (Acarbose)	
				α-Glucosidase inhibitor	77.9 ± 4.2	16.4 ± 0.9 (Acarbose)	
31.			Chrysophanol	α-Glucosidase inhibitor	212.0 ± 4.3	16.4 ± 0.9 (Acarbose)	
32.	*Rheum turkestanicum*	Root	Physcion	α-Glucosidase inhibitor	228.0 ± 5.2	16.4 ± 0.9 (Acarbose)	(Dehghan, Salehi, and Amiri 2018)
33.	*Rhus coriaria*	Leaves	Penta-*O*-galloyl-β-glucopyranose	α-Amylase inhibitor	6.32 ± 0.18	10.69 ± 0.50 (acarbose)	(Gök et al., 2020)
				α-Glucosidase inhibitor	4.10 ± 0.10	0.12 ± 0.01 (Acarbose)	
34.			Amentoflavone		11.30 ± 0.70		
35.			Agathisflavone		11.40 ± 0.90		
36.	*Arcytophyllum thymifolium*	Aerial parts	Iridoid asperulosidic acid	α-Amylase inhibitor	69.4 ± 3.1	26.3 ± 1.2 (Acarbose)	(Milella et al., 2016)
37.			Rhamnetin		73.9 ± 5.9		
38.	*Quercus gilva*	Leaves	Tiliroside	α-Glucosidase inhibitor	28.36 ± 0.11 mM	13.90 ± 0.01 mM (Quercetin)	(Indrianingsih et al., 2015)
39.			Catechin		168.60 ± 5.15 mM		
40.			Epicatechin		920.60 ± 10.10 mM		
41.	*Musa* spp. (Baxijiao)	Flowers	9-(4′-hydroxyphenyl)-2-methoxyphenalen-1-one	α-Glucosidase inhibitor	0.013 mM	1.54 mM (Acarbose)	(Sheng et al., 2014)
42.			Daucosterol		0.42 mM		
43.			β-sitosterol		0.685 mM		
44.			Ferulic acid		6.47 mM		
45.			Vanillic acid		11.92 mM		

Table 1. (Continued)

Compound reference No	Plant name	Plant part used	Compound name	Activity	IC_{50} Value (µM)		Reference article
46.	*Hylotelephium erythrostictum*		2-(3′,4′-dihydroxyphenyl)-2,3-dihydro-4,6-dihydroxy-2-(methoxy)-3-benzofuranone	α-Glucosidase inhibitor	1.8	822.9 (Acarbose)	(Quan et al., 2020)
47			Quercetin		230.3		
48.			Apigenin		365.4		
49.			Diosmetin		382.8		
50.			Kaempferol		420.5		
51.			Kaempferide		646.7		
52.			Rhamnocitrin		731.1		
53.	*Quercus coccifera*	Bark	(-)-8- Chlorocatechin	α-Glucosidase inhibitor	43.60 ± 0.67 µg/mL	50.45 ± 0.20 µg/mL (Acarbose)	(Sari et al., 2019)
54.	*Combretum quadrangulare*	Leaves	6,8,3′,5′-Tetrabromokumatakenin	α-Glucosidase inhibitor	30.5 ± 1.9	332.5 (Acarbose)	(Dao et al., 2021)
55.			6,8,5′-Tribromoayanin		87.1 ± 2.3		
56.			Luteolin		97.7 ± 1.7		
57.			Apigenin		130.8 ± 3.9		
58.			Gardenin D		188.0 ± 3.1		
59.			Mearnsetin		205.3 ± 5.6		
60.			Rhamnocitrin		206.7 ± 2.6		
61.			Ayanin		245.3 ± 3.7		
62.			8-Bromokumatakenin		275.0 ± 4.5		
63.			Myricetin-3,7,30, 50 -tetramethyl ether		282.0 ± 2.9		
64.			*ent*-atisane-3-oxo-16β,17-acetonide		69.62		

Compound reference No	Plant name	Plant part used	Compound name	Activity	IC_{50} Value (µM)		Reference article
65.			*ent*-3α-acetoxy-16β,17-dihydroxyatisane	α-Glucosidase inhibitor	102.18		
66.	*Euphorbia antiquorum*	Aerial parts	Ingol 12-acetate		115.23	332.5 (Acarbose)	(C. L. Tran et al., 2021)
67.			*ent*-1α,3α,16β,17-tetrahydroxyatisane		125.20		
68.			ethyl *ent*-3,4- seco-4,16β,17-trihydroxyatisane-3-carboxylate		130.80		
69.			Calliter penone		156.14		
70.	*Mangifera indica*	Seed Kernel	1, 2, 3, 4, 6- penta-*O*-galloyl-α-D-glucoside	α-Glucosidase inhibitor	0.07 ± 0.10	0.11 ± 0.01 (Acarbose)	(Yang et al., 2020)
71.			1, 2, 3, 4, 6-penta-*O*-galloyl-β-D-glucoside		0.60 ± 0.36		
72.	*Liparis nervosa*	Whole grass	7S, 7'S, 8R, 8'R-icariol A_2	α-Glucosidase inhibitor	43.76 ± 2.03	273.12 ± 11.84 (Acarbose)	(Liu et al., 2021)
73.			Sinapaldehyde		98.81 ± 0.99		
74.			Erigeside 2		145.88 ± 3.54		
75.	*Angelica decursiva*	Whole plants	3'(R)-*O*-acetyl-40 (S)-*O*-tigloylkhellactone	α-Glucosidase inhibitor	93.39 ± 0.99	201 ± 1.02 (Acarbose)	(Yousof Ali, Jung, and Choi 2015)
76.			cis-3'-acetyl-4'-angeloylkhellactone		264.26 ± 1.08		
77.			Decursinol		65.29 ± 0.81	183.29 ±1.02 (Acarbcse)	(Ali et al., 2016)
78.			4-hydroxy Pd-C-III		77.30 ± 1.07		
79.			4′-methoxy Pd-C-I		89.19 ± 0.77		
80.			Decursidin		79.09 ± 0.11		
81.			2′-isopropyl psoralene		85.82 ± 0.99		
82.			Umbelliferone 6- carboxylic acid		172.10 ± 0.19		

Table 1. (Continued)

Compound reference No	Plant name	Plant part used	Compound name	Activity	IC_{50} Value (µM)		Reference article
83.	*Celastrus paniculatus*	Seeds	1α,9β-Dibenzoyloxy-2β-acetoxy-6β-cinnamoyloxy-4β-hydroxyldihydro-β-agarofuran	α-Glucosidase inhibitor	35.60 ± 0.843	52.87 ± 0.224 (Acarbose)	(Sasikumar et al., 2018)
84.			1α-Acetoxy-6β,9α-dibenzoyloxy-8α-cinnamoyloxy-4β-hydroxydihydro-β-agarofuran		36.54 ± 0.173		
85.			1α,9β-Dibenzoyloxy-6β-cinnamoyloxy-4β-hydroxydihydro-β-agarofuran		39.56 ± 0.761		
86.			1α,6β,8β,15-Tetraacetoxy-9α-benzoyloxy-4β-hydroxydihydro-β-agarofuran		42.58 ± 0.209		
87.			1α,6β,9β-Tribenzoyloxy-4β-hydroxydihydro-β-agarofuran		44.83 ± 0.453		
88.			1α,9β-Dibenzoyloxy-4β-hydroxydihydro-β-agarofuran		45. 84 ± 0.356		
89.	*Morus alba*	Branches	Kuwanon G	α-Glucosidase inhibitor	1.44 ± 0.11	350.9 ± 17.94 (Acarbose)	(Kwon et al., 2022)
90.			Oxyresveratrol		1.86 ± 0.20		
91.			Kuwanon C		14.75 ± 0.88		
92.			Norartocarpetin		31.95 ± 1.72		
93.			Moracin M		32.43 ± 1.65		

Compound reference No	Plant name	Plant part used	Compound name	Activity	IC_{50} Value (µM)		Reference article
94.			Dihydromorin		47.35 ± 2.25		
95.	*Curcuma longa*	Root	Bisdemethoxycurcumin	α-Glucosidase inhibitor	12.5 ± 0.2	2.50 ± 0.02 (Genistein)	(Kalaycıoğlu, Gazioğlu, and Erim 2017)
96.			Curcumin		21.1 ± 0.3		
97.			Demethoxycurcumin		26.4 ± 0.2		
98.	*Mangifera mekongensis*	Bark	Ambonic acid	α-Glucosidase inhibitor	1.2	214.5 (Acarbose)	(Nguyen et al., 2016)
99.			Mekongsterol B		2.5		
100.			Mangiferonic acid		13.2		
101.			Mangiferolic acid		16.7		
102.			β-sitosteryl-3- O-β-D-glucopyranosyl-6′-O-palmitate		21.1		
103.			Mekongsterols A		27.7		
104.			Ambolic acid		112.0		
105.	*Livistona chinensis*	Fruits	4′,4″-dihydroxy-3,3′,3″-triethoxy-7,9′:7′,9-diepoxy-4,8″-oxy-8,8′-sesquineo-lignan-7″,9″-diol	α-Glucosidase inhibitor	5.71 ± 0.17	61:34 ± 1.02 (Acarbose)	(Yuwei Wang et al., 2021)
106.			4′,4″-dihydroxy-3,3′,3″,5,5′ -pentamethoxy-7,9′:7′,9-diepoxy-4,8″-oxy-8,8′-sesquineo-lignan-7″,9″-di		19.65 ± 0.21		
107.			4′,4″ -dihydroxy-3,3′,3″,5,5′,5″-hexamethoxy-7,9′:7′,9-diepoxy-4,8″-oxy-8,8′-sesquineolignan-7″,9″-diol		22.73 ± 1.07		
108.			Epicatechin		24.03 ± 0.38		
109.			Variecolorquinones A		29.61 ± 0.40		

Table 1. (Continued)

Compound reference No	Plant name	Plant part used	Compound name	Activity	IC_{50} Value (µM)		Reference article
110.	*Salacia chinensis*	Stems	30-Hydroxylup-20(29)-en-3-one	α-Glucosidase inhibitor	211.5	214.51 (Acarbose)	(Truc et al., 2019)
111.			Lup-20(29)-ene-3β,30-diol		246.8		
112.	*Cichorium intybus*	Seeds	Diacetate derivative of cichoridiol (18R,19-20(30)-taraxasten-3,21R-diacetate)	α-Gucosidase inhibitor	10 ± 0.62	425 ± 8.14 (Deoxynojirimycin)	(Atta-ur-Rahman et al., 2008)
113.			18R,19-20(30)-taraxasten-3,21R-diol (Cichoridiol)		51.9 ± 1.1		
114.			Vanillic acid		69 ± 0.008		
115.			Friedelin		321 ± 8.04		

The percentage of inhibition has been determined according to Equation **1**:

$$\text{Inhibition (\%)} = \left(1 - \frac{A-a}{B-b}\right) \times 100 \quad \textbf{(1)}$$

where A is the absorbance of the compound with enzyme, B is the absorbance of the control without compound, a is the absorbance of the compound blank without enzyme, and b is the absorbance of the blank control without compound and enzyme. The 50% inhibitory concentration of the compounds was calculated and compared with the reference standard.

Plant-Based Bioactive Compounds and Their Diabetic Management

Compounds isolated from medicinal plants such as *Calendula officinalis, Callistemon rigidus, Cyperus rotundus, Wedelia trilobata, Rheum turkestanicum, Rhus coriaria, Arcytophyllum thymifolium, Quercus gilva, Musa* spp, *Hylotelephium erythrostictum, Quercus coccifera, Combretum quadrangulare, Euphorbia antiquorum, Mangifera indica, Liparis nervosa, Angelica decursiva, Celastrus paniculatus, Morus alba, Curcuma longa, Mangifera mekongensis, Livistona chinensis Salacia chinensis* and *Cichorium intybus* have been reviewed in this chapter. The compounds listed in Table 1 have significant α-glucosidase and α-amylase inhibitory activities.

Olennikov et al. have discovered an inhibitory effect on α-amylase in the ethanolic extract and the soluble fraction in the ethyl acetate of the leaves of *Calendula officinalis*. Twenty-five compounds, including six phenolic acid glucosides, five phenylpropanoids, five coumarins, and nine flavonoids, have been isolated from the crude extract fractions. Among them, compounds **1, 2, 3** and **4** have shown strong inhibitory effects on *Aspergillus niger* α-amylase with IC_{50} values 5.72, 5.92, 8.79, and 14.04 μM, respectively compared to acarbose (IC_{50} = 14.78 μM). Compounds **5-16** have exhibited α-amylase inhibition of -amylase with IC_{50} values between 15.45 and 89.85 μg/mL (Olennikov and Kashchenko 2014).

In a study conducted by Kobayashi et al., two compounds (**17** and **18**) have been isolated from the stem bark of *Callistemon rigidus* that exhibit inhibitory effects on α-amylase in isolated mouse plasma. The extraction was carried out using methanol, and the residue obtained was dissolved in water and successively divided into chloroform, ethyl acetate, and n-butanol.

Compounds **17** and **18** have IC_{50} values of 90.5 and 457.0 mM, respectively, which are less active compared to acarbose (IC_{50} = 45.4 mM) (Kobayashi et al., 2006).

Using phytochemical fractionation of the methanol extract of *Cyperus rotundus*, Tran et al. have isolated compound **19** along with three stilbene dimers, **20**, **21** and **22**. Among them, compound **19** has inhibited only α-amylase with an IC_{50} value of 24.2 ± 1.1 μM compared to acarbose (IC_{50} = 776.1 ± 36.7 μM), whereas compounds **21** and **22** have inhibited α–glucosidase with IC_{50} values of 94.3 ± 6.8 and 168.1 ± 12.5 μM, respectively compared to acarbose (IC_{50} = 2060 ± 97.5 μM). Compound **20** has inhibited both α-glucosidase (IC_{50} = 210.5 ± 17.3 μM compared to the acarbose IC_{50} value of 2060 ± 97.5 μM) and α-amylase (IC_{50}= 21.7 ± 1.4 μM compared to the acarbose IC_{50} value of 776.1 ± 36.7 μM) (H. H. T. Tran et al., 2014).

A study by Luyen et al., has shown that compounds **23**, **24** and **25** isolated from the methanol extract of *Wedelia trilobata* leaves have inhibitory potency against the α-glucosidase enzyme with respective IC_{50} values of 27.54 ± 1.12, 173.78 ± 2.37, and 190.40 ± 2.01 μg/mL (Compared to acarbose IC_{50} of 450.56 ± 2.31 μg/mL). Furthermore, compounds **25** and **24** have shown inhibitory activity against α-amylase with IC_{50} values of 52.08 ± 0.56 and 181.97 ± 2.62 μg/mL, respectively compared to acarbose (IC_{50} = 6.78 ± 0.32 μg/mL). The IC_{50} values of two other compounds **26** and **27** (87.10 ± 1.89 and 112.20 ± 2.87 μg/mL) isolated from leaves of *Wedelia trilobata* have exhibited inhibition against the α-amylase enzyme compared to acarbose (IC_{50} = 6.78 ± 0.32 μg/mL). (Luyen et al., 2019).

Five compounds (**28-32**) with α-glucosidase and α-amylase inhibitory activity have been isolated and identified by Dehghan et al., from the ethyl acetate extract of roots of *Rheum turkestanicum*. Among them, compound **28** has exhibited similar inhibitory activity against α-amylase and α-glucosidase, with IC_{50} values of 46.4 ± 1.5 and 17.0 ± 1.0 μM respectively, compared to those of acarbose (IC_{50} values of 47.4 ± 1.1 and 16.4 ± 0.9 μM). Furthermore, **29** and **30** with IC_{50} values of 42.5 ± 1.4 μM and 77.9 ± 4.2 μM respectively, have shown inhibitory effects against α-glucosidase, while they showed α-amylase inhibitory activity of -amylase with IC_{50} values of 184.7 ± 4.0 and 107.5 ± 3.6 μM respectively. Compounds **31** and **32** have shown only inhibitory activities against α-glucosidase enzyme (IC_{50} = 212.0 ± 4.3 and 228.0 ± 5.2 μM respectively) (Dehghan, Salehi, and Amiri 2018).

Using activity-guided isolation, Gök et al. have isolated three active compounds (**33**, **34** and **35**) from the leaves and fruits of *Rhus coriaria* and all have inhibited α-glucosidase with IC_{50} values of 4.10 ± 0.10, 11.30 ± 0.70, and 11.40 ± 0.90 μM, respectively compared to acarbose (IC_{50} = 0.12 ± 0.01 μM). Furthermore, compound **33** has inhibited α-amylase enzyme with an IC_{50} of 6.32 ± 0.18 μM compared to an acarbose IC_{50} value of 10.69 ± 0.50 μM (Gök et al., 2020).

Milella et al. have isolated compounds **36** and **37** from the aerial parts of *Arcytophyllum thymifolium* and both compounds have exhibited lower α-amylase inhibitory activity (IC_{50} = 69.4 ± 3.1 and 73.9 ± 5.9 μM respectively) compared to acarbose (IC_{50}= 26.3 ± 1.2 μM) (Milella et al., 2016).

Indrianingsih et al. have isolated three compounds (**38**, **39** and **40**) from the methanolic extract of the leaves of *Quercus gilva*. Among them, the highest α-glucosidase inhibitory activity of -glucosidase has been obtained for compound **38** with an IC_{50} of 28.36 ± 0.11 mM, followed by compounds **39** and **40** with IC_{50} values of 168.60 ± 5.15 and 920.60 ± 10.10 mM, respectively (compared to the standard quercetin standard IC_{50} = 13.90 ± 0.01 mM) (Indrianingsih et al., 2015).

Five *Bacillus stearothermophilus* α-glucosidase inhibitor compounds (**41-45**) have been isolated from *Musa* spp. (Baxijiao) flowers by Sheng et al. The IC_{50} values of the compounds ranged between 0.013 and 11.92 mM. Compared to acarbose (IC_{50} of 1.54 mM), compound **41** has shown a strong α-glucosidase inhibitory activity of -glucosidase (IC_{50} = 0.013 mM) (Sheng et al., 2014).

A study carried out by Quan et al. has shown that compounds **46-52** isolated from the ethyl acetate extract of *Hylotelephium erythrostictum* have inhibitory activities against α-glucosidase enzyme with IC_{50} values in the range of 1.8 to 731.1 μM. Among them, compound **46** has shown significant α-glucosidase inhibitory activity of -glucosidase with an IC_{50} value of 1.8 μM than acarbose (IC_{50}= 822.9 μM) (Quan et al., 2020).

Sari et al., have isolated compound **53** from methanol extract of *Quercus coccifera* which has shown moderate inhibitory activity of *Saccharomyces cerevisiae* α-glucosidase inhibitory activity (IC_{50} = 43.60 ± 0.67 μg/mL), compared to acarbose (IC_{50}= 50.45 ± 0.20 μg/mL) (Sari et al., 2019).

Sixteen flavones have been isolated by Dao et al. from the leaves of *Combretum quadrangulare*. Among them, compounds **54-63** have exhibited α-glucosidase inhibitory activities of -glucosidase with IC_{50} values ranging between 30.5 and 282.0 μM, which were more potent than acarbose (IC_{50} value 332.5 μM) (Dao et al., 2021).

Six potent α-glucosidase inhibitors (**64-69**) have been isolated from the aerial parts of *Euphorbia antiquorum* by Tran et al. Among them, compound **64** has shown the highest α-glucosidase inhibitory activity with an IC_{50} value of 69.62 μM compared to acarbose, (IC_{50} of 332.5 μM). Compounds **65**, **66**, **67**, **68** and **69** have also shown potent inhibitory effects against α-glucosidase where the IC_{50} values are in the range of 102.08 to 156.14 μM (C. L. Tran et al., 2021).

Yang et al. have isolated two α-glucosidase inhibitors (**70** and **71**) from *Mangifera indica* seed kernel with IC_{50} values of 0.07 ± 0.10 and 0.60 ± 0.36 μM respectively, compared to acarbose (IC_{50} value of 0.11 ± 0.01 μM) (Yang et al., 2020).

Eleven phenylpropanoids have been isolated by Liu et al., from the whole grass of *Liparis nervosa*. Among them, only three compounds (**72**, **73** and **74**) have been identified as potent α-glucosidase inhibitors with IC_{50} values of 43.76 ± 2.03, 98.81 ± 0.99, and 145.88 ± 3.54 μM respectively compared to acarbose (IC_{50} = 273.12 ± 11.84 μM) (Liu et al., 2021).

Ali et al., have reported that the bioactivity-guided fractionation of the methanol extract of the entire plant, *Angelica decursiva* yielded seven compounds which exhibited α-glucosidase inhibitory activity. Among them, compounds **75** and **76** possessed IC_{50} values of 93.39 ± 0.99 μM and 264.26 ± 1.08 μM respectively compared to acarbose (IC_{50} value of 201 ± 1.02 μM) (Yousof Ali, Jung and Choi 2015). In another study, six natural coumarins, **77-82** isolated from *A. deursiva*, have exhibited potent inhibitory activities against α-glucosidase with IC_{50} values ranging between 65.29 ± 0.81 and 172.10 ± 0.19 μM compared to acarbose (IC_{50} value of 183.29 ±1.02 μM) (Ali et al., 2016).

Six dihydro-β-agarofuran sesquiterpenoids have been identified by Sasikumar et al. identified six dihydro--agarofuran sesquiterpenoids, from *Celastrus paniculatus* which exhibited moderate α-glucosidase inhibition. The molecular coupling study has been supported by the observed α-glucosidase inhibition of compounds **83**, **84**, **85**, **86**, **87** and **88** and the IC_{50} values were in the range of 35.60 ± 0.843 to 45.84 ± 0.356 μM compared to acarbose with an IC_{50} value of 52.87 ± 0.224 μM (Sasikumar et al., 2018).

Compounds **89-94** have been isolated from *Morus alba* by Kwon et al. All compounds have shown inhibitory effects against α-glucosidase with IC_{50} values ranging from 1.44 ± 0.11 to 47.35 ± 2.25 μM. Compounds **89** and **90** have shown significant inhibitory activity against α-glucosidase with IC_{50} values of 1.44 ± 0.11 and 1.86 ± 0.20, μM respectively compared to acarbose (IC_{50} value of 350.9 ± 17.94 μM) (Kwon et al., 2022).

Kalaycolu et al., have isolated three curcuminoids, **95**, **96** and **97** from the root of *Curcuma longa* that exhibited α-glucosidase inhibitory activity with IC_{50} values of 12.5 ± 0.2, 21.1 ± 0.3, and 26.4 ± 0.2 μM respectively compared to the reference standard (IC_{50} value of 2.50 ± 0.02 μM) (Kalaycıoğlu, Gazioğlu, and Erim 2017).

A study conducted on the n-hexane fraction of *Mangifera mekongensis* by Nguyen et al. has reported α-glucosidase inhibitory activity of -glucosidase with an IC_{50} value of 17.1μg/mL. Two steroids (**99** and **103**) along with five compounds **(98**, **100**, **101**, **102**, and **104)** isolated from the bark of *Mangifera mekongensis* have shown α-glucosidase inhibitory activities. Compared to acarbose (IC_{50} value of 214.5 μM), the seven compounds (**98**-**104**) have demonstrated α-glucosidase inhibitory activities of -glucosidase, with IC_{50} values ranging from IC_{50} values of 1.2 to 112.0 μM. Among them, compounds **98** and **99** have exhibited significant inhibition against α-glucosidase with IC_{50} values of 2.5μM and 1.2μM respectively (Nguyen et al., 2016).

Wang et al. have isolated twenty-two compounds from fruits of *Livistona chinensis* that possess α-glucosidase inhibitory activity with IC_{50} values ranging between 5.71 ± 0.17 and 29.61 ± 0.40 μM. Among them, compound **105** has shown significant α-glucosidase inhibitory activity of -glucosidase (IC_{50} value of 5.71 ± 0.17 μM) compared to acarbose (IC_{50} value of 61.34 ± 1.02 μM) (Yuwei Wang et al., 2021).

Compounds **110** and **111** isolated by Truc et al., from the stems of *Salacia chinensis* have shown α-glucosidase inhibitory activity with IC_{50} values of 211.5 and 246.8 μM, respectively compared to the acarbose (IC_{50} of 214.51 μM) (Truc et al., 2019).

Compounds **112**, **113**, **114** and **115** are triterpenoids which have been isolated from *Cichorium intybus* by Rahman et al. The diacetate derivative of compound **113** (compound **112**) has exhibited more potent α-glucosidase inhibitory activity (IC_{50} value of 10 ± 0.62 μM) than its parent compound **113** (IC_{50} value of 51.9 ± 1.1 μM). Compound **114** has also inhibited α-glucosidase, with an IC_{50} value of 69 ± 0.008 μM. In this study, deoxynojirimycin was used as standard inhibitor (IC_{50} value of 425 ± 8.14 μM) (Atta-ur-Rahman et al., 2008).

Inhibitory Mechanisms of Anti α-Amylase and Anti α-Glucosidase Compounds

Kinetic studies conducted on plant-based α-amylase and α-glucosidase inhibitors have shown competitive, non-competitive, and mixed inhibition-type mechanisms toward the corresponding substrates. Compounds **38** and **39** have shown an uncompetitive α-glucosidase inhibition, and compound **40** has exhibited noncompetitive inhibition. Compounds **45**, **53**, **58**, **59**, **66** and **70** have demonstrated a non-competitive mechanism of inhibition (Indrianingsih et al., 2015), (Sheng et al., 2014), (Sari et al., 2019), (Dao et al., 2021), (C. L. Tran et al., 2021), (Yang et al., 2020).

The kinetics of enzyme inhibition has revealed that compounds **43**, **44**, **46**, **71**, **78**, **80**, **81** and **82** have shown competitive α-glucosidase inhibition of -glucosidase (Sheng et al., 2014), (Quan et al., 2020), (Yang et al., 2020), (Ali et al., 2016). On the contrary, the inhibitory activity of compounds **77**, **79**, **89**, **90**, **91**, **92**, **93** and **94** have shown mixed-type α-glucosidase inhibition (Ali et al., 2016) (Kwon et al., 2022). The quercetin standard has shown a mixed inhibitory type, while acarbose and deoxynojirimycin have shown a competitive inhibitory type.

Conclusion

Natural resources continue to be considered as strong possibilities for drug discovery and are essential to drug development initiatives. In addition, many therapeutic herbs offer a rich source of bioactive compounds that have potent pharmacological effects, but are remarkably free of adverse side effects. In the current chapter, an effort has been made to provide an overview of plant-based antidiabetic compounds, which may be beneficial to health professionals, researchers, and academics working in the fields of pharmacology and therapeutics. Therefore, investigating the mechanisms of action of natural substances, particularly those that have promising activity, may aid in the development of better anti-diabetic drugs or serve as a foundation for the creation of improved anti-diabetic molecules utilising medicinal chemistry techniques. To better understand the mechanisms of action of antidiabetic compounds at the cellular and molecular level, more research must be done.

References

Afrisham, R., Aberomand, M., Ghaffari, M. A., Siahpoosh, A., and Jamalan, M. (2015). Inhibitory Effect of Heracleum persicum and Ziziphus jujuba on Activity of Alpha-Amylase. *Journal of Botany*, 2015.

Alam, S., Sarker, M. M. R., Sultana, T. N., Chowdhury, M. N. R., Rashid, M. A., Chaity, N. I., Zhao, C., Xiao, J., Hafez, E. E., Khan, S. A., and Mohamed, I. N. (2022). Antidiabetic phytochemicals from medicinal plants: prospective candidates for discovery and development.*Frontiers in endocrinology*, 13.

Ali, M. Y., Jannat, S., Jung, H. A., Jeong, H. O., Chung, H. Y., and Choi, J. S. (2016). Coumarins from Angelica decursiva inhibit α-glucosidase activity and protein tyrosine phosphatase 1B. *Chemico-Biological Interactions*, 252, pp. 93-101.

Arumugam, G., Manjula, P., and Paari, N. (2013). A review: Anti diabetic medicinal plants used for diabetes mellitus. *Journal of Acute Disease*, 2(3), pp. 196-200.

Bailey, C. J., and Day, C. (1989). Traditional plant medicines as treatments for diabetes. *Diabetes care*, 12(8), pp. 553-564.

Dao, T. B. N., Nguyen, T. M. T., Nguyen, V. Q., Tran, T. M. D., Tran, N. M. A., Nguyen, C. H., Nguyen, T. H. T., Nguyen, H. H., Sichaem, J., Tran, C. L., and Duong, T. H. (2021). Flavones from Combretum quadrangulare growing in Vietnam and their alpha-glucosidase inhibitory activity. *Molecules*, 26(9), p. 2531.

Dehghan, H., Salehi, P., and Amiri, M. S. (2018). Bioassay-guided purification of α-amylase, α-glucosidase inhibitors and DPPH radical scavengers from roots of Rheum turkestanicum. *Industrial Crops and Products*, 117, pp. 303-309.

Gök, H. N., Deliorman Orhan, D., Gürbüz, İ., and Aslan, M. (2020). Activity-guided isolation of α-amylase, α-glucosidase, and pancreatic lipase inhibitory compounds from Rhus coriaria L. *Journal of Food Science*, 85(10), pp. 3220-3228.

Indrianingsih, A. W., Tachibana, S., Dewi, R. T., and Itoh, K. (2015). Antioxidant and α-glucosidase inhibitor activities of natural compounds isolated from Quercus gilva Blume leaves. *Asian Pacific Journal of Tropical Biomedicine*, 5(9), pp. 748-755.

Jhong, C. H., Riyaphan, J., Lin, S. H., Chia, Y. C., and Weng, C. F. (2015). S creening alpha-glucosidase and alpha-amylase inhibitors from natural compounds by molecular docking in silico. *Biofactors*, 41(4), pp. 242-251.

Kalaycıoğlu, Z., Gazioğlu, I., and Erim, F. B. (2017). Comparison of antioxidant, anticholinesterase, and antidiabetic activities of three curcuminoids isolated from Curcuma longa L. *Natural Product Research*, 31(24), pp. 2914-2917.

Kambale, E. K., Quetin-Leclercq, J., Memvanga, P. B., and Beloqui, A. (2022). An Overview of Herbal-Based Antidiabetic Drug Delivery Systems: Focus on Lipid-and Inorganic-Based Nanoformulations. *Pharmaceutics*, 14(10), p. 2135.

Khan, V., Najmi, A. K., Akhtar, M., Aqil, M., Mujeeb, M., and Pillai, K. K. (2012). A pharmacological appraisal of medicinal plants with antidiabetic potential. *Journal of pharmacy & bioallied sciences*, 4(1), p. 27.

Kim, K. T., Rioux, L. E., and Turgeon, S. L. (2014). Alpha-amylase and alpha-glucosidase inhibition is differentially modulated by fucoidan obtained from Fucus vesiculosus and Ascophyllum nodosum. *Phytochemistry*, 98, pp. 27-33.

Kobayashi, K., Ishihara, T., Khono, E., Miyase, T., and Yoshizaki, F. (2006). Constituents of stem bark of Callistemon rigidus showing inhibitory effects on mouse α-amylase activity. *Biological and Pharmaceutical Bulletin*, 29(6), pp. 1275-1277.

Kumar, S., Narwal, S., Kumar, V., and Prakash, O. (2011). [alpha]-glucosidase inhibitors from plants: A natural approach to treat diabetes. *Pharmacognosy reviews*, 5(9), p. 19.

Kwon, R. H., Thaku, N., Timalsina, B., Park, S. E., Choi, J. S., and Jung, H. A. (2022). Inhibition mechanism of components isolated from Morus alba branches on diabetes and diabetic complications via experimental and molecular docking analyses. *Antioxidants*, 11(2), p. 383.

Liu, L., Zou, M., Yin, Q., Zhang, Z., and Zhang, X. (2021). Phenylpropanoids from Liparis nervosa and their *in vitro* antioxidant and α-glucosidase inhibitory activities. *Medicinal Chemistry Research*, 30, pp. 1005-1010.

Luyen, N. T., Binh, P. T., Tham, P. T., Hung, T. M., Dang, N. H., Dat, N. T., and Thao, N. P. (2019). Wedtrilosides A and B, two new diterpenoid glycosides from the leaves of Wedelia trilobata (L.) Hitchc. with α-amylase and α-glucosidase inhibitory activities. *Bioorganic Chemistry*, 85, pp. 319-324.

Meuleneire, F. (2008). Management of diabetic foot ulcers using dressings with Safetac: a review of case studies. *Wounds UK*, 4(4), pp. 16-30.

Milella, L., Milazzo, S., De Leo, M., Vera Saltos, M. B., Faraone, I., Tuccinardi, T., Lapillo, M., De Tommasi, N., and Braca, A. (2016). α-Glucosidase and α-amylase inhibitors from Arcytophyllum thymifolium. *Journal of Natural Products*, 79(8), pp. 2104-2112.

Modak, M., Dixit, P., Londhe, J., Ghaskadbi, S., and Devasagayam, T. P. A. (2007). Indian herbs and herbal drugs used for the treatment of diabetes.

Nguyen, H. X., Le, T. C., Do, T. N. V., Le, T. H., Nguyen, N. T., and Nguyen, M. T. T. (2016). α-Glucosidase inhibitors from the bark of Mangifera mekongensis. *Chemistry Central Journal*, 10, pp. 1-6.

Olennikov, D. N. and Kashchenko, N. I. (2014). Componential profile and amylase inhibiting activity of phenolic compounds from Calendula officinalis L. leaves. *The Scientific World Journal*, 2014.

Ozougwu, J. C., Obimba, K. C., Belonwu, C. D., and Unakalamba, C. B. (2013). The pathogenesis and pathophysiology of type 1 and type 2 diabetes mellitus. *J Physiol Pathophysiol*, 4(4), pp. 46-57.

Patil, R., Patil, R., Ahirwar, B., and Ahirwar, D. (2011). Current status of Indian medicinal plants with antidiabetic potential: a review. *Asian Pacific Journal of Tropical Biomedicine*, 1(2), pp. S291-S298.

Quan, Y. S., Zhang, X. Y., Yin, X. M., Wang, S. H., and Jin, L. L. (2020). Potential α-glucosidase inhibitor from Hylotelephium erythrostictum. *Bioorganic & Medicinal Chemistry Letters*, 30(24), p. 127665

Rasouli, H., Hosseini-Ghazvini, S. M. B., Adibi, H., and Khodarahmi, R. (2017). Differential α-amylase/α-glucosidase inhibitory activities of plant-derived phenolic compounds: a virtual screening perspective for the treatment of obesity and diabetes. *Food & function*, 8(5), pp. 1942-1954.

Rasouli, H., Yarani, R., Pociot, F., and Popović-Djordjević, J. (2020). Anti-diabetic potential of plant alkaloids: Revisiting current findings and future perspectives. *Pharmacological research*, 155, p. 104723.

Salehi, B., Ata, A., V. Anil Kumar, N., Sharopov, F., Ramirez-Alarcon, K., Ruiz-Ortega, A., Abdulmajid Ayatollahi, S., Valere Tsouh Fokou, P., Kobarfard, F., Amiruddin Zakaria, Z., and Iriti, M. (2019). Antidiabetic potential of medicinal plants and their active components. *Biomolecules*, 9(10), p. 551.

Sales, P. M., Souza, P. M., Simeoni, L. A., Magalhães, P. O., and Silveira, D. (2012). α-Amylase inhibitors: a review of raw material and isolated compounds from plant source. *Journal of Pharmacy & Pharmaceutical Sciences*, 15(1), pp. 141-183.

Sari, S., Barut, B., Özel, A., Kuruüzüm-Uz, A., and Şöhretoğlu, D. (2019). Tyrosinase and α-glucosidase inhibitory potential of compounds isolated from Quercus coccifera bark: *in vitro* and in silico perspectives. *Bioorganic Chemistry*, 86, pp. 296-304.

Sasikumar, P., Sharathna, P., Prabha, B., Varughese, S., Kumar, A., Sivan, V. V., Sherin, D. R., Suresh, E., Manojkumar, T. K., and Radhakrishnan, K. V. (2018). Dihydro-β-agarofuran sesquiterpenoids from the seeds of Celastrus paniculatus Willd. and their α-glucosidase inhibitory activity. *Phytochemistry Letters*, 26, pp. 1-8.

Sheng, Z., Dai, H., Pan, S., Wang, H., Hu, Y., and Ma, W. (2014). Isolation and characterization of an α-glucosidase inhibitor from Musa spp. (Baxijiao) flowers. *Molecules*, 19(7), pp. 10563-10573.

Singab, A. N., Youssef, F. S., and Ashour, M. L. (2014). Medicinal plants with potential antidiabetic activity and their assessment. *Med Aromat Plants*, 3(151), pp. 2167-0412.

Svensson, B. (1988). Regional distant sequence homology between amylases, α-glucosidases and transglucanosylases. *FEBS letters*, 230(1-2), pp. 72-76.

Tran, C. L., Dao, T. B. N., Tran, T. N., Mai, D. T., Tran, T. M. D., Tran, N. M. A., Dang, V. S., Vo, T. X., Duong, T. H., and Sichaem, J. (2021). Alpha glucosidase inhibitory diterpenes from Euphorbia antiquorum growing in Vietnam. *Molecules*, 26(8), p. 2257.

Tran, H. H. T., Nguyen, M. C., Le, H. T., Nguyen, T. L., Pham, T. B., Chau, V. M., Nguyen, H. N., and Nguyen, T. D. (2014). Inhibitors of α-glucosidase and α-amylase from Cyperus rotundus. *Pharmaceutical biology*, 52(1), pp. 74-77.

Truc, D. T. T., Vy, C. T. H., Phu, D. H., Hoang, N. M., and Nhan, N. T. (2019). Lupan-type triterpenoids from the stems of Salacia chinensis L. (Celastraceae) and their α-glucosidase inhibitory activities. *Vietnam Journal of Chemistry*, 57(4), pp. 433-437.

Truscheit, E., Frommer, W., Junge, B., Müller, L., Schmidt, D. D., and Wingender, W. (1981). Chemistry and biochemistry of microbial α-glucosidase inhibitors. *Angewandte Chemie International Edition in English*, 20(9), pp. 744-761.

Wang, Y., Xiang, L., Wang, C., Tang, C., and He, X. (2013). Antidiabetic and antioxidant effects and phytochemicals of mulberry fruit (Morus alba L.) polyphenol enhanced extract. *PloS one*, 8(7), p. e71144.

Wang, Y., Zhai, J., Yang, D., Han, N., Liu, Z., Liu, Z., Li, S., and Yin, J. (2021). Antioxidant, anti-inflammatory, and antidiabetic activities of bioactive compounds from the fruits of Livistona chinensis based on network pharmacology prediction. *Oxidative Medicine and Cellular Longevity*, 2021, pp. 1-21.

Yang, D., Chen, X., Liu, X., Han, N., Liu, Z., Li, S., Zhai, J., and Yin, J. (2020). Antioxidant and α-glucosidase inhibitory activities guided isolation and identification of components from mango seed kernel. *Oxidative Medicine and Cellular Longevity*, 2020.

Yousof Ali, M., Jung, H. A., and Choi, J. S. (2015). Anti-diabetic and anti-Alzheimer's disease activities of Angelica decursiva. *Archives of pharmacal research*, 38, pp. 2216-2227.

Zareen, S., Choudhary, M. I., Akhtar, M. N., and Khan, S. N. (2008). α-Glucosidase inhibitory activity of triterpenoids from Cichorium intybus. *Journal of Natural Products*, 71(5), pp. 910-913.

Zulcafli, A. S., Lim, C., Ling, A. P., Chye, S., and Koh, R. (2020). Focus: Plant-based Medicine and Pharmacology: Antidiabetic Potential of Syzygium sp.: An Overview. *The Yale journal of biology and medicine*, 93(2), p. 307.

Chapter 5

Phytochemicals as Anti-Diabetic Agents

Anugrah Michael[1]
Aniket Singh[1]
and Arpita Roy*

[1]Department of Biotechnology, School of Engineering & Technology,
Sharda University, Greater Noida, India

Abstract

One of the major diseases on the planet, diabetes mellitus, is becoming more common and its fatality rate is increasing. Serious health consequences result from not following the glucose intake guidelines. Although conventional hypoglycemic medications tend to be beneficial, they often have ramifications. Therefore, medicinal herbs may serve as a supplemental source of antidiabetic experts. With a focus on preclinical and clinical studies, we have collected data on the antidiabetic potential of various plants. The favourable capability is provided by the coordinated and consolidated activity of its metabolic profile of naturally dynamic mixes.

Keywords: medicinal herbs, diabetes, preclinical, metabolic profile, antidiabetic

---

* Corresponding Author's Email: arbt2014@gmail.com.

In: Antidiabetic Plants
Editor: Arpita Roy
ISBN: 979-8-88697-957-2

Introduction

Diabetes mellitus (DM), a clinical illness particularised to uncontrolled hyperglycemia caused by the protection of a lack of insulin or by a cell from insulin function. It affects 16 million people in the United States and more than 200 million people worldwide, making it the most common endocrine disorder (Wadkar et al., 2008; Debra HJ, 1991). Due to its high prevalence, depressing outlook, and high mortality, diabetes is now the 'third enemy' of humanity, behind cancer and cardiovascular diseases (Li et al., 2004). By 2030, the number may reach 366 million, meaning that one in ten people will likely have diabetes as a result of an unhealthy lifestyle and insufficient exercise. This prediction was made by the WHO (Wild et al., 2004, Kaul et al., 2013). It corresponds to when a body cannot control its glucose levels, a continuing illness that is rapidly spreading and threatens human wellness around the world due to the recurrence of cases studied and significant increases in therapeutic expenditures. Furthermore, the astonishing assumptions it makes about the future of humanity and the nation's economy are dangerous. Type I and II are the two classifications of DM (Kerru et al., 2018). Type 2 diabetes alone contributes to more than 80% of all reported diabetic conditions. Diabetes in general, including both types, can cause neuropathy, long-term illness with higher chances of the patient dying early; it also adds up a huge cost and mental trauma for the person and their family. Type 1 diabetes mellitus (IDDM) is insulin dependent, which means that the body. Children and young adults are more likely to experience it. Type I corresponds to 5-10% of the total cases. Most people are affected by Type-2, accounting for 90-95% of cases of diabetes, noninsulin-dependent diabetic mellitus (NIDDM), in which the body does not produce enough insulin or uses the released insulin improperly. Due to the growing elderly population, increased prevalence of obesity, and increasingly sedentary lifestyles, type 2 diabetes is given another name, adult-onset diabetes, approaching epidemic levels (Forouhi et al., 2010). Diabetes that occurs during pregnancy is called gestational diabetes. Its cause is still unknown; however, the development of gestational diabetes is thought to be influenced by excessive proinsulin and some people theorize that this may stress beta cells. Progesterone, cortisol, prolactin, human placental lactogen, and oestrogen are all found in high concentrations and may have an effect on peripheral insulin sensitivity and beta cell function, according to some (Kuhl et al., 1984).

For people with type 2, daily insulin combinations are essential to prevent catabolic outflow that can otherwise result in diabetic ketoacidosis, coma, and death. To manage the excessive arrival of glucagon or combat its increase in hepatic glucose and ketone production, there are virtually no Langerhans islets of Langerhans in the pancreas. In addition, there is a shortage to amount of insulin given.

Deficiency could be due to exogenous synthetic substances of the climate or diet, viral disease, or immunological factors such as a problem of the immune system in hereditarily weak people. Non-insulin-subordinate diabetes mellitus (NIDDM, otherwise called Type II or development beginning) occurs overwhelmingly in more experienced individuals, for example 16.8% of people over 65 years of age in the US have NIDDM, and it is frequently associated with heftiness. NIDDM addresses various diabetic states in which they are typically low in number compared to a-phones and insulin discharge is generally adequate to interfere with ketogenic activities of glucagon, however, not to prevent hyperglycemia. The basal rate of hepatic glucose creation is increased in subjects with NIDDM and this is strongly correlated with the level of fasting hyperglycemia. This increased rate of glucose discharge by the liver is the result of impaired hepatic aversion to insulin, decreased insulin emission through impeded β-cell responsiveness to glucose, and increased glucagon discharge through a decreased glucose capacity to suppress glucagon. The proficiency in glucose take-up by fringe tissues is likewise hindered due to a blend of diminished insulin discharge and imperfect cell insulin activity (insulin obstruction). Receptor-interceded insulin obstruction could be a result of different elements, including expanded serine threonine phosphorylation of the receptor with diminished tyrosine phosphorylation, receptor desensitisation, receptor and acquired underlying deformities in the insulin receptor (Chaudhary et al., 2018).

The theory has been mentioned in Ayurveda by Sushruta, and diabetes has long been recognised to exist. Its medication has been around for more than 80 years. In the first century AD, the Greek physician Aeretaeus coined the term "diabetes". One of the main hotspots for another drug or a potential to create another drug is thought to be plant materials that are used as traditional diabetes treatment. For diabetes, as well as for some other diseases, traditional practitioners emphasise phytochemicals derived from plant sources. More than 400 plants are currently used to produce hypoglycemia effects, and in each and every one of these cases, the claims made by experts or clients are reasonable and complete. In this way, a valid logical evaluation, plant selection through pharmacological tests, followed by substance inspections, is crucial. The main form of treatment consisted of the use of plants before insulin and oral hypoglycemic medications were developed (Wadkar et al., 2008).

Management of Diabetes

Early detection is the key to successfully managing diabetes; without early diagnosis and treatment, the more likely the outcomes for their health will be. This means that places where vital medical services are provided should have easy access to diagnostics such as blood glucose testing. Patients will occasionally need professional evaluation or therapy for entanglements, and hence laid-up frameworks for reference and reference back-reference are necessary. Managing lipids and pulse to reduce cardiovascular risk and other complications, managing blood sugar through a combination of diet, exercise and prescription of medications or routinely checking for ill effects on eyes, kidneys, and feet to facilitate prior diagnosis are some interventions for people with DM. Using rules and norms, the board can be strengthened. Regarding the board of coordinated noncommunicable diseases (NCDs), efforts should be made to further create limits with respect to the termination and treatment of diabetes to provide better results (Roglic et al., 2016). Instead of screening entire populations for diabetes, important consideration groups should concentrate their efforts on early detection, lifestyle counseling, and targeted treatment of risk factors among those susceptible to diabetes and cardiovascular disease (Forouhi et al., 2010).

Recent Regulatory Developments

Natural medications, as characterised by administrative measures, comprise only those customary prescriptions, which essentially use therapeutic plant arrangements for treatment. The WHO has characterized customary medication (counting home-grown drugs) as containing restorative practises that have been present, nearly for a few years, before the turn of events and spread of current medication and others that are still being used. As of late, the FDA and EMEA have taken a strong fascination, evaluated the administrative systems overseeing the turn of events, and utilisation of herbal medication. This distinct fascination has given a critical fillip to the regular items industry and has fundamentally reduced the passage hindrances for botanicals and related items. India and China obviously enjoy a characteristic advantage over the others. Furthermore, uncontrolled diabetes causes numerous persistent confusions, such as visual impairment, cardiovascular breakdown, and renal disappointment. Research into new hypoglycemic and possibly antidiabetic specialists is progressing at a rapid rate in an effort to stop this alarming medical condition. The profile of home-grown plants that impact hypoglycemia is of particular interest in the current survey. Leguminoseae, Lamiaceae, Liliaceae, Cucurbitaceae, Asteraceae, Moraceae, Rosaceae, Euphorbiaceae, etc. are some of the plant families with the strongest hypoglycemic effects. An additional factor that helps to reduce or even eliminate diabetic entanglements could be more advanced glucose homeostasis (Chauhan et al., 2010).

Molecular Mechanism Involved in Diabetes

Insulin is a peptide chemical that manages the degree of glucose in the blood by directing the digestion of sugars, fats, and proteins in the objective tissues, and albeit numerous substantial cells express insulin receptors. The impact of insulin is immediate on skeletal muscle, liver and adipocytes and these tissues. A significant and unmistakable job in metabolic equilibrium that requires the presence of exceptional insulin flagging pathways. For example, insulin upgrades glucose usage in skeletal muscles and the capacity to overabundance in liver by expanding glucose transport and glycogen union, while in the liver insulin actuates the course of glycogen arrangement and increases the quality articulation. Similarly, it has an impact on systems that cause sugar to range from decreased insulin emission to diminished insulin activity to coordinate neurological impacts (Sulaiman et al., 2019, Jwad et al., 2022).

The transport of glucose is stimulated by insulin, and absorption to tissue is a critical mechanism for maintaining glucose homeostasis. In the insulin-animated condition, skeletal muscle serves as the primary site for glucose elimination. Insulin increases skeletal muscle glucose transport by directing the important insulin-directed glucose carrier glucose carrier 4 (GLUT4) from intracellular vesicles to the PM layer, as well as transverse tubules. The decrease in glucose absorption by insulin activity is most likely due to changed Glut4 dealing capacity or lower Glut4 capacity (Choi et al., 2010).

Insulin Receptor Signaling

Insulin receptors have built-in tyrosine kinase activities. Insulin that binds to the insulin receptor causes it to become autophosphorylated. Insulin receptor substrate proteins (IRS) are then phosphorylated by the phosphorylated receptor on tyrosine accumulations. Since tyrosine phosphorylation occurs infrequently (0.03% of total amino-corrosive phosphorylation) in mammalian cells, it is recognised as a component of the insulin receptor (Kuhl et al., 1998). Phosphorylated IRS enrols an assortment of SH2 space-containing proteins to start a perplexing flagging fountain. One of these proteins, phosphotidylinisitol-3'- Gracious kinase (PI3K) intervenes in the vast majority of metabolic activities by enacting various serine/threonine kinases or the mammalian objective of rapamycin (mTOR). Akt/PBB activates glucose intake into the cell, advances the glycogen combination, smothers liver gluconeogenesis, increases unsaturated fat and fatty substance blend, and suppresses lipolysis in fat tissue (Chang et al., 2010).

Insulin labelling is the result of a series of events that begin with receptor binding to insulin on the cell surface, followed by receptor autophosphorylation, activation of receptor tyrosine kinases, and substrate tyrosine phosphorylation of the insulin receptor (IRS), including IRS1, IRS2, IRS3, IRS4, Gab1 and Shc. Phosphatidylinositol 4,5-bisphosphate (PIP2) and layer phospholipids are phosphorylated at the 3 'position' by phosphoinositide 3-kinase (PI3K) after IRS are restricted to the enzyme's regulatory subunit through the Src homology 2 (SH2) regions. Insulin-intervened Glut4 is moved from intracellular vesicles to the plasma film by phosphorylating the 160 kDa substrate (AS160) of activated Akt. Furthermore, PKC activation is also involved in the direction of Glut4 migration under the influence of insulin. However, protein tyrosine phosphatases (PTPs), which are a large set of proteins, also dephosphorylate and inactivate the insulin receptor (IR), having opposing effects on insulin activity and glucose digestion. The balance between phosphorylation and dephosphorylation is what ultimately limits the physiological rule of insulin activity. In particular, the PI3K pathway plays a major role in the insulin flagging process, essential for the metabolic effects of insulin on glucose transport and Glu4 translocation (Chang et al., 2010).

Action of Insulin

The activation of blood glucose uptake by tissues, especially muscle and fat, is one of the key functions. Unambiguous glucose carrier proteins that are added to the plasma layer of cells act as a barrier to spread of this by working with dissemination. When glucose binds to the carrier in its outward-facing configuration, the carrier protein undergoes a conformational change and transports glucose within the cell. The carrier is then reused according to its original layout. Molecular cloning research efforts over the past 10 years have led to the recognition that a quality group of glucose carriers – referred to as GLUT1 through GLUT7 in the request in which they were cloned – participate in glucose transport. GLUT1-5 and GLUT7 encode functional glucose carriers, while GLUT6 is a pseudogene, which interferes with glucose transport. Numerous studies have focused on the potential role that glucose carriers may play in the development of diabetes.

Diabetes is represented by three important pathologic cycles.

1) There is a defect in insulin secretion; pancreatic cell may play a role in altered glucose detection, which contributes to impaired insulin secretion.
2) The glucose yield is not adequately expanded. In the liver, GLUT2 plays an important role, while GLUT1 plays a less important one. It has been suggested that the intracellular organelle GLUT7 participates in gluconeogenesis. However, insulin does not play a strong regulatory role in hepatic glucose transport (as opposed to liver glucose digestion).
3) Instead, insulin dramatically activates both glucose transport and use in peripheral tissues, such as muscle and fat cells. A key pathogenic factor for both NIDDM and IDDM is impaired glucose utilisation in these tissues. In these tissues, GLUT4 plays an important role in the transport of glucose, while GLUT1 plays a supporting role.

Since its greatest effects occur in 10 minutes, insulin swiftly activates glucose transport of glucose in fat and muscle cells. The baseline state, which is devoid of insulin, is characterised by a relationship between GLUT4 glucose transporters and the explicit film vesicles. Insulin binds to its receptor in the plasma layer, initiating a series of events that cause GLUT4 carrier vesicles to travel or grow to the plasma layer, where they dock, merge, an activation or opening step occurs, and glucose enters the cell. A constant cycle of GLUT4 carrier reuse occurs between endosomes and the plasma film during this particular contact. Insulin accelerates the exocytotic rate and possibly recruits carriers from another intracellular pool. Diabetes could make any of these strategies less effective (Kahn et al., 1996).

Present Antidiabetic Drugs

Presently accessible remedial options include dietary adjustment, oral hypoglycemics, and insulin infusions. Numerous normal items and home-made prescriptions have been suggested for the treatment of diabetes (Jung et al., 2006). Insulin is a chemical emitted by Langerhans in the pancreas. Starch uptake is basically heavily influenced by insulin. The lack in beta cells happens in an individual due to the utilitarian problem.

Oral Hypoglycemic Drugs

These medications control blood glucose levels by decreasing them and are taken by mouth. The central downside of hormonal therapy is daily infusions. Subsequently, the search for orally dynamic drugs began. Table 1 provides details about the classification of drugs.

Table 1. Classification of drugs

Class	Generation	Examples
Sulfonylureas	2nd generation	Glibenclamide, Glipizide, Gliclazide.
	1st generation	Tolbutamide, Chlorpropamide, Acetohexamide, Tolazamide.
Biguanides	-	Phenformin, Metformin
Miscellaneous	-	(I) Acarbose, (II) Guar gum

I. Sulfonylureas

They activate receptors in pancreatic islet cells to release insulin reserve to glucose. This does not improve insulin production or work in people who are completely insulin dependent, and for a successful course of treatment, it is likely that approximately 30% of participants with normal cell function also have diabetes.

II. Biguanides

Despite the fact that they do not trigger insulin release, their action depends on the existence of some insulin. Smother liver gluconeogenesis and glucose production. By enhancing anaerobic glycolysis, mitochondrial respiratory chain-advanced fringe glucose utilisation. Limit your intake of B12, amino acids, other hexoses, glucose, and other sugars.

III. Other drugs

(i) Acarbose is a complex oligosaccharide that reversibly inhibits α-glucosidases, the final compounds involved in the processing of starches on the brush border of the small gastrointestinal mucosa. mild hypoglycemia and can be utilized as a supplement to help people with severe diabetes refrain from eating. Tooting is the real result of them.

(ii) Guar gum: This dietary fibre (polysaccharide) is derived from Guar beans in the Indian group, forming a thick gel-like substance in the presence of water. It helps relieve back gastric exhaustion, gastroenteritis travel, and starch assimilation when taken shortly before or together with food (Wadkar et al., 2008).

Glucose is reduced with oral sulfonylureas such as glimepiride and glyburide, which primarily work by increasing the secretion of Langerhans insulin in the islet. This is done by closing potassium channels that are subordinate to adenosine triphosphate by inhibiting the receptor for sulfonylurea receptor in cells. Resulting in cell depolarisation, causing a flood of Ca2+ and the provision of stored insulin from the secretory granules. This component only functions when insulin is nearby (Defronzo and Ralph, 1999; Inzucchi et al., 2002). Biguanides, another type of oral hypoglycemic drug, work by increasing insulin-stimulated sugar uptake and use, reducing hepatic gluconeogenesis and restoring peripheral tissue resistance of peripheral tissues to insulin. However, biguanides are ineffective in insulin deficiency. Metformin serves as the best example of this group.

Glucosidase inhibitors, including acarbose and miglitol, prevent specific proteins from breaking down starches in the small intestine. Most of the time, this team of hypoglycemic experts works by slowing the rate at which sugars are absorbed by the body. Acarbose also restricts to the carbohydrate-restricting region and prevents the hydrolysis of pancreatic -amylase and -glucosidase proteins into monosaccharides. Resulting in slower retention and drop in postprandial glucose levels (Lebovitz and Harold, 1997; Koski and

Renee, 2004). Nonsulfonylurea secretagogues, which include meglitinide and repaglinide, work similarly to sulfonylureas in increasing insulin release from active cells, are the last category of oral hypoglycemic agents. But this group of oral anti-diabetic medications has connections to various cell receptors (Mayerson et al., 2002). The primary method of managing diabetes is the use of manufactured oral hypoglycemic drugs in conjunction with insulin, but this method does not completely reversing the course of the disease's complications and is further undermined by the fact that the drugs also have observable side effects (Rao et al., 2010). The use of these oral hypoglycemic medications has been linked to a number of drawbacks, including drug opposition (decreased effectiveness) and adverse effects. Like, around 44% of patients experience adequacy loss after 6 years of treatment, while medications that increase blood sugar are considered to be unprepared to address hyperlipidemia (Dey et al., 2002). The search for more modern antidiabetic medications from natural sources continues (Wadkar et al., 2008) due to the few restrictions associated with the use of currently manufactured antidiabetic tranquilizers.

Precautions with an Oral Hypoglycemic Agent

Although hypoglycemia can occur when using sulfonylurea compounds, the frequency of these occurrences is much lower than when insulin is used. When dealing with kidney diseases, biguanide should not be used. The related shortcomings of insulin and oral hypoglycemic medications have sparked interest in the examination of other sources that are antagonistic to diabetic movement. Numerous studies have investigated possible plant medications that could be used to treat diabetes mellitus. Traditional clinical writing has not included home-made diabetes treatments. Plants have definite commitments to the management of diabetes mellitus (Jaleel et al., 2006). Oral hypoglycemic specialists have made significant strides in the treatment of diabetes, but because currently developed drugs have some drawbacks, research for more advanced drugs continues. Recently, interest in the use of plant remedies has increased. Ayurvedic prescriptions are made from plant materials, either as a single medication or in combination with other substances, in contrast to manufactured drugs, which are more deadly and prone to side effects. Various portions have been used for their glucose-lowering effects in traditional structures, including fenugreek (Trigonella foenum-gracecum), Gudmar, Jambul, and Karela (Momordica charantia)

(Gymnema sylvestre). Gymnemic acids 1 through 4, as well as guarmarin, have been shown to have antidiabetic effects (Resmi et al., 2001).

Current IDDM treatment focusses on revelations that a concentrate of the meat pancreata could effectively reduce blood glucose levels in pancrectomized canines. Their use of a pancreatic concentrate in a human diabetic in 1922 denoted the main use of the pancreatic antidiabetic guideline, insulin, in the treatment of DM. Few unique arrangements, cow-like, porcine, and human insulin, are currently accessible, including long-acting or lente structures, and a routine of daily infusions addresses the ongoing norm of IDDM treatment for IDDM (CK et al., 1999).

Medicinal Plants for Diabetes

Some healing plants have recently been found to adapt to treating diabetes in general and are used in observational treatments for diabetes and hyperlipidemia. Diabetes and the problems it causes remain a serious clinical problem despite the availability of effective antidiabetic medications on the market. The ability of these plants to restore the function of pancreatic tissues by increasing insulin production, to prevent glucose uptake through the gastrointestinal tract, or to support metabolites in insulin subordinate cycles is all attributed to their antihyperglycemic effects (Marles et al., 1995).

Although there are more than 450 species with hypoglycemic effects that have been described, the possibility of discovering new anti-diabetic drugs from everyday plants remains attractive due to the presence of compounds that have safe and effective effects for diabetes mellitus. Glycosides, alkaloids, terpenoids, flavonoids, and carotenoids are just a few of the substances found in numerous plant species that are frequently cited as having antidiabetic effects. Information about each species will be retained for future viewings and presented sequentially. Things like general organic and ordered information, global circulation, trial studies, and activity systems will be included in this information. Traditional plant remedies for diabetes are still widely used around the world, despite the existence of effective anti-diabetic medications on the market. Generally speaking, natural remedies and ingredients from one's own garden are believed to be less toxic and unaffected by side effects than synthetic ones. The WHO recommends the importance of hypoglycemic agents of plant origin used in conventional medicine. Due to their capacity to restore the function of pancreatic tissues by increasing insulin production or lowering glucose retention of glucose during digestion, these plants are believed to have antihyperglycemic effects. Therefore, treatment with herbal remedies significantly affects the reduction of glucose-level variability and cell protection. Although there is typically very little organic information on the precise mechanisms of activity in the treatment of diabetes, it has been discovered that the vast majority of plants contain substances such as glycosides, alkaloids, terpenoids, flavonoids, etc. that are often mistaken for having antidiabetic effects. Since diabetes mellitus presents numerous difficulties for both medical professionals and patients, the search for alternative treatments will continue on a global scale (Malviya et al., 2010).

The study of conventional anti-diabetic plants will be the best course of action. This will help to develop locally accessible elective prescription drugs for the treatment of diabetes in underdeveloped countries, as well as the commercial advancement of novel organic hypoglycemic specialists and antidiabetic treatment assistants. The destruction of tropical rainforests results in the loss of a significant regular resource for anticipated new medications, including the supply of actual plants, their microbial plasm, which would be necessary for the hereditary improvement of developed assortments and tissue societies, and their constituents, which could act as new medications or models for future treatments. More than 33% of all plant-derived drugs come from species found in tropical rainforests. It would be ideal if the financial viability of creating new medicines from essential rainforest species could act as a motivator for conservation and management. The urgency of developing the momentum level of research on plant-based diabetes medications is highlighted by the rate at which the Amazon rainforest is being destroyed and the serious need for elective diabetes prescriptions around the world. This is undoubtedly the motivation for the many audits on anti-diabetic plants that have been distributed over the past few years.

The initial step expected to speed up antidiabetic plant research is to gather a more extensive survey of antidiabetic plants than has recently been distributed, which is being achieved in the current work. Then, high-need plants should be chosen from the general rundown. The rules for high-need might differ starting with one analyst and then onto the next, in view of their specific advantages, public and institutional wellbeing objectives, and geographic area. In any case, the accompanying general rules might be helpful:

1. Customary use in at least one nation.
2. Tentatively resolved hypoglycemic movement.
3. Absence of definite data on hypoglycemic components.

4. Trial proof for low harm.
5. Organic overflow.

Along these lines, plants which show extraordinary commitment, however, are as of now under broad examination, would be barred from this rundown, in spite of the fact that they might be of incredible interest to clinical analysts. In excess of 1200 types of plants are currently being used to treat DM, half as customary cures and half as trial specialists read up on their hypoglycemic impacts. More than 80% of these conventional cures concentrated pharmacologically were shown to have hypoglycemic movement, demonstrating the benefit of concentrating on customary cures as a hotspot for new hypoglycemic specialists. However, further investigation uncovered an incredible array of hypoglycemic impact systems, not of which are highly valuable. More than 33% of the multitude of plants depicted here have been accounted for to be harmful, stressing the requirement for a painstakingly arranged logical examination to recognize those hypoglycemic plants with genuine restorative viability and well-being (Marles et al., 1995). The antidiabetic effects are attributed to a phytochemical cocktail or to isolated plant parts. Alkaloids, phenolic acids, flavonoids, glycosides, saponins, polysaccharides, stilbenes, and tannins are the phytochemicals that are responsible most frequently for antidiabetic effects. The medicinal effects of phytochemicals include glucose metabolism, insulin release, cell stimulation, activation of the NF-kB pathway, inhibition of gluconeogenic substances, ROS protection & guidance of lipid metabolism (Salehi et al., 2019).

Antidiabetic Potential of Plants

Alangium lamarckii

Alangium lamarckii of the Alangiaceae family, found near gardens in southern part of India. The leaves of *Alangium lamarckii* showed a significant antidiabetic property. In the Koski and R. study, Biguanides do not increase insulin discharge. They advance tissue glucose intake and decrease liver glucose production, thus delivering an antihyperglycemic result and not a sugar-lowering effect (Kumar et al., 2016). Phytochemical analysis of *A. lamarckii* has shown the presence of different classes of substance compounds, viz. Alkaloids, terpenoids, steroids, tannins, phenols, etc. (Kumar et al., 2016). Some authors detailed that alkaloids, flavonoids, steroids/terpenoids, and phenolic compounds are known to be bioactive antidiabetic standards.

Aloe barbadensis

The Asphodelaceae family includes the ancient healing plant known as aloe vera. It has approximately 400 different varieties, is distributed in several different countries, and contains a wealth of bioactive ingredients, such as carbohydrates, polyphenols, peptides, sterols, and tannins, among others. Aloe vera has a wide range of natural benefits, including reducing inflammation, cellular support, antidiabetic action, and more. Because liver glycogenesis and liver gluconeogenesis catalysts are activated and restricted, Govindarajan et al. were able to identify the primary fundamental mechanisms of the Aloe vera carb fraction (AVCF) in the treatment of DM. Based on the findings, AVCF can be used as an adjuvant and has impressive normal antidiabetic viability (Govindarajan et al., 2021). Aloe Vera was effective in treating STZ-induced diabetic ulcers by lowering blood glucose, increasing plasma insulin levels, and reducing oxidative stress. It also reduces provocative reactions in STZ-activated diabetic model by suppressing the production of fiery intermediaries (Haghani et al., 2022).

Berberis vulgaris

Berberis vulgaris is commonly known as barberry and it belongs to the Berberidaceae family Berberidaceae. It is the family of spiked deciduous evergreen bushes, with yellow wood and yellow blossoms, and consists of 190 species. Meliani et al. studied plasma glucose reduced the impact of the root bark of *B. vulgaris*. Saponins and watery concentrates during the main day of streptozotocin (STZ)-diabetic rodents caused a huge decrease in blood glucose level. The saponin concentrate of root bark showed a more notable movement than the fluid concentrate. Saponins are plant metabolites that are notable for antidiabetic movement. The watery concentrate also created critical hypoglycemic outcomes. The action of this division could be due to the presence of tannins, saponins, flavonoids, alkaloids, and steroids components. The saponins and watery concentrates of the root bark of *B. vulgaris* showed critical antihyperglycemic exercises in STZ-prompted diabetic rodents. The results recommend that the hypoglycemic impact was due to the presence of saponins that could affect the remaining beta cells (Meliani et al., 2011). According to these results, Boudjelthia et al. proposed that it is related to the concentrates of tannin and saponin present (Boudjelthia et al., 2017).

Catharanthus roseus

In India and other parts of the world, *Catharanthus roseus*, which belongs to the Apocynaceae family, is known by a variety of names. In some countries, including Brazil, Dominica, Jamaica, Mozambique, Taiwan, Thailand, and the West Indies, heated water decoction of leaves or the entire plant is used to treat diabetes. Recent findings indicate that *C. roseus* leaf powder creates an antihyperglycemic result in STZ-induced diabetic rodents, roseus leaf powder produces an antihyperglycemic effect, lowers total cholesterol and fat levels, and simultaneously increases HDL cholesterol. *C. roseus* has been associated with increased insulin sensitivity and plasma insulin concentration. In another review of the plant leaf, separate dichloromethane methanol was found to exhibit an antagonist effect on hyperglycemic movement in alloxan-induced diabetic rodents (Jayanthi et al., 2010).

Centaurium erythraea

Centaurium erythraea (*C. erythraea*) is a plant that belongs to the Gentillaceae group. This species is generally used in customary Moroccan medication to treat specific diseases such as diabetes, stomach related diseases, hepatitis, asthma, sensitivity, and ailment. The physical portrayal of *C. erythraea* revealed the presence of several classes of optional metabolites, including xanthonoids, terpenoids, flavonoids, phenolic acids, and unsaturated fats (El Menyiy et al., 2021).

Coccinia grandis

Coccinia grandis, also known as the ivy gourd, is consumed as a vegetable in many Asian countries such as India, Sri Lanka, Myanmar, and South East Asian countries such as Laos, Malaysia, and is local in numerous districts of Asia, America, and the Pacific. (Krishna et al., 2012; Ononamadu et al., 2021)), it belongs to the Cucurbitaceae family. A total of seven flavonoid glycosides were isolated from *C. grandis* concentrate and were shown to be powerful α-glucosidase inhibitors, considerably stronger than acarbose, an antidiabetic drug (Wasana et al., 2021).

Eugenia jambolana

Eugenia jambolana, also known as jamun in the Indian subcontinent, has been extensively studied for its antidiabetic properties. In alloxan-induced synthetic diabetics with fasting blood glucose levels between 120 and 250 mg/dl, as well as severely diabetic rabbits (fasting blood glucose levels greater than 250 mg/dl), the oral antihyperglycemic effect of water and ethanolic concentrates was investigated. Water extrication was believed to be more efficient than ethanolic removal in lowering fasting blood glucose and increasing blood glucose in glucose resistance. There was a decrease in fasting blood glucose (38% diabetic; 48% seriously diabetic) and an improvement in blood glucose during a glucose resistance test in diabetic bunnies after treatment of diabetic and seriously diabetic hares each day once with 25mg/kg, separately. Furthermore, both diabetic and severely diabetic bunnies had increased plasma insulin levels (Kumar et al., 2016).

Hibiscus esculentus

The effects of *Hibiscus esculentus* extricate on the lipid and glucose profiles of diabetic rodents were examined. We were able to induce diabetes in rodents by administering alloxan monohydrate at a dose of 120 mg/kg. The plant is a rich source of phytochemicals, for example, phenolic compounds, triterpenes, and phytosterols with hostile oxidation (Akbari et al., 2016). The hypoglycemic action of okra is primarily due to the presence of polysaccharides such as gelatin, gum, cellulose, and hemicellulose. The polysaccharides present in Hibiscus can dilemma bile acids in the digestive system and speed up their discharge by limiting bile corrosive reuse (Hajian et al., 2016).

Helicteres isora

Antihyperglycemic activity of root extracts from *Helicteres isora* Linn root extracts in rats with diabetes caused by alloxan. (Sterculiaceae) was examined and a possible mechanism was addressed to decrease blood sugar level. In alloxan-induced diabetic rats, blood glucose levels decreased by 69.13%. These beneficial effects were supported by evidence from histological examinations of the liver, pancreas, and kidney (Venkatesh et al., 2010).

Gymnema sylvestre

Gymnema sylvestre, often known as Gurmar from the milkweed family (Famiy; asclepiadaceae), is a hard woody bark that contains plant from tropical parts of Africa and India that has shown significant antidiabetic activity (Joseph et al., 2013). In the study by joseph et al. the rodent was injected with alloxan monohydrate into their body cavity, which is disintegrated in clean ordinary saline at a portion of around 150 mg for each kg of body weight. The function of cytotoxins such as alloxan is to damage insulin-producing beta cells causing a decrease in insulin levels, which paves the way for decreased uptake by tissue and leads to an "synthetic diabetes" like condition similar to 'synthetic diabetes' (Joseph et al., 2013, Subramaniyan et al., 2014)). Other studies show that the leaves of *Gymnema sylvestre* increase glucose use by coordinating the movement of chemicals responsible for glucose use by subordinate insulin pathways, leading to phosphorylase action, decrease in gluconeogenic chemicals, and sorbitol dehydrogenase protein (Mall et al., 2009; Subramaniyan et al., 2014). Parijit k et al. have shown that corrosive atoms from *Gymnema* leaves fill the receptors on the absorptive layers of the digestive tract and decrease glucose retention, causing low glucose levels (Kanetkar et al., 2007).

Momordica charantia

Momordica charantia, another name for the sick gourd known for his antidiabetic properties, is known in India and in few African nations. The combination of steroidal saponins (charantin), insulin-like polypeptides, and alkaloids has been reported to be the glucose-lowering metabolites of *M. charantia* (Kumar et al., 2010). A variety of phytochemicals have been isolated, but the exact ingredients responsible for the hypoglycemic/ antihyperglycemic actions are still unknown. Triterpene, proteid, steroid, alkaloid, inorganic, lipid, and phenolic compounds are thought to be the main components of bitter melon that are responsible for its antidiabetic effects (Harinantenaina et al., 2006; Tan et al., 2015; Chang et al., 2006). Charantin, polypeptide-p, and vicine are three significant mixtures that are recognised as glucose lowering agents. A small number of glycosides have been found in the stem and foods grown from the ground that belong to the genera of cucurbitane-type triterpenoids (Liu et al., 2009; Harinantenaina et al., 2006; Li et al., 2007). Four triterpenoids, in particular, have AMP-initiated protein kinase action, which is a potential hypoglycemic tool of *M. charantia* (Tan et al., 2008).

Ocimum sanctum

Ocimum sanctum, more generally, Tulsi has been used for millennia in Ayurveda for its different mending properties. The ethanolic concentrate of *O. sanctum* L. fundamentally decreases blood glucose, glycosylated hemoglobin, and urea with a corresponding expansion in glycogen, hemoglobin, and protein in streptozotocin-prompted diabetic rats. The antidiabetic property of tulsi is correlated with its stimulatory effects on physiological pathways of insulin discharge (Grover et al., 2005). Cower et al. proposed that treatment with O. sanctum separate for 30 days from typical rodents taken care of with fructose for 30 days essentially reduced serum glucose level (Gholap et al., 2004) on examination with control bunch. Chattopadyay also revealed that oral organisation of alcoholic concentrate of O. sanctum L. prompted checked glucose lowering (Chattopadhyay et al., 1993) in typical glucose-taking care of hyperglycemic and streptozotocin-actuated diabetic rodents. Additionally, the concentrate potentiates the activity of exogenous insulin in typical rodents. The action of the concentrate was 91.55 and 70.43% of that of Tolbutamide in typical and diabetic rodents, separately (Patil et al., 2011).

Syzygium cumini

Syzygium cumini has a place with restorative plants most frequently suggested as a complementary treatment in type 2 diabetes. The plant was widely considered during the most recent 125 years; around 100 case reports were currently accounted for before the disclosure of insulin. The best investigations used *S. cumini* seed powder or all the more frequently a watery or alcoholic concentrate thereof. Common concentrate doses were 100-200 mg/kg of creatures (rodent, mouse, hare) that were well to the portion levels given in the early case reports (VSS et al., 2018). Glycaemic levels were estimated in typical and exploratory rodents at beginning and at the 1, 5, 10 and 15 days of treatment. Streptozotocin-actuated diabetic rodents showed a huge expansion in glucose levels in contrast to ordinary rodents. The oral organisation of the derivation of ethyl acetic acid and methanol extricates showed a critical reduction in glucose levels. Mycaminose at a portion level of 50 mg/kg also shows a huge reduction in glucose level. Standard medication, glibenclamide, decreased glucose level in 15 days of treatment (Helmstädter and Axel, 2008). Altogether, according to a report, it is revealed that if *Syzygium cumini* presents its antidiabetic impact, this might be related with intensifies found in its seeds in contrast to leaves (Kumar et al., 2010, Oliveira et al., 2005).

Trigonella foenum

In both healthy and alloxan-diabetic rats, the hypoglycemic effects of the alcoholic and aqueous extracts of the *Trigonella foenum-graecum* leaf were examined. The results indicate that the aqueous extract of leaves administered orally and intraperitoneally has a hypoglycemic effect in neither normal nor alloxan-induced hyperglycemic rats (Abdel et al., 1997). Administration of *Trigonella foenum* seed extract to experimental diabetic rats multiple times over the course of six weeks has been shown to lower blood sugar, blood lipid levels, and hemorheological properties (Xue et al., 2007).

Vinca rosea

An herbaceous subshrub called Vinca rosea is also known as Madagascar periwinkle. It is cultivated primarily for the anticancer properties of its alkaloids. Alkaloids and tannins are the two groups of chemicals in vinca that are active (Jaleel et al., 2006). In a study conducted, 14 days of alloxan-induced diabetes in rats were used to examine plant extracts in methanol (500 mg/kg). Pancreatic cell regeneration in diabetic rats was also attributed to methanolic extracts, which substantially improved body weight and lipid profile measurements. Studies on histopathology support the idea that methanolic Vinca rosea extracts may help the pancreas as a probable mechanism for their antidiabetic effect (Ahmed et al., 2010).

Future Prospects

The development of new components for the prescription of diabetes has been largely fueled by advances in traditional medicine research. Numerous auxiliary plants ought to have been examined for suitability in people. Most reports neglected to include the full names of the flavours, the definition process, and the arrangement techniques. Most of the clinical primer strategies were improperly organised, leading to generally dubious revelations. More beneficial clinical tests are valid for additional endorsement, as is proper. However, attempts were made to represent the antidiabetic dynamic norms of antidiabetic plants. Furthermore, in the future, the depicted support plants may be helpful in the arrangement of new sane food assortments with antidiabetic properties or to prevent the hyperglycemic effects of particular food assortments, such as those abundant in essential carbohydrates.

Conclusion

Research initiatives in traditional medicine have largely fuelled the development of new prescription ingredients. Numerous auxiliary plants should have been examined for compatibility with particular people. In the vast majority of reports, the course of action, arranging techniques, and the power name of the flavours were all left out. Most of the clinical primer strategies were poorly organised, frequently resulting in dubious revelations.

More useful clinical examinations are legitimate for additional approval when performed correctly. However, attempts were made to represent antidiabetic dynamic norms from anti-diabetic plants. Furthermore, in the future, the depicted support plants may be helpful in the arrangement of new sane food assortments with antidiabetic properties or to prevent the hyperglycemic effects of particular food assortments, such as those abundant in essential carbohydrates.

References

Ahmed, M.F., Kazim, S.M., Ghori, S.S., Mehjabeen, S.S., Ahmed, S.R., Ali, S.M. and Ibrahim, M., 2010. Antidiabetic activity of Vinca rosea extracts in alloxan-induced diabetic rats. *International Journal of Endocrinology, 2010.*

Akbari, F., Shahinfard, N., Mirhoseini, M., Shirzad, H., Heidarian, E., Hajian, S. and Rafieian-Kopaei, M., 2016. Impacts of Hibiscus esculentus extract on glucose and lipid profile of diabetic rats. *Journal of nephropharmacology*, *5*(2), p.80.

Astiti, M.A., Jittmittraphap, A., Leaungwutiwong, P., Chutiwitoonchai, N., Pripdeevech, P., Mahidol, C., Ruchirawat, S. and Kittakoop, P., 2021. LC-QTOF-MS/MS based molecular networking approach for the isolation of α-glucosidase inhibitors and virucidal agents from Coccinia grandis (L.) Voigt. *Foods*, *10*(12), p.3041.

Boudjelthia, K., Hammadi, K., Kouidri, M. and Djebli, N., 2017. Evaluation of antidiabetic activity of two plants Berberis vulgaris and Zygophyllum geslini. *J. Phys. Chem. Biophys*, *7*(1), pp.1-7.

Chang, C.I., Chen, C.R., Liao, Y.W., Cheng, H.L., Chen, Y.C. and Chou, C.H., 2006. Cucurbitane-Type Triterpenoids from Momordica c harantia. *Journal of natural products*, *69*(8), pp.1168-1171.

Chang, Y.C. and Chuang, L.M., 2010. The role of oxidative stress in the pathogenesis of type 2 diabetes: from molecular mechanism to clinical implication. *American journal of translational research*, *2*(3), p.316.

Chattopadhyay, R.R., 1993. Hypoglycemic effect of Ocimum sanctum leaf extract in normal and streptozotocin diabetic rats. *Indian journal of experimental biology*, *31*(11), pp.891-893.

Chaudhary, N. and Tyagi, N., 2018. Diabetes mellitus: An Overview. *International Journal of Research and Development in Pharmacy & Life Sciences*, *7*(4), pp.3030-3033.

Chauhan, A., Sharma, P.K., Srivastava, P., Kumar, N. and Dudhe, R., 2010. Plants having potential antidiabetic activity: a review. *Der Pharmacia Lettre*, *2*(3), pp.369-387.

Choi, K. and Kim, Y.B., 2010. Molecular mechanism of insulin resistance in obesity and type 2 diabetes. *The Korean journal of internal medicine*, *25*(2), p.119.

Debra, H.J., 1991. Management of Diabetes Mellitus. Perspective of care across the life span.

DeFronzo, R.A., 1999. Pharmacologic therapy for type 2 diabetes mellitus. *Annals of internal medicine*, *131*(4), pp.281-303.

Dey, L., Attele, A.S. and Yuan, C.S., 2002. Alternative therapies for type 2 diabetes. *Alternative medicine review*, *7*(1), pp.45-58.

El Menyiy, N., Guaouguaou, F.E., El Baaboua, A., El Omari, N., Taha, D., Salhi, N., Shariati, M.A., Aanniz, T., Benali, T., Zengin, G. and El-Shazly, M., 2021. Phytochemical properties, biological activities and medicinal use of Centaurium erythraea Rafn. *Journal of Ethnopharmacology*, *276*, p.114171.

Forouhi, N.G. and Wareham, N.J., 2010. Epidemiology of diabetes. *Medicine*, *38*(11), pp.602-606.

Gholap, S. and Kar, A., 2004. Hypoglycaemic effects of some plant extracts are possibly mediated through inhibition in corticosteroid concentration. *Die Pharmazie-An International Journal of Pharmaceutical Sciences*, *59*(11), pp.876-878.

Govindarajan, S., Babu, S.N., Vijayalakshmi, M.A., Manohar, P. and Noor, A., 2021. Aloe vera carbohydrates regulate glucose metabolism through improved glycogen synthesis and downregulation of hepatic gluconeogenesis in diabetic rats. *Journal of Ethnopharmacology*, *281*, p.114556.

Grover, J.K. and Yadav, S.P., 2004. Pharmacological actions and potential uses of Momordica charantia: A review. *Journal of ethnopharmacology*, *93*(1), pp.123-132.

Grover, J.K., Vats, V. and Yadav, S.S., 2005. Pterocarpus marsupium extract (Vijayasar) prevented the alteration in metabolic patterns induced in the normal rat by feeding an adequate diet containing fructose as sole carbohydrate. *Diabetes, Obesity and Metabolism*, *7*(4), pp.414-420.

Haghani, F., Arabnezhad, M.R., Mohammadi, S. and Ghaffarian-Bahraman, A., 2022. Aloe vera and streptozotocin-induced diabetes mellitus. *Revista Brasileira de Farmacognosia*, *32*(2), pp.174-187.

Hajian, S., Asgary, S., Rafieian-Kopaei, M., Sahebkar, A., Goli-Malekabady, N. and Rashidi, B., 2016. Hibiscus esculentus seed and mucilage beneficial effects in reducing complications of diabetes in streptozotocin-induced diabetic rats. *Annals of Research in Antioxidants*, *1*(2).

Harinantenaina, L., Tanaka, M., Takaoka, S., Oda, M., Mogami, O., Uchida, M. and Asakawa, Y., 2006. Momordica charantia constituents and antidiabetic screening of the isolated major compounds. *Chemical and Pharmaceutical Bulletin*, *54*(7), pp.1017-1021.

Harinantenaina, L., Tanaka, M., Takaoka, S., Oda, M., Mogami, O., Uchida, M. and Asakawa, Y., 2006. Momordica charantia constituents and antidiabetic screening of the isolated major compounds. *Chemical and Pharmaceutical Bulletin*, *54*(7), pp.1017-1021.

Helmstädter, A., 2008. Syzygium cumini (L.) SKEELS (Myrtaceae) against diabetes–125 years of research. *Die Pharmazie-An International Journal of Pharmaceutical Sciences*, *63*(2), pp.91-101.

Inzucchi, S.E., 2002. Oral antihyperglycemic therapy for type 2 diabetes: scientific review. *Jama*, *287*(3), pp.360-372.

Jaleel, C.A., Gopi, R., Lakshmanan, G.A. and Panneerselvam, R., 2006. Triadimefon induced changes in the antioxidant metabolism and ajmalicine production in Catharanthus roseus (L.) G. Don. *Plant Science*, *171*(2), pp.271-276.

Jayanthi, M., Sowbala, N., Rajalakshmi, G., Kanagavalli, U. and Sivakumar, V., 2010. Study of anti hyperglycemic effect of Catharanthus roseus in alloxan induced diabetic rats. *Int J Pharm Pharm Sci*, *2*(4), pp.114-6.

Joseph, B. and Jini, D., 2013. Antidiabetic effects of Momordica charantia (bitter melon) and its medicinal potency. *Asian pacific journal of tropical disease*, *3*(2), pp.93-102.

Jung, M., Park, M., Lee, H.C., Kang, Y.H., Kang, E.S. and Kim, S.K., 2006. Antidiabetic agents from medicinal plants. *Current medicinal chemistry*, *13*(10), pp.1203-1218.

Jwad, S.M. and AL-Fatlawi, H.Y., 2022. Types of Diabetes and their Effect on the Immune System. *J. Adv. Pharm. Pract*, *4*, pp.21-30.

Kanetkar, P., Singhal, R. and Kamat, M., 2007. Gymnema sylvestre: a memoir. *Journal of clinical biochemistry and nutrition*, *41*(2), pp.77-81.

Kahn, B.B., 1996. Glucose transport: pivotal step in insulin action. *Diabetes*, *45*(11), pp.1644-1654.

Kaul, K., Tarr, J.M., Ahmad, S.I., Kohner, E.M. and Chibber, R., 2013. Introduction to diabetes mellitus. *Diabetes: an old disease, a new insight*, pp.1-11.

Krishna, R.B., Reddy, S.R., Javangula, H., Swapna, D. and Reddy, K.J., 2012. Isolation and characterization of gymnemic acid from Gymnema sylvestre R. Br. in control of diabetes. *Int J Life Science Pharma Research*, *2*, pp.L1-9.

Kelm, M.A., Nair, M.G., Strasburg, G.M. and DeWitt, D.L., 2000. Antioxidant and cyclooxygenase inhibitory phenolic compounds from Ocimum sanctum Linn. *Phytomedicine*, *7*(1), pp.7-13.

Kerru, N., Singh-Pillay, A., Awolade, P. and Singh, P., 2018. Current anti-diabetic agents and their molecular targets: A review. *European Journal of Medicinal Chemistry*, *152*, pp.436-488.

Koski, R.R., 2004. Oral antidiabetic agents: A comparative review. *Journal of pharmacy practice*, *17*(1), pp.39-48.

Kuhl, C., 1998. Etiology and pathogenesis of gestational diabetes. *Diabetes care*, *21*, p.B19.

Kumar, A., Ilavarasan, R., Jayachandran, T., Deecaraman, M., Aravindan, P., Padmanabhan, N. and Krishan, M.R.V., 2008. Anti-diabetic activity of Syzygium cumini and its isolated compound against streptozotocin-induced diabetic rats. *Journal of Medicinal Plants Research*, *2*(9), pp.246-249.

Kumar, D.S., Sharathnath, K.V., Yogeswaran, P., Harani, A., Sudhakar, K., Sudha, P. and Banji, D., 2010. A medicinal potency of Momordica charantia. *International Journal of Pharmaceutical Sciences Review and Research*, *1*(2), pp.95-100.

Kumar, R., Pate, D.K., Prasad, S.K., Sairam, K. and Hemalatha, S., 2011. Antidiabetic activity of alcoholic leaves extract of Alangium lamarckii Thwaites on streptozotocin–nicotinamide induced type 2 diabetic rats. *Asian Pacific journal of tropical medicine*, *4*(11), pp.904-909.

Kumar, V., 2016. Importance of Alangium salviifolium and its pharmacological update. *European Journal of Medicinal Plants*, *12*(4), p.1.

Lebovitz, H.E., 1997. Alpha-glucosidase inhibitors. *Endocrinology and metabolism clinics of North America*, *26*(3), pp.539-551.

Li, Q.Y., Chen, H.B., Liu, Z.M., Wang, B. and Zhao, Y.Y., 2007. Cucurbitane triterpenoids from Momordica charantia. *Magnetic Resonance in Chemistry*, *45*(6), pp.451-456.

Li, W.L., Zheng, H.C., Bukuru, J. and De Kimpe, N., 2004. Natural medicines used in the traditional Chinese medical system for therapy of diabetes mellitus. *Journal of ethnopharmacology*, *92*(1), pp.1-21.

Liu, J.Q., Chen, J.C., Wang, C.F. and Qiu, M.H., 2009. New cucurbitane triterpenoids and steroidal glycoside from Momordica charantia. *Molecules*, *14*(12), pp.4804-4813.

Mall, G.K., Mishra, P.K. and Prakash, V., 2009. Antidiabetic and hypolipidemic activity of Gymnema sylvestre in alloxan induced diabetic rats. *Global Journal of Biotechnology & Biochemistry*, *4*(1), pp.37-42.

Malviya, N., Jain, S. and Malviya, S.A.P.N.A., 2010. Antidiabetic potential of medicinal plants. *Acta pol pharm*, *67*(2), pp.113-118.

Marles, R.J. and Farnsworth, N.R., 1995. Antidiabetic plants and their active constituents. *Phytomedicine*, *2*(2), pp.137-189.

Marles, R.J. and Farnsworth, N.R., 1995. Antidiabetic plants and their active constituents. *Phytomedicine*, *2*(2), pp.137-189.

Mayerson, A.B. and Inzucchi, S.E., 2002. Type 2 diabetes therapy: a pathophysiologically based approach. *Postgraduate medicine*, *111*(3), pp.83-95.

Meliani, N., Dib, M.E.A., Allali, H. and Tabti, B., 2011. Hypoglycaemic effect of Berberis vulgaris L. in normal and streptozotocin-induced diabetic rats. *Asian Pacific journal of tropical biomedicine*, *1*(6), pp.468-471.

Oliveira, A.C.P., Endringer, D.C., Amorim, L.A.S., Maria das Graças, L.B. and Coelho, M.M., 2005. Effect of the extracts and fractions of Baccharis trimera and Syzygium cumini on glycaemia of diabetic and non-diabetic mice. *Journal of ethnopharmacology*, *102*(3), pp.465-469.

Ononamadu, C. and Ibrahim, A., 2021. Molecular docking and prediction of ADME/ drug-likeness properties of potentially active antidiabetic compounds isolated from aqueous-methanol extracts of Gymnema sylvestre and Combretum micranthum. *BioTechnologia*, *102*(1), pp.85-99.

Patil, R., Patil, R., Ahirwar, B. and Ahirwar, D., 2011. Isolation and characterization of anti-diabetic component (bioactivity—guided fractionation) from Ocimum sanctum L. (Lamiaceae) aerial part. *Asian Pacific journal of tropical medicine*, *4*(4), pp.278-282.

Rai, V.A., Iyer, U. and Mani, U.V., 1997. Effect of Tulasi (Ocimum sanctum) leaf powder supplementation on blood sugar levels, serum lipids and tissues lipids in diabetic rats. *Plant foods for human nutrition*, *50*, pp.9-16.

Raman, A. and Lau, C., 1996. Anti-diabetic properties and phytochemistry of Momordica charantia L. (Cucurbitaceae). *Phytomedicine*, *2*(4), pp.349-362.

Rao, M.U., Sreenivasulu, M., Chengaiah, B., Reddy, K.J. and Chetty, C.M., 2010. Herbal medicines for diabetes mellitus: a review. *Int J PharmTech Res*, *2*(3), pp.1883-1892.

Rasineni, K., Bellamkonda, R., Singareddy, S.R. and Desireddy, S., 2010. Antihyper-glycemic activity of Catharanthus roseus leaf powder in streptozotocin-induced diabetic rats. *Pharmacognosy research*, *2*(3), p.195.

Resmi, C.R., Fathima, A., Sinilal, B. and Latha, M.S., 2001. Antidiabetic effect of a herbal drug in alloxan-diabetic rats. *INDIAN DRUGS-BOMBAY-*, *38*(6), pp.319-322.

Roglic, G., 2016. WHO Global report on diabetes: A summary. *International Journal of Noncommunicable Diseases*, *1*(1), p.3.

Salehi, B., Ata, A., V. Anil Kumar, N., Sharopov, F., Ramirez-Alarcon, K., Ruiz-Ortega, A., Abdulmajid Ayatollahi, S., Valere Tsouh Fokou, P., Kobarfard, F., Amiruddin Zakaria, Z. and Iriti, M., 2019. Antidiabetic potential of medicinal plants and their active components. *Biomolecules*, *9*(10), p.551.

Subramaniyan, V. and Srinivasan, P., 2014. Gymnema sylvestre: A Key for Diabetes Management A Review. *Pharmacology & Toxicology Research*, *1*, pp.1-10.

Sulaiman, M.K., 2019. Diabetic nephropathy: recent advances in pathophysiology and challenges in dietary management. *Diabetology & metabolic syndrome*, *11*, pp.1-5.

Tan, M.J., Ye, J.M., Turner, N., Hohnen-Behrens, C., Ke, C.Q., Tang, C.P., Chen, T., Weiss, H.C., Gesing, E.R., Rowland, A. and James, D.E., 2008. Antidiabetic activities of triterpenoids isolated from bitter melon associated with activation of the AMPK pathway. *Chemistry & biology*, *15*(3), pp.263-273.

Tan, E.S., Abdullah, A. and Kassim, N.K., Antioxidant and Anti-diabetic Properties of Bitter Gourd (Momordica charantia) Fruit.

Vats, V., Yadav, S.P. and Grover, J.K., 2004. Ethanolic extract of Ocimum sanctum leaves partially attenuates streptozotocin-induced alterations in glycogen content and carbohydrate metabolism in rats. *Journal of ethnopharmacology*, *90*(1), pp.155-160.

Venkatesh, S., Madhava Reddy, B., Dayanand Reddy, G., Mullangi, R. and Lakshman, M., 2010. Antihyperglycemic and hypolipidemic effects of Helicteres isora roots in alloxan-induced diabetic rats: a possible mechanism of action. *Journal of natural medicines*, *64*, pp.295-304.

VSS, P., Adapa, D., Vana, D.R., Choudhury, A., Jahangir, M.A. and Chatterjee, A., 2018. Nutritional components relevant to type-2-diabetes: Dietary sources, metabolic functions and glycaemic effects. *Journal of Research in Medical and Dental Science*, *6*(5), pp.52-75.

Wadkar, K.A., Magdum, C.S., Patil, S.S. and Naikwade, N.S., 2008. Antidiabetic potential and Indian medicinal plants. *Journal of herbal medicine and toxicology*, *2*(1), pp.45-50.

Wasana, K.G.P., Attanayake, A.P., Weerarathna, T.P. and Jayatilaka, K.A.P.W., 2021. Efficacy and safety of a herbal drug of Coccinia grandis (Linn.) Voigt in patients with type 2 diabetes mellitus: A double blind randomized placebo controlled clinical trial. *Phytomedicine*, *81*, p.153431.

Wild, S., Roglic, G., Green, A., Sicree, R. and King, H., 2004. Global prevalence of diabetes: estimates for the year 2000 and projections for 2030. *Diabetes care*, *27*(5), pp.1047-1053.

Xue, W.L., Li, X.S., Zhang, J., Liu, Y.H., Wang, Z.L. and Zhang, R.J., 2007. Effect of Trigonella foenum-graecum (fenugreek) extract on blood glucose, blood lipid and hemorheological properties in streptozotocin-induced diabetic rats. *Asia Pac J Clin Nutr*, *16*(Suppl 1), pp.422-6.

Zulcafli, A.S., Lim, C., Ling, A.P., Chye, S. and Koh, R., 2020. Focus: Plant-based Medicine and Pharmacology: Antidiabetic Potential of Syzygium sp.: An Overview. *The Yale journal of biology and medicine*, *93*(2), p.307.

Chapter 6

The Usefulness of Aloe Vera in the Management of Diabetes

Faruk Alam[1]
Ruhul Amin[1,*]
Biplab Kumar Dey[1]
Ronald Darwin[2]
Rahul Kanaoujiya[3]
Jithendar Reddy Mandhadi[1]
and T. Chandra Shekar[1]

[1]Faculty of Pharmaceutical Science, Assam down town University, Panikhaiti, Guwahati, Assam, India
[2]Pharmacology, School of Pharmaceutical Sciences, Vels Institute of Science Technology & Advanced Studies, Chennai, India
[3]Synthetic Inorganic and Metallo Organic Research Laboratory, Department of Chemistry, University of Allahabad, Uttar Pradesh, Prayagraj, India

Abstract

In medium and low-income nations like India, in which the burden of the disease has increased significantly in the last few decades and is likely to continue to increase in the next few decades, diabetes itself has emerged as a substantial threat to the healthcare system on a worldwide scale. Several conditions may be remedied with the use of aloe vera gel. Drinking aloe vera juice has been established to lower blood pressure and improve blood glucose levels, making it an excellent therapy for diabetes.

* Corresponding Author's Email: ruhulglp18@gmail.com.

In: Antidiabetic Plants
Editor: Arpita Roy
ISBN: 979-8-88697-957-2

Although some research has raised concerns about the safety and effectiveness of aloe vera or its components, especially when applied in a variety of doses, other studies have found no evidence to support such claims. The goal of this chapter is to identify the biologically active components of aloe vera that have the potential to play a role in the preventive process.

Keywords: diabetes, aloe vera, aloe juice in diabetes, clinical study

Introduction

Diabetes is a chronic disease defined by excessive blood glucose levels that can be caused by abnormalities in insulin manufacturing, insulin function, or both. Diabetes can be prevented by supporting healthy blood glucose levels. Diabetes is increasingly becoming the leading cause of disease, death, and disability across the globe (Deshpande et al., 2008). Diabetes is a worldwide metabolic disease that affects critical biochemical activities in people of all ages. Diabetes-related metabolic problems cause an increase in superoxide formation in mitochondrial endothelial cells of both arteries, also in the myocardium. As a direct result of this, oxidative stress has been associated with the development of micro- and cardiovascular diabetes problems. As a direct result of this, oxidative stress has been associated with the onset of micro- and cardiovascular diabetes problems (Giacco and Brownlee, 2010). This research found that hypoglycemia was more common among adolescents than among adults. In terms of frequency, type 1 diabetes, often known as DM1, is the second most common form of chronic disease seen in young people. Pain and medical bills are mainly due to complications and deaths caused by diabetes. Up to $174 billion is spent each year on diabetes-related care in the United States, where 9.1% of the population suffers from the disease. (2020). Although there is effective medication, you will need to find a happy medium between insulin dosage, diet, and exercise, and you will benefit from hearing how effectively you are managing your blood sugar levels. Consequently, even the most determined teenager can struggle to establish and maintain such a thorough and rigorous treatment programme consistently. Characteristics of youth, such as originality, longevity, and exceptionality, can be detrimental to an individual's ability to effectively control diabetes. However, better blood sugar management can result from an increased focus on diabetes care, and lower HbA1c concentrations may mitigate the dangers of diabetes complications (2022). Acupuncture, insulin injections, and blood glucose metres are all things that can make compliance more difficult. Despite advances in insulin administration pen and pumps, compliance withdiabetes therapy regimens is challenging for all ages, but teenagers find it more difficult. (Morris et al., 1997). Due to the complexity of the signaling system, adolescents have a hard time achieving and maintaining stable blood glucose levels. Increased insulin resistance has been associated with physiological changes that occur throughout adolescence (Amiel et al., 1986). Physicians may unwittingly raise the burden and restrict health-promoting treatments when tightening blood sugar control regimens to improve results, making compliance harder (Svoren et al., 2007).

Vasculopathy, nephropathy, retinopathy, and neuropathy, chronic kidney disease, and cataracts are all complications of diabetes, and protein glycation is suspected to play a significant role in the development of many diseases (Singh et al., 2014; Amin et al., 2022). Advanced glycation end products (AGEs) are created during the glycation of proteins, and they disrupt the normal structure and function of proteins and enzymes. A sequence of processes, beginning with the Maillard reaction, produces Schiff bases, which are then used to make both fluorescent compounds such as pentosidine and nonfluorescent ones such as carboxymethyl lysine (CML)(Joglekar et al., 2017, Sharma et al., 2015). CML and pentosidine, for example, have been implicated as glycooxidizing damage biomarkers (Haddad et al., 2016). Given the harmful consequences of glycation, it is urgently needed to create protein glycation inhibitors that can help decrease and/or prevent diabetes mellitus problems. In the second half of the 20th century, there was a discernible increase in the number of people who were diagnosed with diabetes. This was mainly attributable to the widespread availability of low-cost, calorie-dense foods in large quantities, as well as the decrease in the amount of regular daily exercise caused by technological advancements (Vlassara and Uribarri, 2014). This chapter will focus on natural diabetes therapy as an alternative to pharmaceutical options due to the many negative effects that diabetic medications can have on the liver's metabolic processes.

The fact that many different types of plants include properties that may be used for medicinal purposes has made it feasible for scientists to develop effective new medications. As a result of the evolution of traditional medicine, aloe vera gel has the potential to treat a wide variety of conditions; hence, the focus of this chapter should be on aloe vera. According to the findings of some research, use has no negative consequences. Plant Aloe vera or its components, while others have raised doubts about their safety and efficacy.

Research is imperative to determine whether or not taking dietary supplements could be an efficient measure to prevent or mitigate the nutritional value. This is commonly because aloe vera is used in several Asian countries and appears to be risk-free. The goal is to isolate the bioactive compounds in Aloe that may play a role in diabetes prevention. Preliminary research suggests that it may be effective against diabetes without causing any undesirable side effects.

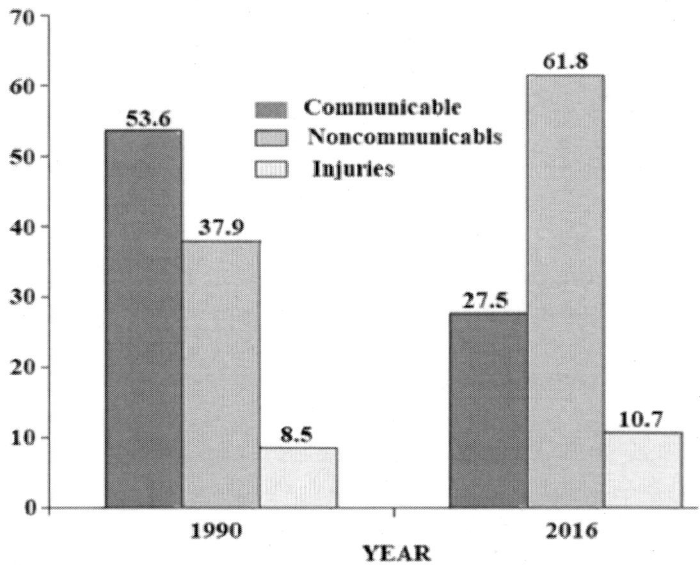

Figure 1. Indicative of the total number of people who died in India during the years 1990 and 2016 (communicable vs. non-communicable vs. injuries).

Burden of Diabetes in India

Diabetes has been more prevalent in India over the past 30 years, as well as in other parts of the world, with India containing a disproportionately large percentage of the total number of cases worldwide. As a result of an epidemiological transition, the patterns of disease in India have changed, with the percentage of total morbidity & premature death changing from communicable, maternal, neonatal, and nutritional disorders (CMNND) to noncommunicable diseases (NCD) and trauma. This change occurred due to an increase in the prevalence of non-communicable diseases in India. In India in 1990, CMNND was responsible for 61% of all DALY, 30% of all NCDs, and 9 percent of all injuries. Due to significant epidemiological changes in India over the course of several years, the proportion of DALYs attributable to CMNNDs in general fell to 33% in 2016, while the proportion attributable to NCDs and injuries rose to 55 and 11%, respectively (Figure 1). When looking at the main individual causes of DALY in India, most NCDs have risen in rank since 1990, with diabetes showing a notable increase, moving from 35th position in 1990 to 13th place in 2016; this represents a four-fold increase in disease burden or the DALY rate. In other words, diabetes has become four times more prevalent in India. (Dall et al., 2014).

According to the 2017 research, "India: Health of the Nation's States' - the India State-Level Disease Burden Initiative, the percentage of deaths caused by NCDs increased from 37.9% in 1990 to 61.82% in 2016. There are four primary NCDs: cardiovascular disease (CVD), cancer, chronic lung disease (CRD), and diabetes; and the four main behavioural risk factors for each of these diseases are poor eating habits, insufficient physical activity, tobacco and alcohol use, and excessive sitting.

Figure 2 shows the precise percentage changes in the Disability Adjusted Life Years (DALY) number for the main individual causes of these NCDs among women from 1990 to 2016.

Management of Diabetes

Due to India's enormous population, Type I diabetes mellitus (DM1) accounts for 5% of all occurrences. Type II diabetes mellitus (DM2) often begins around 57. Mental and social development is crucial now. Young parents are struggling to find work as children acclimate to regular routines and school. DM1 Parents and young patients must adjust their lifestyles for strict surveillance and therapy (Chiang et al., 2018). According to a recent statistical report, type II diabetes is the most common chronic illness. If DM2 is poorly administered, it may cause microvascular, macrovascular, and other problems. The complications of type 2 diabetes are the leading cause of death and disability. (Chawla et al., 2016). Although insulin and oral antihyperglycemic medications such as thiazolidinedione, sulfonylurea, biguanide, alpha-glucosidase inhibitors, meglitinide, and DPP-4 inhibitors are the cornerstones of DM2 therapy, their efficacy and side effects are significant (Chaudhury et al., 2017).

Chemical drugs now used to manage blood sugar levels can cause liver damage, weight gain, and increased risk of various cardiovascular diseases (Garcia-Compean et al., 2009). Furthermore, long-term use of diabetes medications may cause kidney damage and increase the risk of cancer by 1.3 times. Therapy and prediabetes therapy and prevention, on the other hand, are critical to improving well-being and reducing economic expenses (Garcia-Compean et al., 2009).

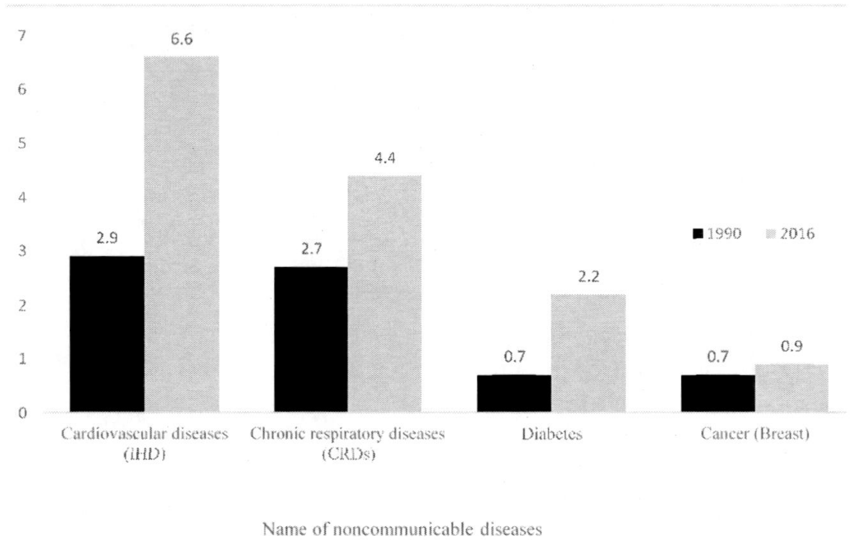

Figure 2. Proportion of changes in the number of DALYs.

As a result, more effective and safer antihyperglycemic drugs are needed. Multiple antihyperglycemic medications with various mechanisms are often used to treat patients with type 2 diabetes patients effectively (Nathan et al., 2009). T2DM is a progressive condition characterised by a steady loss of in-cell activity until it is exhausted, at which point sufficient glycaemic control cannot be supported with a rational combination of oral treatments, which requires the use of insulin as the only therapy. Nutrition-basedtreatment is advocated as an alternative therapy since it has less potential for side effects and is much more maintainable. (Shrivastava et al., 2013).

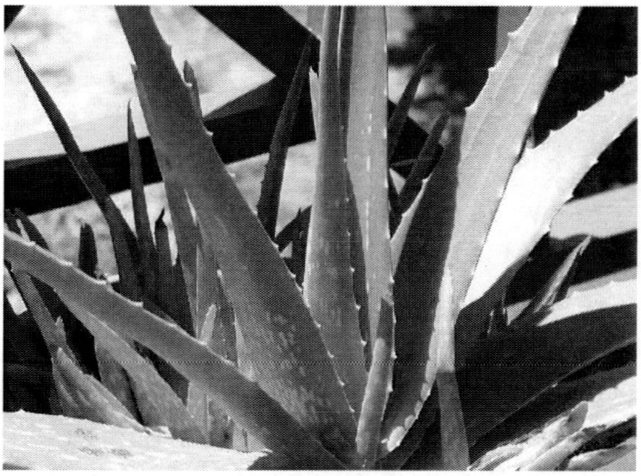

Figure 3. *Aloe vera* Plant.

Using medicinal plants to treat diabetes is preferable to using synthetic medications due to their safety and effectiveness. Blood glucose levels may be reduced due to antioxidants and vitamins E and C contained in plants, as well as flavonoids, tannins, alkaloids, and other plant compounds (Kooti et al., 2016). Aloe vera (L.) Burm., (Figure 3) f. The products (Aloe *barbadensis* Mill; Family-Asphodelaceae; Figure 3) have been used for thousands of years and our fascination with them only appears to grow. Traditional uses of this plant, which originated in the East African/Mediterranean region, can be traced back to 4000 BC, when Egyptians, Assyrians and Mediterranean people all employed it. It was first published in 1650 and then again in 1742 in the London Pharmacopoeia and the London Dispensatory. By 1820, in the United States Pharmacopoeia; by 1867, in the British Pharmacopoeia; and by 1959, it had been included in the FDA's list of approved food additives (Habtemariam, 2017). Today, aloe vera is a commercial plant that is widely used in the food, beverage, pharmaceutical, herbal, and cosmetic sectors.

Description of the Plant

Attributes

Genus Aloe; Asphodelaceae family; Perennial life cycle propagation strategy Suggestion: Tropical and Mediterranean are the countries or regions of origin. Attractive Flowers and Textural Play Value If consumed, it has low toxicity. When properly prepared, it can be used medicinally and in beverages. Height: 1ft. 0in. up to 2ft. 0in. Width: 0ft. 6in. up to 1ft. 0in are dimensions.

Herbaceous, perennial, succulent and Poisonous; Habit: upright; medium growth medium, low maintenance; medium texture.

Flowers

There are golden or yellow flowers, orange flowers, and crimson or burgundy flowers. A raceme is a kind of inflorescence that can be seen on flowers. Worth a gardener in terms of flowers being spectacular; Spring and winter are the seasons during which flower blossoms. The tubular is the form of the flower. The size of the flower can vary from 1 to 3 inches. The elongated terminal clusters of red or yellow orange flowers make up the floral description of this plant. On a stem that is about 3 feet tall, there are pendulous blossoms that are densely packed together. Flowers are only seen in mature plants and may bloom an infinite number of times throughout the course of a plant's lifetime.

Leaves

Green, blue, and grey or silver may be seen in the leaves. The texture of the leaf is fleshy and smooth; Gardener value: Showy Simple leaf type; Rosulate leaf arrangement, lanceolate leaf form, and serrate leaf margins are characteristics of this plant's leaf arrangement. There are no hairs present; Length of leaf is greater than 6 inches; breadth of leaf between 1 and 3 inches Details on the leaf: Plant that lives for many years and has basal leaves that are thick, succulent, and pointed with small white teeth around the edge. The maximum length of the leaves that may develop is around 45 centimetres. They are fragile and easy to shatter, and the insides have a sap that looks like a gel.

Effects of *Aloe* Juice on Diabetes

Potential benefits in the treatment of diabetes come from anecdotal reports that its consumption increases blood sugar levels. Additionally, research has connected Aloe with a reduction in the patient's blood lipid level (fat) level (Deora and Venkatraman, 2022a). There is a substantial quantity of these particles. In certain people with type II diabetes, or perhaps growth slows, severe hepatitis, and wound repair in the blood accelerates (liver infection). Diabetic ulcers and sores on the legs are common and recovery from them is more labour intensive than in those without the disease. This may also indicate

Table 1. Chemicals isolated from leaf pulp and exudates (Sánchez et al., 2020)

Effects	Compounds	Category
Contribution to the digestive process (biochemical catalysts) in the breakdown of fatty and sugary substances.	In several biochemical reactions, enzymes such as amylases, lipases, alkaline phosphatases, cellulases, catalases, and peroxidases play crucial roles.	Enzymes
Bradykinins are deactivated (anti-inflammatory)	enzymes like carboxypeptidases and brady kinases	
Antitumor	Lectins	
Antioxidants	αα-tocopherol, B-1,2,6,12, C, A (β-carotene), folic acid, and E Choline	vitamins
Function as an enzyme. Few acts as antioxidants	Cu, Zn, K, Na, Ca, Se, Mn, Mg, Cr and Fe	Minerals
Massive purification. Small amounts: intestinal absorption aid, effective antimicrobials, powerful analgesics.	Anthrone-C-glycosides, chromones, aloeemodin-9-anthrone, lsobarbaloin, and barbaloin are all components of echinacea.	Anthraquinone
Wound Healing and anti-inflammatory action	Auxins, gibberellins	Hormones
Anti-inflammatory and antibacterial	Aspirin-like composite	Salicylic acid
Anthrone-C-glycosides, chromones, aloeemodin-9-anthrone, lsobarbaloin, and barbaloin are all components of echinacea.	It has 20 of the 22 amino acids that are not necessary and seven of the eight amino acids that are necessary.	Amino acids
Increase the penetration of other substances.	Topical applications include inactive substances.	Lignin
Anti-inflammatory	Cholesterolβ-sitosterol, campestral and lupeol.	Sterols
Analgesic and Antiseptic	Lupeol	
Antiseptic and Cleansing	Soapy substances	Saponins
Immunomodulators	Mono- and polysaccharides (glucose and fructose) (glucomannans and polyominoes)	Sugars
Moisturizer	Glumannan	

that total cholesterol is improving and that cholesterol levels are decreasing (Sharma et al., 2021). The anti-diabetic action of *A. vera* has been the subject of several published clinical studies. The potential to improve blood sugar levels in diabetics has been widely studied (Haghani et al., 2022). Because aloe vera supplements have the potential to reduce blood gushing and improve transmission to the farthest point, it is possible that diabetic patients who suffer from limbic neuropathy might benefit from using them (numbness in the hands and feet). Aloe vera is beneficial for people with diabetes. Researchers found that Aloe, when extracted regularly into the container structure, reduced glucose levels and damaged low-density lipoprotein cholesterol more effectively than sham treatment, without causing any of the side effects (Alinejad-Mofrad et al., 2015b). According to Blue Shield Integral and Elective Health, regular use of 5-15 millilitres of Aloe juice (double the recommended daily amount) has been shown to reduce blood glucose and cholesterol levels in both animals and humans. There are potent plant components in aloe that can reduce pain, increase tissue growth, and accelerate recovery. Polysaccharides, such as acetylmannan, have been used for centuries as analgesics and therapeutics, and can also increase blood flow and oxygenation. The Aloe vera plant contains a unique molecule called allantoin. Having a soothing and pain-relieving quality due to its stickiness, it is very effective (Alinejad-Mofrad et al., 2015b). Regular use of Aloe in the treatment of diabetes can help with a variety of difficulties, including ulcers, wounds, and infections, due to its high oxidant content (Table 1). Figure 4 shows the different chemical constituents and their structures present in Aloe vera.

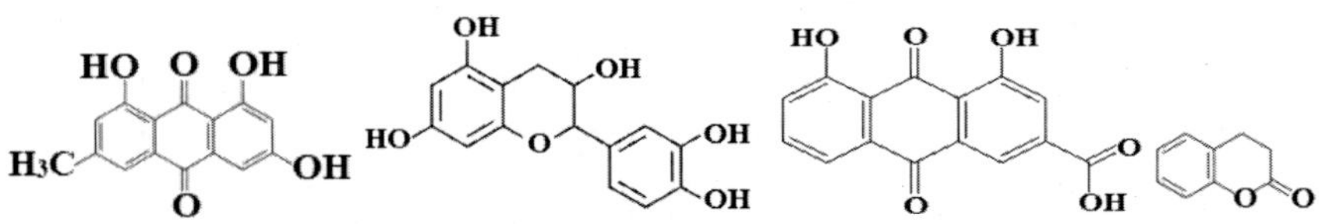

Emodin Cianidanol Rhein 3,4-dihydrocoumarin

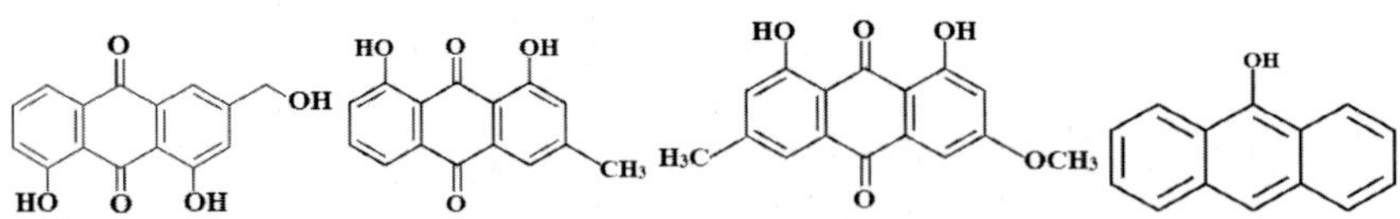

Aloe-emodin ChrysophanolPhyscionAnthranol

Figure 4. (Continued).

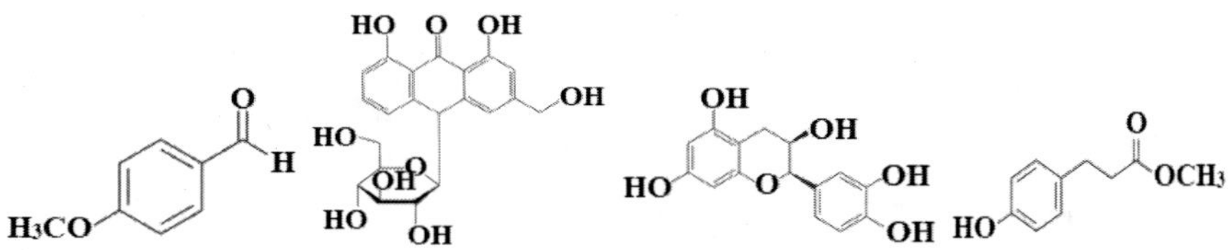

4-Methoxy Aloin B (-)-Epicatechin Methyl 3-(4-benzaldehyde hydroxyphenyl) propionate

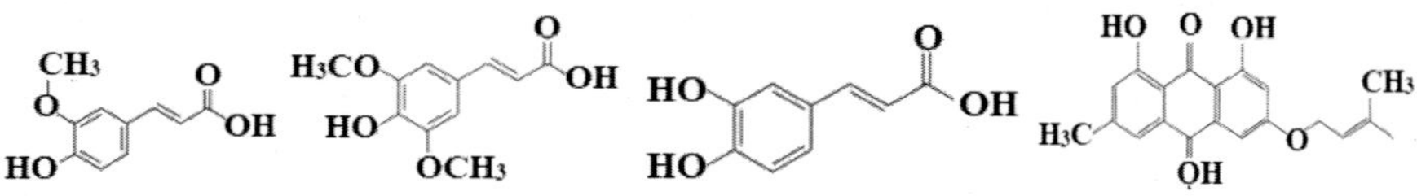

Ferulic acid Sinapic acid Caffeic acid Madagascine

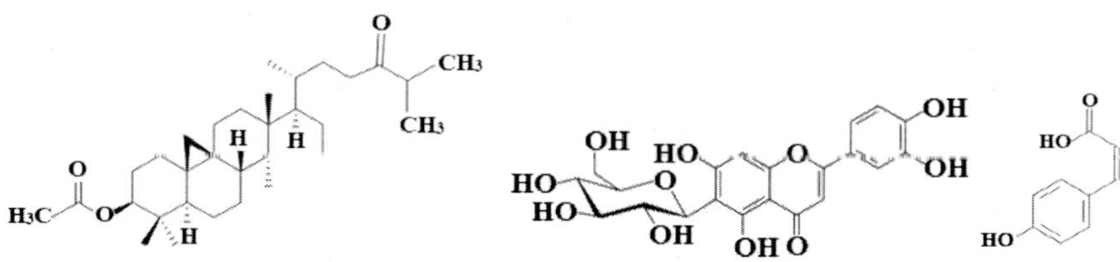

24-Methylenecycloartanol Isoorientin *cis-p*-Coumaric acid

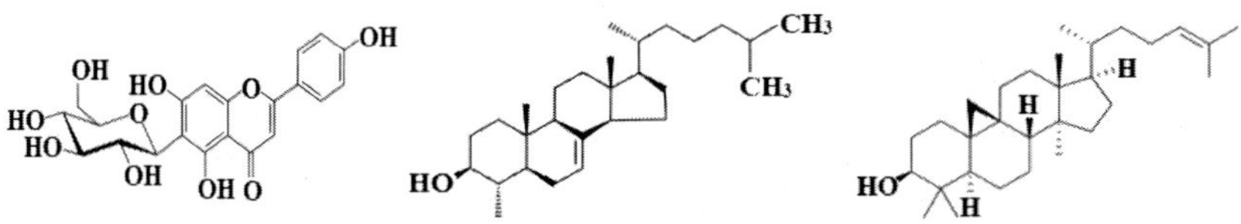

Isovitexin Lophenol Cycloartanol

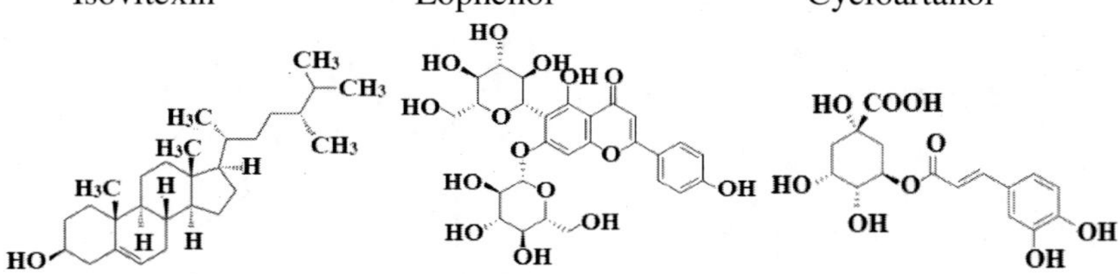

Campesterol Saponarin Chlorogenic acid

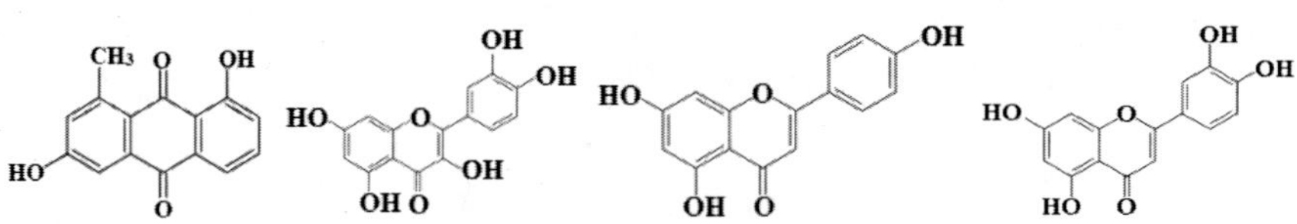

Aloesaponarin-II Quercetin Apigenin Luteolin

Figure 4. (Continued).

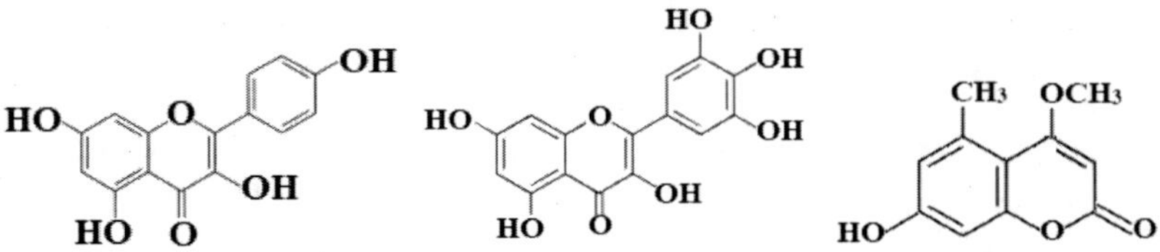

Kaempferol Myricetin 7-Hydroxy-4-methoxy- 5-methylchromen-2-one

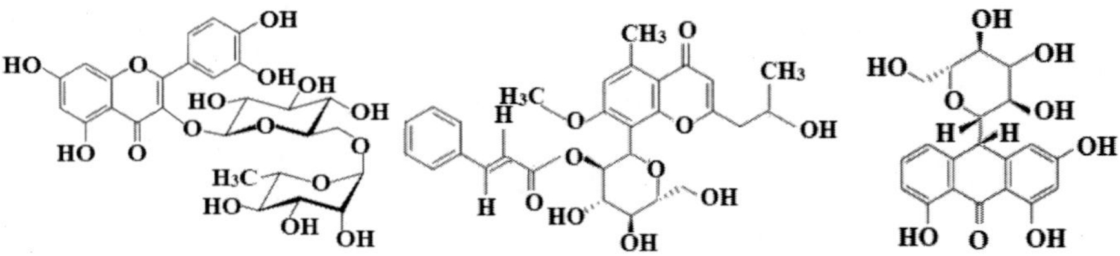

Rutin Methyl Aloesinyl cinnamate Barbaloin

Figure 4. Chemical Constituents and Structure.

Aloe for Diabetes Mellitus

Studies conducted by scientists have revealed that drinking *A. vera* juice can help decrease blood pressure and improve sugar levels, which are both symptoms of diabetes. Furthermore, there was a reduction in inflammation associated with acute hepatitis disease and wounds healed more rapidly (Alinejad-Mofrad et al., 2015b). There are many different types of acids, including acetic acid, citric acid, gallic acid, cinnamic acid, fumaric acid, lactic acid, vanillic acid, oxalic acid, vanillin, lactic acid, L-malic acid, isocitric acid, and isosorbide acid. This includes the acids 2,5-dihydro benzoic acid and salicylaldehyde. To name a few: 1- (2-dihydroxy-6-methyl- phenyl) (2,4-dihydroxy-6-methyl- phenyl) geranyloxyemodin; P-cresol; catechol; lectins; mannans; anthraquinones; '-2- (1-phenyl-1Hpyrazol-4-yl) ethan-1-one' (R) - 3- (4-Hydroxyphenyl) 2 (MeAc) -panoic acid, Geranyloxyemodin, Lectins, P-cresol, Catechol, and other phenolic compounds ethyl 2-oxo-3,4-dihydro chromene, 1,2,8-trihydroxy-6-methyl anthracene-9,10-dione, -3-carboxylate Many biological activities can be attributed to Figure-4 (Yongchaiyudha et al., 1996a). Aloe juice has become more popular and you may have seen it on the supermarket shelves. But what is exactly right? Is it also good for your health? Many inferred medicinal benefits that have been circulating in the Internet media, one of which is that it is beneficial for those with diabetes (Roger Williams et al., 2020). Here is a look at the research on the effects of aloe juice on glucose levels in diabetics. It is used in hot and arid locations such as the Mediterranean, Middle East, India, and Africa. Aloe is grown in Florida,

Texas, and Arizona in the United States. The plant is tasty and its leaves have an obvious gel that aids in water storage. You may be familiar with Aloe gel, which is often used to treat sunburn (Sharma et al., 2021). This comparable gel is used to make aloe juice. Squeezing or pressing an Aloe leaf extracts the gel, which is then sieved before being diluted with water to form a thick and sticky fluid. Organ damage from excessive glucose levels can occur if the condition is not managed. Today in the world, 382 million people suffer from diabetes, and most of them have type II. People with diabetes are more likely to try alternative treatments than those without the disease.

Aloe Vera in Type I and Type-II Diabetes

Your body's resistance to insulin is the underlying cause of diabetes (high blood sugar or glucose). The Mayo Clinic reports that diabetics are more likely to have heart failure or stroke, as well as damage to their nerves, poor circulation, the need for small repairs, impaired vision, and even infection (Chari et al., 2006). The Aloe plant has been used medicinally for thousands of years, both externally and internally, and there is some evidence that it may help reduce glucose levels. Your primary care provider (PCP) can tell you whether you are a good candidate to use Aloe to alleviate diabetes symptoms (Susana Oteng et al., 2019). Diabetes may take many forms, including the following. Patients with type I (also known as T1D) and type II diabetes (also known as T2D) have bodies that are unable to manufacture sufficient amounts of insulin and are thus wholly dependent on insulin injections. Type II diabetes, which affects mostly adults, is caused by cells' failure to use insulin.

Effects on Hyperglycemia

Long-term metabolic imbalances associated with diabetes mellitus can increase the probability of developing cardiovascular disease. Hyperglycemia manifests itself in increased urine, thirst, and appetite (Becheva and Kirkova-Bogdanova, 2022). Several studies have examined the effect of several plants on the reduction of blood sugar. *Trigonella foenum-graecum, Ipomoea batatas* (sweet potato), *Momordica carantia* (bitter gourd) and *Cinnamomum verum* (Almalki et al., 2019, Jung et al., 2006).

Several research initiatives have shown that some species of A. vera have anti-diabetic effects (Rashidi et al., 2013, Taghizadeh et al., 2016). This plant's blood glucose lowering method could be related to its involvement in increasing glucose metabolism or its antioxidant activity, which decreases peroxide and oxidative damage (Hashempur et al., 2015). Some of these processes will be examined in further detail in the sections that follow.

Antihyperglycemic Studies in Animals

The research found that A. vera had an antioxidant impact in lowering blood glucose. For four weeks, the mice received the following treatments: Streptozotocin alone (STZ), STZ plus *Withania somnifera* extract (20mg/kg), STZ plus *A. vera* extract (32 mg / kg) and STZ plus *W. somnifera* and *A. vera* extract together. Compared to the control group, diabetic mice had significantly higher plasma glucose levels (Rajasekaran et al., 2005).

In diabetic mice, researchers found oxidative damage to the cortex and hippocampi, in addition to severe impairment of motor and cognitive behavioralskills. Two alcoholic extracts were shown to be more effective than one in reducing plasma glucose levels. Furthermore, extracts may induce a significant decrease in oxidative damage to brain regions, which would then enhance poor motor and cognitive behavioural abilities (Parihar et al., 2004).

Blood sugar levels were not affected in nondiabetic rats given A. vera gel (10ml/kg) or leaf pulp (500mg/kg) by oral administration in a separate study (that is, the group with normal blood glucose levels) (Okyar et al., 2001).

Rajasekaran et al. (2004) gave rats 200 and 300mg/kg ofalcoholic aloe vera preparations for 21 days. Normal/fasted, oral glucose loaded and STZ-induced diabetic rats were grouped. Non-diabetic rats fasted. Normal and fasting rats' blood glucose levels of normal and fasting rats and glucose tolerance were influenced by different extracts. The glucose metabolism of STZ-induced diabetic rats was investigated using these extracts. The results showed that A. vera extracts can reduce blood glucose levels in high-glucose animals without harming control rats. (Rajasekaran et al., 2004).

The aloe vera gel produced lophenol (4,19-cyclolanostan-3-ol) and phytosterols of cycloartenol (9,19-cyclolanostan-3-ol). A. vera gel phytosterols have been studied for their anti-obesity and anti-diabetic effects. A study examined obese, type II diabetic Zucker diabetic fatty rats (ZDF). These rats received a 60% fat HFD. ZDF rats received 25 g kg-1 phytosterols daily for 44 days. (Misawa et al., 2008).

Phytosterols reduced random blood glucose, hyperglycemia, HbA1c, serum free fatty acid and TG levels, but not total cholesterol or abdominal fat tissue weight. Phytosterols can cure hyperlipidemia, hyperglycemia, obesity, and the development of visceral fat (Saito et al., 2012).

Another research gave ZDF rats lophenol and cycloartenol orally to test their behaviour. In addition to previous results, this study found that phytosterols might lower serum levels of monocyte chemotactic protein1 levels and liver gene expression levels of gluconeogenic enzymes (G-6-Pase and PEPCK), lipogenic enzymes (ACC and FAS) and SREBP1. They may increase blood adiponectin and liver glycolysis enzyme mRNA (like GK). The mentioned research also showed that the in the liver of ACO, CPT1, and PPAR expression increased. These findings show a change in genes for glucose and lipid metabolism. These phytosterols prevented and mitigated metabolic problems related to obesity and diabetes in rats. Obesity and diabetes cause metabolic problems. (Misawa et al., 2012b).

Another research examined how phytosterols affect peroxisome proliferator-activated receptors (PPAR). Fatp1, Acox1, Cpt1 and Hmgcs2 were up-regulated after 12 weeks, while ApoCIII was down-regulated. Compared to HFD controls. In rats, lophenol and cycloartenol could activate PPAR transcription. A quantitative gene expression investigation in diet-induced obese mice (DIO) demonstrated that phytosterols enhance liver fatty acid metabolism. (Misawa et al., 2012a).

Another study gave mice 55 mg/kg STZ daily to cause diabetes. After one week, individuals with blood glucose levels above 250 mg/dl were separated into three groups: 300 mg / kg of A. vera extract, 150 mg / kg, and 1 mg / kg of lisinopril. Renal glutathione increased in the first group after seven weeks. The extract of A. vera at 300 mg/kg may reduce oxidative stress, which contributes to diabetic nephropathy. A. vera extract had a greater impact on diabetes-induced nephropathy and renal oxidative stress than lisinopril. Another study gave mice 55 mg/kg STZ daily to cause diabetes. After one week, individuals with blood glucose levels above 250 mg/dl were separated into three groups: 300 mg / kg of A. vera extract, 150 mg / kg of, and 1 mg/kg lisinopril. Renal glutathione increased in the first group after seven weeks. A. vera extract at 300 mg / kg can reduce oxidative stress, which contributes to diabetic nephropathy. The extract of A. vera had a greater impact on diabetes-induced nephropathy and renal oxidative stress than lisinopril (Arora et al., 2019).

Clinical Studies

In a 2009 study, Yagi et al. investigated the impact of high molecular weight (AHM) fractions of A. vera L. on type II diabetes patients. AHM fractions were obtained by passing water through the gel part of A. vera. They looked at 15 people with type II diabetes whose blood sugar levels were not under control despite the use of oral antihyperglycemic drugs (nine men and six women) (metformin 500 mg and glibenclamide 5 mg; each twice daily). All patients received 0.05 grammes (two tablespoonfuls) of AHM three times a day for a period of 12 weeks, in addition to the diabetes drugs they were already taking. The levels of alanine aminotransferase, aspartate aminotransferase, and creatinine did not change, demonstrating that this drug is safe for the liver and kidneys to consume. Fasting blood glucose, triglyceride, and hemoglobin A1C levels were also reduced (El-Shemy et al., 2010).

According to the findings of the study, A. vera may reduce both blood glucose levels and the effects of glucose on diabetics through several different mechanisms. These mechanisms include a reduction in gluconeogenesis and lipogenesis in the liver, as well as an increase in glycolysis (Deora and Venkatraman, 2022b). Furthermore, A. vera has the ability to modify the expression of several genes that are involved in the metabolism of both glucose and lipids. Furthermore, PPAR transcription activity has been linked to the presence of A. vera. According to the research findings, two phytosterols that were extracted from aloe vera gel, namely lophenol and cycloartenol, play an important role in the anti-diabetic activities of the plant.

Oxidative stress has been linked to the development of several diabetes problems. One of the most essential anti-diabetic processes is the antioxidant properties of A. vera, which have been found in a variety of plant constituents (e.g., phenol, flavonoid, and vitamins C and E). Furthermore, A. vera has been shown that A. vera has anti-diabetic benefits in hyperglycemic patients (Tanaka et al., 2015).

However, this effect was not observed in circumstances where normal blood glucose levels were present. This provides evidence that the herb is antihyperglycemic rather than hypoglycemic in nature. Because hypoglycemia remains the most significant adverse effect of diabetic medications, the fact that A. vera does not affect normal blood glucose levels is an advantage, even though it is a drawback (Suksomboon et al., 2016). As a result, the beneficial benefits of A. vera on diabetes mellitus have been shown in several trials among individuals who also suffered from concurrent diseases such as obesity and hyperlipidemia (Table 2).

Table 2. Research on the clinical effectiveness of A. vera in the treatment of DM

Study type	Dose	Duration	Results	References
Animal studies (male rats)	200 and 300mg/kg orally	21 days	Levels of glucose in the blood (3 hours while taking A. vera with glucose)	(Rajasekaran et al., 2006)
Animal studies (Diabeticfatty rats aged: 6-w)	25μg/kg/day. For 44 consecutive days, daily one dose	6 weeks	MCP1 level ↑ Serum adiponectin level ↑ PPARα	(Saito et al., 2012)
Animal study (rats)	300mg/kg Aloe extract	7 weeks	↓Diabetic nephropathy	(Arora et al., 2019)
Double-blind placebo-	300mg A. vera leaf gel	2 months	↓ Fasting blood glucose,	(Huseini et al., 2012)
Double-blind studies (45 patients with metabolic disorders)	Capsule with 500 mg dose, two times in a day	8 weeks	↓Glucose levels, C-LDL, and ↓ TC	(Alinejad-Mofrad et al., 2015a)
Clinical trials (50 and 22	One tablespoonful of A. vera	At least 2weeks	↓ Blood sugar and ↓TG	(Yongchaiyudha et al., 1996b)
Clinical trials (30 subjects)	100-200mg of A. vera gel powder	12 weeks	↓ Levels of FBG, PPG,	(Choudhary et al., 2014)
Clinical trials-T2DM	Two tablespoonfuls (0.05gr)	12 weeks	↓ FBG, HbA1C and TG	(El-Shemy et al., 2010)
RCT- (136 obese patients with prediabetic orearly diabetic patients)	Capsule with 147mg A. vera gel	8 weeks	↓ FBS, and ↑insulin levels	(Choi et al., 2013)

Discussion

The growing prevalence of type 1 diabetes in the world might be due to several factors. The accelerator and cell stress hypotheses suggest that several nonspecific environmental factors, such as obesity, rapid growth, infections, dietary deficiencies, or psychological stress, can cause pancreatic cells to become exhausted and fail, eventually failing due to secondary autoimmune destruction. There was a considerable gap in these models where a plausible biological mechanism linking cell stress and autoimmunity was lacking. Recent discoveries of HIPs suggest that there may be a causal link between the two. Fatigued cells are believed to be the source of peptides, which can act as powerful neoantigens in a susceptible host and trigger cell-specific autoimmunity. This idea is similar to what happens in the development of celiac disease, where immune-dominant peptides also undergo post-translational modifications. However, HIPs are the remnants of insulin and other cellular hormone breakdown, and therefore are real neo autoantigens, while these peptides are produced from hundreds of proteins present in wheat, rye, barley and oats (gliadins, glutenins, hordein, scaling, and avenins).

It is believed that Aloe species have a better level of physiological activity (World Health Organisation, 1999). Among the more than 75 bioactive chemicals discovered so far include vitamins, minerals, carbohydrates, amino acids, anthraquinones, enzymes, lignin, saponins, and salicylic acid. Researchers believe that anthraquinones, and especially barbaloin, handle the bitter taste and laxative effect of the exudate formed by the leaves. Barbaloin, a polyphenol antioxidant, has been associated with free radical-mediated cytotoxicity and lipid peroxidation. Carotenoids, steroids, terpenes, and phytosterols have been linked to a role in fragrance and colour. The gel of aloe vera plants holds a variety of polysaccharides, including acetyl mannan. Plants have a wide range of biologically active chemicals that can have a wide variety of impacts on living things. Is it true? In a number of respects, yes. Vera's antitumor, antiarthritic, antirheumatic, anticancer, and anti-diabetic properties are only a few of its many medical benefits. A. vera has been used to treat a variety of conditions, including constipation, gastrointestinal problems, and deficiencies in the immune system deficits.

Aloe has been used for millennia as a traditional medicine in many regions of the world, including Latin America and the Arabian Peninsula, for the treatment and control of diabetes (DM). Aloe may help to lower chronic hyperglycemia and blood lipids, prevent diabetes, and prevent cardiovascular problems, according to studies conducted in both humans and animals. There are several potential explanations for why aloe can help diabetics. One is that aloe extract is rich in antioxidants. Aloe's antioxidant capabilities, such as its ability to inhibit free radical generation and increase cellular thiol status, are well established. In addition, its ability to boost glutathione S-transferase activity has been shown. Scientists discovered that the antioxidant abilities of aloe reduced serum MDA levels and increased GSH and SOD levels. Damage to pancreatic beta cells has recently been studied in relation to oxidative stress. Therefore, while oxidative stress plays a role in the development of diabetes, antioxidants such as aloe can have a true antidiabetic influence due to their antioxidant abilities. Consuming 100 grammes of Aloe Vera gel and 20 grammes of psyllium husk daily has been shown to reduce both blood sugar and cholesterol levels. All study subjects were between the ages of 35 and 65, and all had atherosclerotic heart disease. Diabetics in this category include those whose fasting blood sugars are within the normal range and another 177 patients who, after two months of treatment, demonstrated the need to discontinue all oral hypoglycemic medications. Independent studies have also been conducted on the effects of aloc vera gel on blood glucose and lipid indicators in diabetics. Seventy-two type 2 diabetic women participated in the study and half of them received a tablespoon of Aloe gel twice a week for six weeks, while the other half received a placebo. Neither serum triglycerides nor blood glucose levels increased, but serum triglycerides and blood glucose levels decreased significantly.

In the second study, patients received glibenclamide and aloe gel or placebo. Serum triglyceride and blood glucose levels were found to be significantly lower in the aloe group. Another case study showed that aloe latex could cause a decrease in blood glucose levels among fasting subjects. Additionally, 60 hyperlipidemic individuals had significant reductions in blood levels of low-density lipoproteins of total cholesterol, triglycerides, and low-density lipoprotein levels after consuming whole leaf Aloe extract for 12 weeks. Therefore, Aloe has a substantial beneficial impact on matters related to diabetes and cardiovascular disease, as shown by early findings of clinical investigations. Numerous studies of the Aloe formulation have been conducted in animal models, with mixed results on hyperglycemia and blood lipids. Two different types of animal tests were conducted. For starters, Aloe latex was administered to mice with alloxan-induced diabetes, and then Aloe gel was administered to rats with streptozotocin-induced diabetes (STZ). Aloe gel, however, has been shown to increase glucose levels in tetraoxane-induced diabetic rats. The anti-diabetic efficacy of processed Aloe gel was also examined in diet-induced obesity (DIO) mice, an animal model with metabolic abnormalities similar to non-insulin-dependent human diabetes, including hyperglycemia, obesity, and insulin resistance. Plasma insulin levels, along with cholesterol, triglyceride, and free fatty acid concentrations, have been shown to be lowered by Aloe gel extract in STZ-induced diabetic rats.

Conclusion

Although diabetes has become a serious public health problem around the world, the situation is especially severe in low- and middle-income countries like India, where the burden has grown dramatically in recent decades and is expected to expand much more quickly in the coming decades. As a result, this has the potential to significantly affect healthcare care costs and death rates among people with diabetes in India. Primary diabetes prevention in prediabetes individuals, early diabetes diagnosis, screening for complications, and providing appropriate medication at all levels of care for those who already have diabetes will play a role in reducing the prevalence of diabetes and its associated consequences.

The plant and its components, such as emodin and phytosterols, may be useful in the treatment of metabolic syndrome in a number of different ways. One effect of these pathways is an increase in glucose metabolism, whereas another is a decrease in oxidative stress-induced damage. Oral administration of A. vera reduces glucose levels in both people and diabetic rats by improving glycoprotein metabolism. Although the exact mechanism of A is unknown, studies are possible to control insulin release from beta pancreatic cells. It has not been determined how vera achieves its anti-diabetic effects. Phytosterols in this plant improve blood lipid profile, glucose tolerance, and glycated hemoglobin (HbA1c) levels. There has been consistent confirmation of these findings in clinical investigations.

References

Alinejad-Mofrad, S., Foadoddini, M., Saadatjoo, S. A., and Shayesteh, M. (2015). Improvement of glucose and lipid profile status with Aloe vera in pre-diabetic subjects: a randomized controlled-trial. *Journal of diabetes & metabolic disorders*, 14, pp. 1-7.

Alinejad-Mofrad, S., Foadoddini, M., Saadatjoo, S. A., and Shayesteh, M. (2015). Improvement of glucose and lipid profile status with Aloe vera in pre-diabetic subjects: a randomized controlled-trial. *Journal of diabetes & metabolic disorders*, 14, pp. 1-7.

Almalki, D. A., Alghamdi, S. A., and Al-Attar, A. M. (2019). Comparative study on the influence of some medicinal plants on diabetes induced by streptozotocin in male rats. *Biomed Research International*, 2019.

Amiel, S. A., Sherwin, R. S., Simonson, D. C., Lauritano, A. A., and Tamborlane, W. V. (1986). Impaired insulin action in puberty. *New England Journal of Medicine*, 315(4), pp. 215-219.

Amin, R., Thalluri, C., Docea, A. O., Sharifi-Rad, J., and Calina, D. (2022). Therapeutic potential of cranberry for kidney health and diseases. *eFood*, 3(5), p. e33.

Arora, M. K., Sarup, Y., Tomar, R., Singh, M., and Kumar, P. (2019). Amelioration of diabetes-induced diabetic nephropathy by Aloe vera: Implication of oxidative stress and hyperlipidemia. *Journal of dietary supplements*, 16(2), pp. 227-244.

Becheva, M. S. V., and Kirkova-Bogdanova, A. G. (2022). Prophylactics of Type 2 Diabetes and Diabetic Foot. *Iranian Journal of Public Health*, 51(10), p. 2370.

Chari, S. T., Smyrk, T. C., Levy, M. J., Topazian, M. D., Takahashi, N., Zhang, L., Clain, J. E., Pearson, R. K., Petersen, B. T., Vege, S. S., and Farnell, M. B. (2006). Diagnosis of autoimmune pancreatitis: the Mayo Clinic experience. *Clinical Gastroenterology and Hepatology*, 4(8), pp. 1010-1016.

Chaudhury, A., Duvoor, C., Reddy Dendi, V. S., Kraleti, S., Chada, A., Ravilla, R., Marco, A., Shekhawat, N. S., Montales, M. T., Kuriakose, K., and Sasapu, A. (2017). Clinical review of antidiabetic drugs: implications for type 2 diabetes mellitus management. *Frontiers in endocrinology*, 8, p. 6.

Chawla, A., Chawla, R., and Jaggi, S. (2016). Microvasular and macrovascular complications in diabetes mellitus: distinct or continuum? *Indian journal of endocrinology and metabolism*, 20(4), p. 546.

Chiang, J. L., Maahs, D. M., Garvey, K. C., Hood, K. K., Laffel, L. M., Weinzimer, S. A., Wolfsdorf, J. I., and Schatz, D. (2018). Type 1 diabetes in children and adolescents: a position statement by the American Diabetes Association. *Diabetes care*, 41(9), pp. 2026-2044.

Choi, H. C., Kim, S. J., Son, K. Y., Oh, B. J., and Cho, B. L. (2013). Metabolic effects of aloe vera gel complex in obese prediabetes and early non-treated diabetic patients: Randomized controlled trial. *Nutrition*, 29(9), pp. 1110-1114.

Choudhary, M., Kochhar, A., and Sangha, J. (2014). Hypoglycemic and hypolipidemic effect of Aloe vera L. in non-insulin dependent diabetics. *Journal of food science and technology*, 51, pp. 90-96.

Dall, T. M., Yang, W., Halder, P., Pang, B., Massoudi, M., Wintfeld, N., Semilla, A. P., Franz, J., and Hogan, P. F. (2014). The economic burden of elevated blood glucose levels in 2012: diagnosed and undiagnosed diabetes, gestational diabetes mellitus, and prediabetes. *Diabetes care*, 37(12), pp. 3172-3179.

Deora, N., and Venkatraman, K. (2022). Aloe vera in diabetic dyslipidemia: Improving blood glucose and lipoprotein levels in pre-clinical and clinical studies. *Journal of Ayurveda and Integrative Medicine*, 13(4), p. 100675.

Deora, N., and Venkatraman, K. (2022). Aloe vera in diabetic dyslipidemia: Improving blood glucose and lipoprotein levels in pre-clinical and clinical studies. *Journal of Ayurveda and Integrative Medicine*, 13(4), p. 100675.

Deshpande, A. D., Harris-Hayes, M., and Schootman, M. (2008). Epidemiology of diabetes and diabetes-related complications. *Physical therapy*, 88(11), pp. 1254-1264.

El-Shemy, H. A., Aboul-Soud, M. A. M., Nassr-Allah, A. A., Aboul-Enein, K. M., Kabash, A., and Yagi, A. (2010). Antitumor properties and modulation of antioxidant enzymes' activity by Aloe vera leaf active principles isolated via supercritical carbon dioxide extraction. *Current medicinal chemistry*, 17(2), pp. 129-138.

Garcia-Compean, D., Jaquez-Quintana, J. O., Gonzalez-Gonzalez, J. A. and Maldonado-Garza, H. (2009). Liver cirrhosis and diabetes: risk factors, pathophysiology, clinical implications and management. *World journal of gastroenterology: WJG*, 15(3), p. 280.

Giacco, F., and Brownlee, M. (2010). Oxidative stress and diabetic complications. *Circulation research*, 107(9), pp. 1058-1070.

Habtemariam, S. (2017). Could we really use aloe vera food supplements to treat diabetes? Quality control issues. *Evidence-Based Complementary and Alternative Medicine*, 2017.

Haddad, M., Knani, I., Bouzidi, H., Berriche, O., Hammami, M., and Kerkeni, M. (2016). Plasma levels of pentosidine, carboxymethyl-lysine, soluble receptor for advanced glycation end products, and metabolic syndrome: the metformin effect. *Disease markers*, 2016.

Haghani, F., Arabnezhad, M. R., Mohammadi, S., and Ghaffarian-Bahraman, A. (2022). Aloe vera and streptozotocin-induced diabetes mellitus. *Revista Brasileira de Farmacognosia*, 32(2), pp. 174-187.

Hashempur, M. H., Heydari, M., Mosavat, S. H., Heydari, S. T., and Shams, M. (2015). Complementary and alternative medicine use in Iranian patients with diabetes mellitus. *Journal of integrative medicine*, 13(5), pp. 319-325.

Huseini, H. F., Kianbakht, S., Hajiaghaee, R., and Dabaghian, F. H. (2011). Anti-hyperglycemic and anti-hypercholesterolemic effects of Aloe vera leaf gel in hyperlipidemic type 2 diabetic patients: a randomized double-blind placebo-controlled clinical trial. *Planta medica*, pp. 311-316.

Joglekar, M. M., Bavkar, L. N., Sistla, S., and Arvindekar, A. U. (2017). Effective inhibition of protein glycation by combinatorial usage of limonene and aminoguanidine through differential and synergistic mechanisms. *International Journal of Biological Macromolecules*, 99, pp. 563-569.

Jung, M., Park, M., Lee, H. C., Kang, Y. H., Kang, E. S., and Kim, S. (2006). Antidiabetic agents from medicinal plants. *Current medicinal chemistry*, 13(10), pp. 1203-1218.

Kooti, W., Farokhipour, M., Asadzadeh, Z., Ashtary-Larky, D., and Asadi-Samani, M. (2016). The role of medicinal plants in the treatment of diabetes: a systematic review. *Electronic physician*, 8(1), p. 1832.

Misawa, E., Tanaka, M., Nabeshima, K., Nomaguchi, K., Yamada, M., Toida, T., and Iwatsuki, K. (2012). Administration of dried Aloe vera gel powder reduced body fat mass in diet-induced obesity (DIO) rats. *Journal of nutritional science and vitaminology*, 58(3), pp. 195-201.

Misawa, E., Tanaka, M., Nomaguchi, K., Nabeshima, K., Yamada, M., Toida, T., and Iwatsuki, K. (2012). Oral ingestion of Aloe vera phytosterols alters hepatic gene expression profiles and ameliorates obesity-associated metabolic disorders in Zucker diabetic fatty rats. *Journal of agricultural and food chemistry*, 60(11), pp. 2799-2806.

Misawa, E., Tanaka, M., Nomaguchi, K., Yamada, M., Toida, T., Takase, M., Iwatsuki, K., and Kawada, T. (2008). Administration of phytosterols isolated from Aloe vera gel reduce visceral fat mass and improve hyperglycemia in Zucker diabetic fatty (ZDF) rats. *Obesity research & clinical practice*, 2(4), pp. 239-245.

Morris, A. D., Boyle, D. I., McMahon, A. D., Greene, S. A., MacDonald, T. M., and Newton, R. W. (1997). Adherence to insulin treatment, glycaemic control, and ketoacidosis in insulin-dependent diabetes mellitus. *The Lancet*, 350(9090), pp. 1505-1510.

Mintah, S. O., Asafo-Agyei, T., Archer, M. A., Junior, P. A. A., Boamah, D., Kumadoh, D., Appiah, A., Ocloo, A., Boakye, Y. D., and Agyare, C. (2019). Medicinal plants for treatment of prevalent diseases. *Pharmacognosy-Medicinal Plants*, pp. 1-19.

Nathan, D. M., Buse, J. B., Davidson, M. B., Ferrannini, E., Holman, R. R., Sherwin, R., and Zinman, B. (2009). Medical management of hyperglycemia in type 2 diabetes: a consensus algorithm for the initiation and adjustment of therapy: a consensus statement of the American Diabetes Association and the European Association for the Study of Diabetes. *Diabetes care*, 32(1), pp. 193-203.

Okyar, A., Can, A., Akev, N., Baktir, G., and Sütlüpinar, N. (2001). Effect of Aloe vera leaves on blood glucose level in type I and type II diabetic rat models. *Phytotherapy Research*, 15(2), pp. 157-161.

Parihar, M. S., Chaudhary, M., Shetty, R., and Hemnani, T. (2004). Susceptibility of hippocampus and cerebral cortex to oxidative damage in streptozotocin treated mice: prevention by extracts of Withania somnifera and Aloe vera. *Journal of clinical neuroscience*, 11(4), pp. 397-402.

Rajasekaran, S., Ravi, K., Sivagnanam, K., and Subramanian, S. (2006). Beneficial effects of Aloe vera leaf gel extract on lipid profile status in rats with streptozotocin diabetes. *Clinical and experimental pharmacology and physiology*, 33(3), pp. 232-237.

Rajasekaran, S., Sivagnanam, K., Ravi, K., and Subramanian, S. (2004). Hypoglycemic effect of Aloe vera gel on streptozotocin-induced diabetes in experimental rats. *Journal of Medicinal food*, 7(1), pp. 61-66.

Rajasekaran, S., Sivagnanam, K., and Subramanian, S. (2005). Antioxidant effect of Aloe vera gel extract in streptozotocin-induced diabetes in rats. *Pharmacol Rep*, 57(1), pp. 90-96.

Rashidi, A. A., Mirhashemi, S. M., Taghizadeh, M., and Sarkhail, P. (2013). Iranian medicinal plants for diabetes mellitus: a systematic review. *Pakistan journal of biological sciences: PJBS*, 16(9), pp. 401-411.

Roger Williams, M. D., Taylor-Robinson, S. D., and Lim, A. K. (2020). The Effect of Aloe Vera Juice on Liver Enzymes and Hepatic Structure in a Healthy Population. *Integrative Medicine*, 19(3), pp. 30-34.

Saito, M., Tanaka, M., Misawa, E., Yamada, M., Yamauchi, K., and Iwatsuki, K. (2012). Aloe vera gel extract attenuates ethanol-induced hepatic lipid accumulation by suppressing the expression of lipogenic genes in mice. *Bioscience, biotechnology, and biochemistry*, 76(11), pp. 2049-2054.

Sánchez, M., González-Burgos, E., Iglesias, I., and Gómez-Serranillos, M. P. (2020). Pharmacological update properties of Aloe vera and its major active constituents. *Molecules*, 25(6), p. 1324.

Sharma, C., Kaur, A., Thind, S. S., Singh, B., and Raina, S. (2015). Advanced glycation End-products (AGEs): an emerging concern for processed food industries. *Journal of food science and technology*, 52, pp. 7561-7576.

Sharma, M. K., Chauhan, J., Kumar, M., Joshi, C. K., Sharma, S., and Lai, C. (2021). Prospects of Aloe vera and its Bioactive Compounds in Diabetes: Critical Review. *Journal of Pure and Applied Microbiology*, 15(4), pp. 1781-1798.

Shrivastava, S. R., Shrivastava, P. S., and Ramasamy, J. (2013). Role of self-care in management of diabetes mellitus. *Journal of diabetes & Metabolic disorders*, 12(1), pp. 1-5.

Singh, V. P., Bali, A., Singh, N., and Jaggi, A. S. (2014). Advanced glycation end products and diabetic complications. *The Korean journal of physiology & pharmacology: official journal of the Korean Physiological Society and the Korean Society of Pharmacology*, 18(1), p. 1.

Suksomboon, N., Poolsup, N., and Punthanitisarn, S. (2016). Effect of Aloe vera on glycaemic control in prediabetes and type 2 diabetes: a systematic review and meta-analysis. *Journal of clinical pharmacy and therapeutics*, 41(2), pp. 180-188.

Svoren, B. M., Volkening, L. K., Butler, D. A., Moreland, E. C., Anderson, B. J., and Laffel, L. M. (2007). Temporal trends in the treatment of pediatric type 1 diabetes and impact on acute outcomes. *The Journal of pediatrics*, 150(3), pp. 279-285.

Taghizadeh, M., Rashidi, A. A., Taherian, A. A., Vakili, Z., Sajad Sajadian, M., and Ghardashi, M. (2016). Antidiabetic and antihyperlipidemic effects of ethanol extract of Rosa canina L. fruit on diabetic rats: An experimental study with histopathological evaluations. *Journal of evidence-based complementary & alternative medicine*, 21(4), pp. NP25-NP30.

Tanaka, M., Misawa, E., Yamauchi, K., Abe, F., and Ishizaki, C. (2015). Effects of plant sterols derived from Aloe vera gel on human dermal fibroblasts *in vitro* and on skin condition in Japanese women. *Clinical, cosmetic and investigational dermatology*, pp. 95-104.

Vlassara, H., and Uribarri, J. (2014). Advanced glycation end products (AGE) and diabetes: cause, effect, or both? *Current diabetes reports*, 4, pp. 1-10.

Yongchaiyudha, S., Rungpitarangsi, V., Bunyapraphatsara, N., and Chokechaijaroenporn, O. (1996). Antidiabetic activity of Aloe vera L. juice. I. Clinical trial in new cases of diabetes mellitus. *Phytomedicine*, (3), pp. 241-243.

Chapter 7

Momordica Charantia in Anti-Diabetics: Past, Present and Future

Mohsina Patwekar and Faheem Patwekar*

Luqman College of Pharmacy, Gulbarga, Karnataka, India

Abstract

One of the first known human diseases is diabetes mellitus. DM is one of the most prevalent diseases in both developed and developing countries. The most well-known endocrine disorder, diabetes mellitus, affects hundreds of millions of people around the world and results in more than 1 million deaths each year. Type 1 and type 2 DM are the two subtypes of the disease. When insulin-producing cells are damaged and unable to produce insulin, type 1 diabetes occurs. When the insulin administered is ineffective, type 2 diabetes develops. One of the main functions of the human body is to promote glucose uptake of glucose into cells, where it is used to produce energy. Insulin is a key metabolic hormone that has a variety of other functions. The endocrine pancreas does not create enough insulin, or insulin does not work properly due to which patients have excessive blood glucose levels, which are excreted in urine. The creation of effective and secure anti- diabetic medications continues to be a major issue for contemporary scientific study. Plants and herbal remedies have been used as medicine for centuries. Since ancient times, its fruit has been consumed as a vegetable and is used in folk medicine to cure diabetes mellitus. *Momordica charantia* has been used for a very long time as a food and as a hypoglycemic agent. Up to a third of people with DM are believed to use alternative therapies to lower blood glucose levels. *Momordica charantia* is one plant that has attracted the most attention for its ability to treat diabetes. *Momordica charantia*, a plant native to tropical and subtropical areas of the world and belonging to the *Cucurbitaceae* family, is widely cultivated. There are parts of the *M.*

* Corresponding Author's Email: faheem_ip@rediffmail.com.

charantia extract that structurally resemble animal insulin. The fruits of this medicinal plant contain Charantia, a natural steroidal glycoside that has been shown to have a potential hypoglycemic action. The phytochemical composition and anti- diabetic action of *M. charantia* are discussed in this review.

Keywords *Momordica charantia*, diabetes, past, present

Introduction

One of the oldest human diseases, diabetes mellitus (DM) affects approximately 200 million people worldwide in 2011 (Amos AF et al., 2010). According to WHO data from 2016,422 million people had diabetes in 2014, and the prevalence has increased since 1980 (World Health Organisation 2016). Diabetes increases the risk of developing blindness by 25 times, renal failure by 20 times, gangrene-related amputation 20 times, coronary heart disease by 2 to 6 times, and ischemic brain damage by 2 to 6 times in diabetics. (Wolf SP, 1993) According to the International Diabetics Federation, by 2030, 80% of diabetics worldwide would live in low- and middle-income countries. Diabetics is a chronic metabolic disorder that affects how carbohydrates are metabolised. It can be caused by a complete insulin deficiency (insulin-dependent diabetes mellitus), a reduction in insulin production, or an increase in insulin production combined with resistance (non- insulin-dependent diabetes mellitus). Because fat cells cannot proliferate, function as mitochondria and burn fat, fat accumulation develops in skeletal muscle and the liver, resulting in the insulin resistance linked to obesity. (Heilbornn L et al., 2004) Type 1 diabetes Immune-mediated cell death that is typically followed with total lack of insulin – type 2 diabetes – a gradual decline in insulin release from cells gestational diabetes, and specialised forms of diabetes are the four main types of diabetes. (American Diabetes Association 2018). The main benefits of herbal medications appear to be their affordability, effectiveness, and low frequency of side effects. More than 80% of the world's population, according to the WHO, rely on traditional herbal therapy for their primary health care.

Around the world, a wide variety of plants have been utilised to cure diabetes. In fact, this may be the only available treatment option available for the treatment of patients with diabetes in many regions of the world, especially in developing countries. (Garau et al., 2003) According to botanical research of conventional natural remedies, 1200 species have been used to diagnose and cure hyperglycemia. One of the medicinal plants with hypoglycemic activity that has received extensive research is M. charantia (Figure 1) (family: Cucurbitaceae). It is a climber that is frequently raised for food in South America, Africa, and Asia. It is also grown to a height of 1500 metres in all of India. (Desai and Tatke, 2015). In these studies, different components of M. charantia, including seed, fruit and even the entire plant, were used (Table 1) (Thakur et al., 2010). Knowing the active compounds that have been identified from numerous plant types, the alternative medical system is currently gaining speed. (Baby and Jini, 2011). The development of MC research has led to the identification of a wide range of phytochemicals, including steroids, proteins, vitamins, minerals, flavonoids, and ascorbic acid (Jia et al., 2017). In addition, other biological properties have been confirmed, including antioxidant, hypoglycemic, anticancer, and antibacterial properties. (Nagarani et al., 2014)

Taxonomy

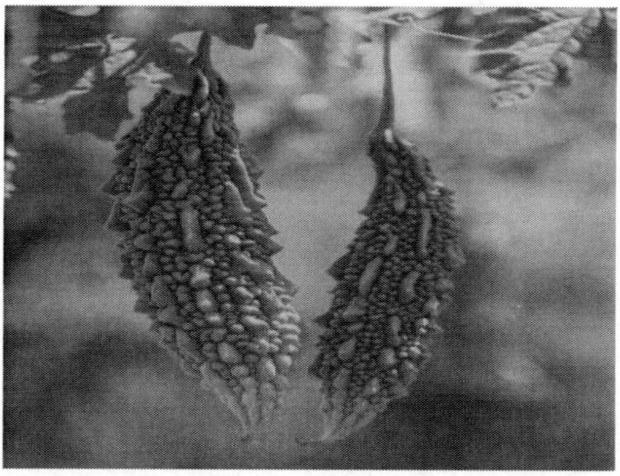

Figure 1. Momordica charantia.

Momordica Charantia (Bitter Gourd)

It is a thin, branching, angled and grooved annual climber that can reach a height of 5 m. The tendrils are simple and thin. Simple, mostly 5-7 lobed leaves with one or two branches on the tendrils. It has simple alternating leaves with 3-7 deeply spaced lobes that are 4-12 cm in diameter. When the fruit is immature, it is light green; as it ripens, it turns orange -yellow. Fruit: cylindrical, spheroid or spindle shaped; typically, warty or ridged; irregularly dehisces into a fleshy capsule with three valves or is indehiscent. The compacted brown seeds are covered with a brilliant red pulp. Male and female flowers are produced separately by each plant. Flowers: Staminate flowers are typically solitary on a bracteate scape, a calyx with five lobed petals which are usually yellow in colour, anthers dissimilar or systematic, with two being dithecal and the other being monothecal, as well as cells that are bent or flexible. It has a distinctive smell and bitter taste. (Singh et al., 1998).

History and Classification of MC

Momordica charantia is used mainly as another treatment for diabetes. The plant thrives in tropical climates and belongs to the Cucurbitaceae family. The bitter melon fruit is cylindrical and light green, resembling a cucumber, and is produced on a vine with green leaves and yellow blooms. Bitter melon extract, often known as vegetable insulin, has a long history of use in America, Asia, and Africa as a hypoglycemic agent. Evidence from in vitro, animal, and various shoddy doses of human research points to the slight hypoglycemic impact of bitter melon and certain of its raw extract. (Joseph and Jini, 2013). Chinese and Ayurvedic physicians have been using M. charantia, often known as bitter melon, as traditional herbal medication for the initial stages of diabetes and high blood glucose levels since ancient times. (Leung et al., 2009). Over the past 70 years, studies demonstrating the effectiveness of bitter gourd in decreasing blood glucose have appeared irregularly in the literature. Since the early 1900s, bitter gourd has been used regularly to treat diabetes and high blood glucose in the Dominican Republic, Puerto Rico, and Cuba. (Joseph and Jini, 2013). Bitter gourd, often known as karela, is said to effectively decrease blood sugar levels in Britain, according to immigrant herbalists. Bitter gourd has been used for a very long time in various traditional Asian medical systems. Bitter gourds are traditionally believed to improve digestion, which can be beneficial for humans with dyspepsia, constipation, and slow digestion. However, it can occasionally aggravate heartburn and ulcers. (Teoh et al., 2010). Ayurveda, an Indian medical system, claims that bitter gourd induces pitta, reduces kuph and vatta and regulates jaundice blood impurities, and fever. In addition, this vegetable is helpful for treating liver conditions, skin condition and other cold symptoms. Diabetes and dysentery are managed in Mexico using the entire plant. The leaf or areal parts are used in Peruvian herbal medicine to cure inflammation of many types, malaria and measles. (Ahmad et al., 2012) In particular, M. charantia is used as a traditional remedy for the treatment of diabetes. Studies have revealed that it includes an ingredient known as 'plant insulin', which has been proved to be quite helpful in reducing blood and urine and blood glucose levels.

Classification of MC

Scientific name: Momordica charantia
Kingdom: Plantae
Division: Magnoliophyte
Family: Cucurbitaceae
Genus: Momordica
Species: Charantia
Duration: Annual
Class: Magnoliopsida

Charantin

The chemical charantin is a combination of stigmasteryl glucoside (Figure 2) and sitosteryl glucoside (Figure 3). Charantin may be used to treat diabetes and may eventually be used in place of other medications. Charantin, a cucurbitane-type triterpinoids characteristic found in M. charantia, may have an anti-diabetic effect. (Desai and Tatke, 2015). According to studies, the substance is superior to the oral hypoglycemic drug tolbutamide in terms of effectiveness. (Pitipanapong et al., 2007) Charantin is made up of a combination of sitosterol beta-d-glucose and 5,25-stigmedin-3beta-glycoside. It has blood sugar-lowering abilities comparable to those of insulin. Charantin is soluble in ether (Yuwai et al., 1991). It is a tasteless and neutral compound, and one of the bioactive compounds, charantin, is found within every plant sector, but is most common in fruits. Charantin lowers blood sugar levels by increasing glycogen production and glucose uptake in fat cells, liver and muscles. In addition, it helps insulin- secreting beta cells repair themselves or create new ones by promoting pancreatic beta cells' production of insulin. Charantin's alcoholic extract was discovered to be a more potent anti-diabetic drug than tolbutamide, which is occasionally used to treat diabetes (Wang et al., 2014).

Table 1. Chemical constituents of *Momordica charantia*

Parts	Structure	Chemical constituents
Plant body	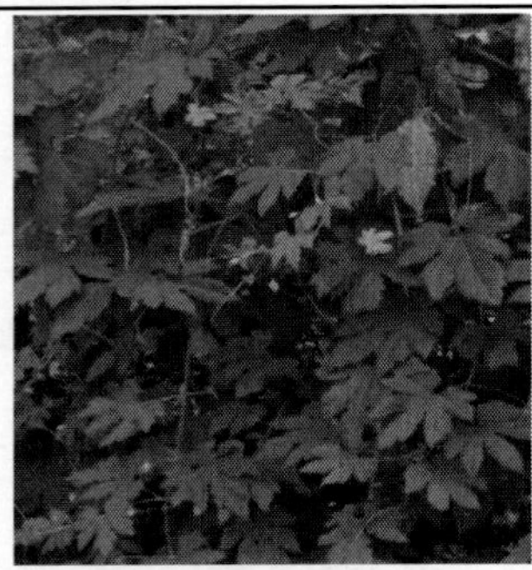	Momordenol, momordicins, momordolol, momorcharins, charantin, charine, cryptoxanthin, cucurbetacins, cucurbitanes, cycloartenols, diosgenin, galacturonic acids, goyaglycosides, goyasaponins, (26-31) The stem and fruit of *M. charantia* are classified as cucurbitane-type triterpinoids and are included in this group. (32, 33)
Seed	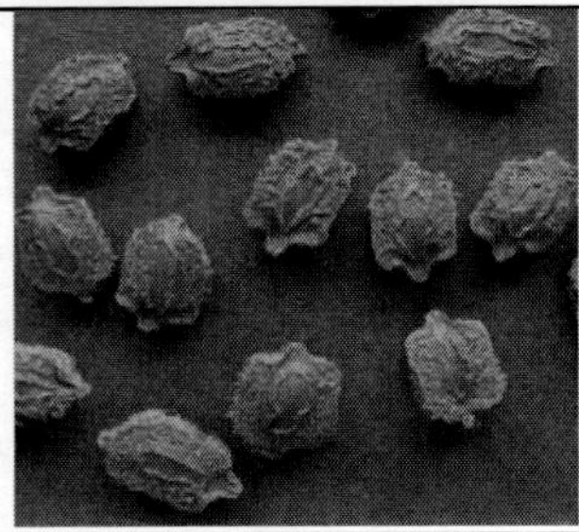	Seeds contain some fatty acids such as myristic, lauric, palmitic, stearic, oleic, linolenic acids and amino acids such as valine, threonine methionine, isoleucine, leucine, phenylalanine, and glutamic acid. Enzyme- Urease

Parts	Structure	Chemical constituents
Fruit	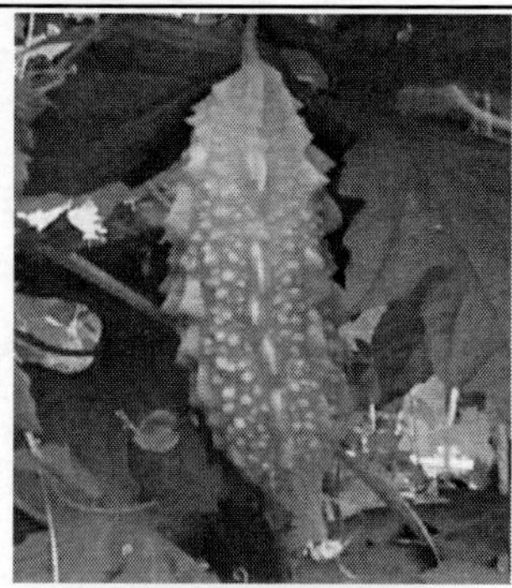	Serine, aspartic acid, threonine, glutamic acid, alanine, pipecolic acid, luteolin are the amino acids present in the fruit of *M. charantia*. Alkaloids, Glycosides, saponins, reducing sugar, resins, phenolic components, fixed oil, steroidmomordicine, protein (polypeptide-p), charantin, ascorbigen, and free acid are all present in the fruit of bitter gourd (Yuwai et al., 1991)
Leaves	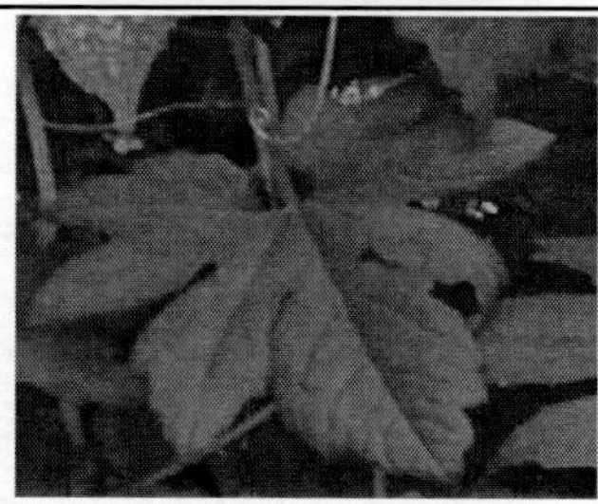	The leaves and the fruit are excellent sources of the vitamin B, as well as magnesium, calcium, phosphorus potassium, and iron which are all nutrients found in the leaves. (Yuwai, et al., 1991)

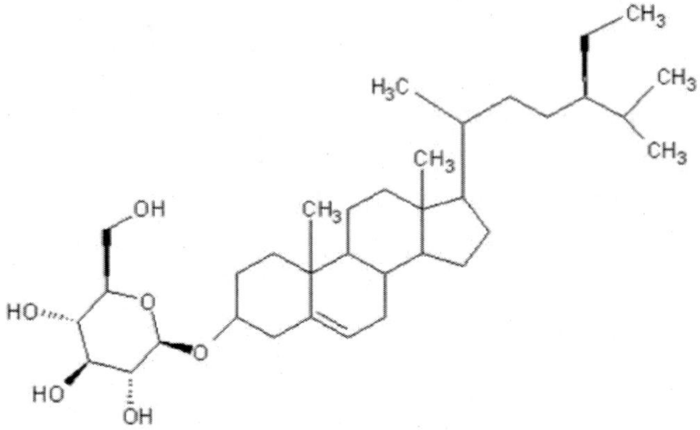

Figure 2. Chemical structure of stigmasteryl glucoside.

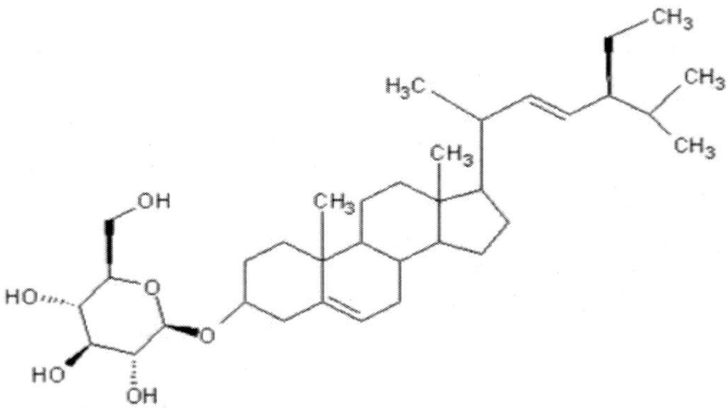

Figure 3. Chemical structure of sitosteryl glucoside.

Polypeptide-p

When M. charantia extract is administered subcutaneously, hypoglycemic protein polypeptide-p, also known as p- insulin, has been found to decrease blood glucose levels in gerbils, langurs, and people. One of the most popular vegetables that naturally control diabetes and include the polypeptide p is bitter melon (Tian, M. et al., 2015). Because p-insulin copies the function of human insulin, it can be used to substitute animal- based insulin in people with type 1 diabetes (Arif et al., 2021).

Other Components

As a result of the binding of two insulin receptors, bitter gourd lectin exhibits an insulin-like action. When operating in ancillary tissues and, like the effects in the brain, decreasing appetite, this lectin reduces blood glucose levels. Lectin is possibly an important factor in the hypoglycemic response that follows the consumption of bitter gourd and may help with the treatment of adult- onset diabetes (Krawinkel and Keding, 2006).

The other significant substance that has been identified in bitter melon seeds is vicine, a glycol alkaloid (Krawinkel and Keding, 2006). When administered intraperitoneally to non- diabetic fasting rats, this pyrimidine nucleoside has been shown to cause hypoglycemia.

Three cucurbitane triterpinoids were studied and found to considerably decrease blood sugar levels in diabetic mice. The structure of two more key compounds that were also investigated and found to be the same were also discovered (Raman and Lau, 1996).

One of the key bioactive compounds of M. charantia is polysaccharides. Polysaccharides of the M. charantia fruit have been shown to have a range of bioactive properties, including anti-inflammatory, immune stimulating, neuroprotective, anti-tumour, and antimicrobial. (Quazi et al., 2022)

Mechanism of the Anti-Diabetic Effect of MC

Momordica charantia is currently one of the most beneficial herbs for the treatment of diabetes, its traditional use is confirmed by contemporary scientific proof of its positive effect. (49, 50) A study of traditional applications of M. charantia in India showed that it is one of the most important plants for decreasing blood sugar glucose levels in diabetic individuals. (Faheem et al., 2021) Today more than 140 studies from around the world have examined the antihyperglycemic and hypoglycemic properties of various extracts and components of M. charantia in both human and animal models (Faheem et al., 2020).

Preservation of islets cells and their functions, suppression of key gluconeogenic enzyme, stimulation of the the key enzyme of HMP pathway, inhibition of intestinal glucose uptake, stimulation of peripheral and skeletal muscle glucose use, hypoglycemia effect and inhibition of adipocyte differentiation are some of the potential mechanisms of the hypoglycemic action of M. charantia and its various extracts and compounds (Figure 3) (Patwekar et al., 2022). Research indicates that M. charantia alters the expression of the PPAR- gene to enhance serum and liver lipid profiles and serum glucose levels. According to similar research, M. charantia protects pancreatic beta cells by reducing the activity of FN-B and MAPK a in MIN6N8 cells. Protein tyrosine phosphatase 1B (PTP1B), a depressive regulator of insulin signaling, may be a therapeutic target for the treatment of type 2 diabetes. (Ahmed et al., 2004)

MC and Glucose Metabolism

The impact of *M. charantia* powder and chloroform extract on glucose and amino acids by skeletal L6 myotubes and sodium (Na+) and potassium (K+) glucose by jejunum brush border membrane vesicles in both age-matched control and STZ- induced diabetic rats has been compared to those of insulin in several studies (Figure 4). The finding demonstrates that N-methylaminoisobutric acid (14C-MeAIB) and 3H- deoxy glucose absorption by skeletal muscle cells can be stimulated by lyophilised fruit juice at 5-10g / ml. The amplitude of these effects was comparable to the results achieved with 100 nmol/L of insulin. The unambiguous findings showed that *M. charantia* has capabilities similar to those of insulin, related to phytoconstituents of *M. charantia* known as V insulin (53) The fruit of *M. charantia* can suppress the action of and glucose-6-phosphatase fructose 1,6 -diphosphates while simultaneously increasing the activity of glucose-6-phosphatase dehydrogenase, according to previous research. (Garau et al., 2003)

Effect of MC Fruit Juice on Myelinated Fibres

The researchers found that the diabetic animal's area was reduced in all phases, having an identical impact on the thickness of the myelin and cross-sectional axon area but having no effect on the unmyelinated axon. There are data that suggest that giving antioxidants to STZ- diabetic rats can stop the onset of functional impairments. In diabetic rats, *M. charantia* treatment can restore normal amounts of myelinated fibres, most likely as a result of lower blood glucose levels. When managing DM and associated complications, the administration of *M. charantia* may be helpful as an adjuvant therapy to reduce oral hypoglycemic medications (Xu et al., 2022).

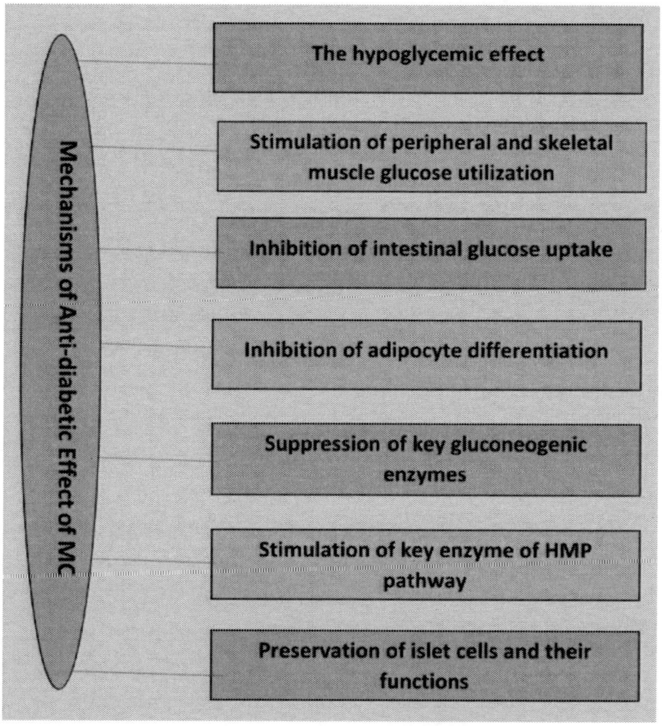

Figure 4. Mechanism of the anti-diabetic effect of MC.

Effect of MC on Lipid Metabolism

Furthermore, *M. charantia* reduced the expression of lipogenic genes in fatty tissue from obese mice developed by a diet, inhibiting lipogenesis and boosting lipid oxidation linked to mitochondrial decoupling. *M. charantia* increased the transport of the amount of fat in mitochondria was reduced by long-chain fatty acids and increased carnitine palmitoyl transfer ase-1 and acyl- CoA dehydrogenase activities in mitochondria of the liver and muscle. Furthermore, it increased adiponectin levels, skeletal muscle, gastrocnemius muscle and the action of UCP3 and 1 uncoupling protein 1 activities, and it decreased obesity. The expression of UCP was also influenced by *M. charantia*. Due to the fact that peripheral adiponectin injection decreases adiposity and increases the expression of UCP1 and UCP3 mRNA in skeletal muscle and brown adipose tissue, respectively. Adiponectin appears to be the way *M. charantia* functions (Wang and Ryu 2015).

Effect of MC on Pancreatic Beta Cells

In neonatal streptozotocin- induced type 2 diabetic rats, the administration of an ethanolic extract of the fruit pulp of *M. charantia* increased islet growth, total area of beta cells, number of beta cells, and insulin levels compared to diabetic rats not receiving treatment. Recovery at different stages is influenced by acetone extracted from the *M. charantia* fruit, which also restores normal beta cell activity. By preserving structural integrity and controlling functions such as hormone synthesis and release, *M. charantia* maintains blood glucose levels in diabetes within the normal range (Xiang et al., 2007).

Streptozotocin-induced fat peroxidation in the mouse pancreas, a rat insulinoma cell line, and islets was significantly decreased by *M. charantia*. Additionally, it decreased streptozotocin-induced apoptosis in rat insulinoma cells, demonstrating the mechanisms of protection of bitter gourd fruit juice for RIN cell, islets, and pancreatic beta cells. Only normal rats experienced a continuous decrease in serum glucose levels after taking *M. charantia* freeze dried powder orally for 2 weeks with and without 0.15%(w/w) cholesterol and 0.5%(w/w) bile acid in the diet (Ahmed et al., 2004).

Compared to diabetics who did not receiving treatment, the fruit juice significantly increased the amount of beta cells in the treated animals with *M. charantia*. Compared to diabetic rats that did not receive *M. charantia* treatment, the number of alpha cells did not change significantly.

Without increasing tissue respiration concurrently, fruit juice increased tissue absorption of glucose. It has been established that an aqueous extract of the immature fruit of *M. charantia* can partially encourage the production of insulin-form isolated beta cells in fat hyperglycemia mice. (Ahmed et al., 2004)

When different extracts of *M. charantia* were administered orally, various patterns of antihyperglycemic effects were observed without changing the insulin response, indicating a mechanism of action that is not dependent on intestinal glucose absorption and probably involves additional pancreatic function. Two substances can be found in *M. charantia*. Hexokinase activity can be inhabited by one of the substances, while glucose uptake may be affected by the other. Both demonstrated glucosuria- lowering abilities. (Tahira and Hussain, 2014).

Conclusion

Diabetes Mellitus is a significant issue for world health that is now spreading like an outbreak. In the current environment, herbal remedies are still used in prevention and treatment. In this review study, the anti- diabetic properties of *Momordica charantia*, often known as bitter melon, have been researched. For an ethnic minority with a high prevalence of diabetes who prefer natural treatment methods due to cultural beliefs. *M. harantia* may be a viable option. The pyrimidine nucleoside, polypeptide-p, plant insulin, charantin, vicine, glycosides, and p-insulin are the components of the karela. In this case, a different author used *Momordica charantia* fruit and leaf extraction. As extraction mediums, ethanol, methanol, and water were utilised. The serum cholesterol level in the diabetic rat was reduced by those derived media as part of their anti- diabetic properties. In conclusion, treating pre- diabetic or diabetics with herbal remedies may be an alternative to oral hypoglycemic effects, since they not only show promise in lowering blood sugar levels, but also in enhancing lipid profiles, controlling high blood pressure, and promoting antioxidant function. However, to assess the quantity and quality of active pharmaceutical ingredients present in the finished products, which must then be tested on a human subject through well- designed clinical trials and confirmed and certified by the relevant regulatory authorities of the country, the ethnopharmaceutical field, which is rapidly expanding, urgently needs validated testing protocols. In general, most scientific research points to the fact that regular consumption of bitter gourd can prevent or treat a number of health- related issues. As a new and promising method, nanoencapsulation of active compounds employing different biocompatible polymers is also necessary to promote their sustained released property and enhanced bioavailability.

Acknowledgment

The authors offer her special thanks to Luqman College of Pharmacy for allowing her to carry out this work. I am particularly grateful for the assistance and coordination support provided by Ruhin Fatema.

References

Ahmad, Z., Zamhuri, K. F., Yaacob, A., Siong, C. H., Selvarajah, M., Ismail, A. and Hakim, M. N., 2012. In vitro anti-diabetic activities and chemical analysis of polypeptide-k and oil isolated from seeds of Momordica charantia (bitter gourd). *Molecules*, *17*(8), pp. 9631-9640.

Ahmed, I., Adeghate, E., Cummings, E., Sharma, A. K. and Singh, J., 2004. Beneficial effects and mechanism of action of Momordica charantia juice in the treatment of streptozotocin-induced diabetes mellitus in rat. *Molecular and cellular biochemistry*, *261*, pp.63-70.

Amos, A. F., McCarty, D. J. and Zimmet, P., 1997. The rising global burden of diabetes and its complications: estimates and projections to the year 2010. *Diabetic medicine*, *14*(S5), pp. S7-S85.

Arif, R., Ahmad, S., Mustafa, G., Mahrosh, H. S., Ali, M., ul Qamar, M. T. and Dar, H. R., 2021. Molecular docking and simulation studies of antidiabetic agents devised from hypoglycemic polypeptide-P of Momordica charantia. *BioMed research international*, *2021*.

Baby, J. and Jini, D., 2011. A medicinal potency of Capparis decidua-a harsh terrain plant. *Research Journal of Phytochemistry*, *5*(1), pp.1-13.

Borri, A., Panunzi, S. and De Gaetano, A., 2019, October. Rapid and ultra-rapid insulin in glycemic control. In *2019 IEEE International Conference on Systems, Man and Cybernetics (SMC)* (pp. 336-341). IEEE.

Desai, S. and Tatke, P., 2015. Charantin: An important lead compound from Momordica charantia for the treatment of diabetes. *Journal of Pharmacognosy and Phytochemistry*, *3*(6), pp.163-166.

Faheem, I. P., Gopalakrishana, B., Mohsina, F. P. and Ahmad, N., 2020. Antidiabetic activity OF FICUS dalhousiae miq leaves ethanolic extract ON streptozotocin induced diabtes IN wistar albino rats. *World Journal Of Pharmaceutical Research*, *10*(1), p.1258.

Faheem, I. P., Gopalakrishna, B., Mohsina, F. P. and Priya, S., 2021. Antidiabetic potential of ethanolic leaf extract of Crataeva magna in streptozotocin-induced diabetic model. *Innovations in Pharmaceuticals and Pharmacotherapy*, *9*, pp.1-7.

Garau, C., Cummings, E., Phoenix, D. A. and Singh, J., 2003. Beneficial effect and mechanism of action of Momordica charantia in the treatment of diabetes mellitus: a mini review. *Dubai Diabetes and Endocrinology Journal*, *11*, pp.46-55.

Heilbronn, L., Smith, S.R. and Ravussin, E., 2004. Failure of fat cell proliferation, mitochondrial function and fat oxidation results in ectopic fat storage, insulin resistance and type II diabetes mellitus. *International journal of obesity*, *28*(4), pp.S12-S21.

Jia, S., Shen, M., Zhang, F. and Xie, J., 2017. Recent advances in Momordica charantia: functional components and biological activities. *International journal of molecular sciences*, *18*(12), p.2555.

Joseph, B. and Jini, D., 2013. Antidiabetic effects of Momordica charantia (bitter melon) and its medicinal potency. *Asian pacific journal of tropical disease*, *3*(2), pp.93-102.

Krawinkel, M. B. and Keding, G. B., 2006. Bitter gourd (Momordica charantia): a dietary approach to hyperglycemia. *Nutrition reviews*, *64*(7), pp.331-337.

Leung, L., Birtwhistle, R., Kotecha, J., Hannah, S. and Cuthbertson, S., 2009. Anti-diabetic and hypoglycaemic effects of Momordica charantia (bitter melon): a mini review. *British Journal of Nutrition*, *102*(12), pp.1703-1708.

Nagarani, G., Abirami, A. and Siddhuraju, P., 2014. Food prospects and nutraceutical attributes of Momordica species: a potential tropical bioresources–a review. *Food Science and Human Wellness*, *3*(3-4), pp.117-126.

Patwekar, M., Patwekar, F., Mezni, A., Sanaullah, S., Fatema, S.R., Almas, U., Ahmad, I., Tirth, V. and Mallick, J., 2022. Assessment of antioxidative and alpha-amylase potential of polyherbal extract. *Evidence-based Complementary and Alternative Medicine*, *2022*.

Pitipanapong, J., Chitprasert, S., Goto, M., Jiratchariyakul, W., Sasaki, M. and Shotipruk, A., 2007. New approach for extraction of charantin from Momordica charantia with pressurized liquid extraction. *Separation and Purification Technology*, *52*(3), pp.416-422.

Quazi, A., Mohsina, F. P., Faheem, I. P. and Priya, S., 2022. Silico ADMET analysis, molecular docking and in vivo anti diabetic activity of polyherbal tea bag formulation in streptozotocin-nicotinamide induced diabetic rats. *International Journal of Health Sciences*, *6*, pp.343-372.

Raman, A. and Lau, C., 1996. Anti-diabetic properties and phytochemistry of Momordica charantia L. (Cucurbitaceae). *Phytomedicine*, *2*(4), pp.349-362.

Singh, A., Singh, S. P. and Bamezai, R., 1998. Momordica charantia (Bitter Gourd) peel, pulp, seed and whole fruit extract inhibits mouse skin papillomagenesis. *Toxicology letters*, *94*(1), pp.37-46.

Tahira, S. and Hussain, F., 2014. Antidiabetic evaluation of Momordica charantia L fruit extracts. *The West Indian Medical Journal*, *63*(4), p.294.

Teoh, S. L., Latiff, A. A. and Das, S., 2010. Histological changes in the kidneys of experimental diabetic rats fed with Momordica charantia (bitter gourd) extract. *Rom. J. Morphol. Embryol*, *51*(1), pp.91-5.

Thakur, G., Pal, K., Mitra, A., Mukherjee, S., Basak, A. and Rousseau, D., 2010. Some common antidiabetic plants of the Indian subcontinent. *Food Reviews International*, *26*(4), pp.364-385.

Tian, M., Zeng, X.Q., Song, H. L., Hu, S. X., Wang, F. J., Zhao, J. and Hu, Z. B., 2015. Molecular diversity and hypoglycemic polypeptide-P content of Momordica charantia in different accessions and different seasons. *Journal of the Science of Food and Agriculture*, *95*(6), pp.1328-1335.

Wang, H. Y., Kan, W. C., Cheng, T. J., Yu, S. H., Chang, L. H. and Chuu, J. J., 2014. Differential anti-diabetic effects and mechanism of action of charantin-rich extract of Taiwanese Momordica charantia between type 1 and type 2 diabetic mice. *Food and Chemical Toxicology*, *69*, pp.347-356.

Wang, J. and Ryu, H. K., 2015. The effects of Momordica charantia on obesity and lipid profiles of mice fed a high-fat diet.*Nutrition research and practice*, *9*(5), pp.489-495.

Wolff, S. P., 1993. Diabetes mellitus and free radicals: free radicals, transition metals and oxidative stress in the aetiology of diabetes mellitus and complications. *British medical bulletin*, *49*(3), pp.642-652.

World Health Organization, 2016. *World Health Organization Global Report on Diabetes*. Geneva: World Health Organization.

Xiang, L., Huang, X., Chen, L., Rao, P. and Ke, L., 2007. The reparative effects of Momordica Charantia Linn. extract on HIT-T15 pancreatic beta-cells. *Asia Pac. J. Clin. Nutr.*, *16*(1), pp.249-252.

Xu, B., Li, Z., Zeng, T., Zhan, J., Wang, S., Ho, C.T. and Li, S., 2022. Bioactives of Momordica charantia as Potential Anti-Diabetic/Hypoglycemic Agents. *Molecules*, *27*(7), p.2175.

Yuwai, K. E., Rao, K. S., Kaluwin, C., Jones, G. P. and Rivett, D. E., 1991. Chemical composition of Momordica charantia L. fruits. *Journal of Agricultural and Food Chemistry*, *39*(10), pp.1762-1763.

Chapter 8

Assessment of the Antidiabetic Properties of *Zanthoxylum Armatum*

Noopur Srivastava[1,*]
Nisha Saxena[2]
and Chhaya Dagar[1]
[1]Department of Chemistry and Biochemistry, Sharda School of Basic Sciences and Research, Sharda University, Greater Noida, Uttar Pradesh, India
[2]Department of Chemistry, M. R. M. College, Lalit Narayan Mithila University, Darbhanga, Bihar, India

Abstract

Z. armatum is a small tree that belongs to the Rutaceace family and is known as Indian Prickly Ash. It shows several medicinal properties such as antioxidative, antitumor, anti-inflammatory, analgesic, antimicrobial, and insecticidal/larvicidal activity. The biologically important compounds are found in the different parts (leaves, bark, flowers, and fruits) of *Z. armatum*. The results reveal that lignans and flavonoids are the principal components in leaves samples, while aporphine alkaloids, lignans and amides are the main constituents in bark samples of this plant. Tambulin, a flavanol isolated from this plant, has shown potent insulin secretory activity.

Keywords: *Z. armatum,* diabetes, tambulin, antidiabetic activity

---

* Corresponding Author's Email: noopursriv@gmail.com.

In: Antidiabetic Plants
Editor: Arpita Roy
ISBN: 979-8-88697-957-2

Introduction

Diabetes, being a lifestyle disease, requires lifelong medication. In such a scenario, the dependence on allopathic medicines creates a burden on the masses. The discipline of herbal medicines is to lend a helping hand. Although cheaper in contrast to the western system of medication, herbal medicines are predominantly dependent on their availability. Among the rich flora of medicinal plants that show anti-diabetic action, *Zanthoxylum armatum* is one such species that has attracted little attention. More than 250 species of *Zanthoxylum* have been reported from all over the world, including Japan, Taiwan, Malaysia, China, Pakistan, Bhutan, Philippines, Nepal, and India. The Indian Himalayan region contains over eleven species of Zanthoxylum, viz. *Z. nitidium, Z. acanthopodium, Z. oxophyllum, Z. armatum, Z. planispinum, Z. budrunga, Z. ovafolium.* Among these, *Z. armatum* and *Z. acanthopodium* have been investigated more (Sekar et al., 2010; Samant et al., 1998).

Z. armatum has been recognised by various names such as 'Winged prickly ash' or 'Toothache tree', local names such as 'Tejphal' in Hindi, 'Tejowati' in Sanskrit, 'Mukhthrubi' in Manipuri and 'Timur' in Nepali. For a long time, the fruits of this plant have been used for the treatment of fever, cold, expulsion worms, and toothache remedy. The main components include amides, lignans, and alkaloids derived from the bark of the plant. It is found up to an altitude of 2,500 m, widely found in Kashmir and the northern part of India.

Z. armatum belongs to the Rutaceae family which is widely used in traditional folk medicine, and possesses anti-inflammatory, antibacterial, hepatoprotective and antidiabetic properties. Detail studies of these species in order to explain medicinal properties are still in the pipeline and are being investigated (Kala et al., 2005).

Chemical Constituents

Phytoconstituents from the stem, bark, and seeds of *Z. armatum* have been found to be of medicinal value. They belong to an array of chemical classes, such as terpenes, flavonoids, alkaloids, steroids, amino acids, glycosides, amides, coumarins, benzenoids, etc. Some important ones are linalool and limonene in substantial amounts from the oil(seeds), armatamide from stem. The essential oil derived from seeds is reported to have more than 20 different constituents (Figure 1) and this was confirmed by GC-MS analysis.(Gupta et al., 2011,Gardener et al., 1995, Bhat et al., 2018) Other functional groups found were in the category of fatty acids, alkenic acids, lignins, phenolics, aromatic and volatile compounds.(Kalia et al., 1999, Sati et al., 2011, Ahmad et al., 1993, Waheed et al., 2011)Asarin, fargesin, zanthonitrile, berberine, L-asarin, L-sesamin, L-planinin, methyl cinnamate, linalyl acetate, citral, geraniol, citral, limonene, sabines, methyl-n-n-nonyl ketone, linalyl acetates, sesquiterpenes are some more components of *Z. armatum.*

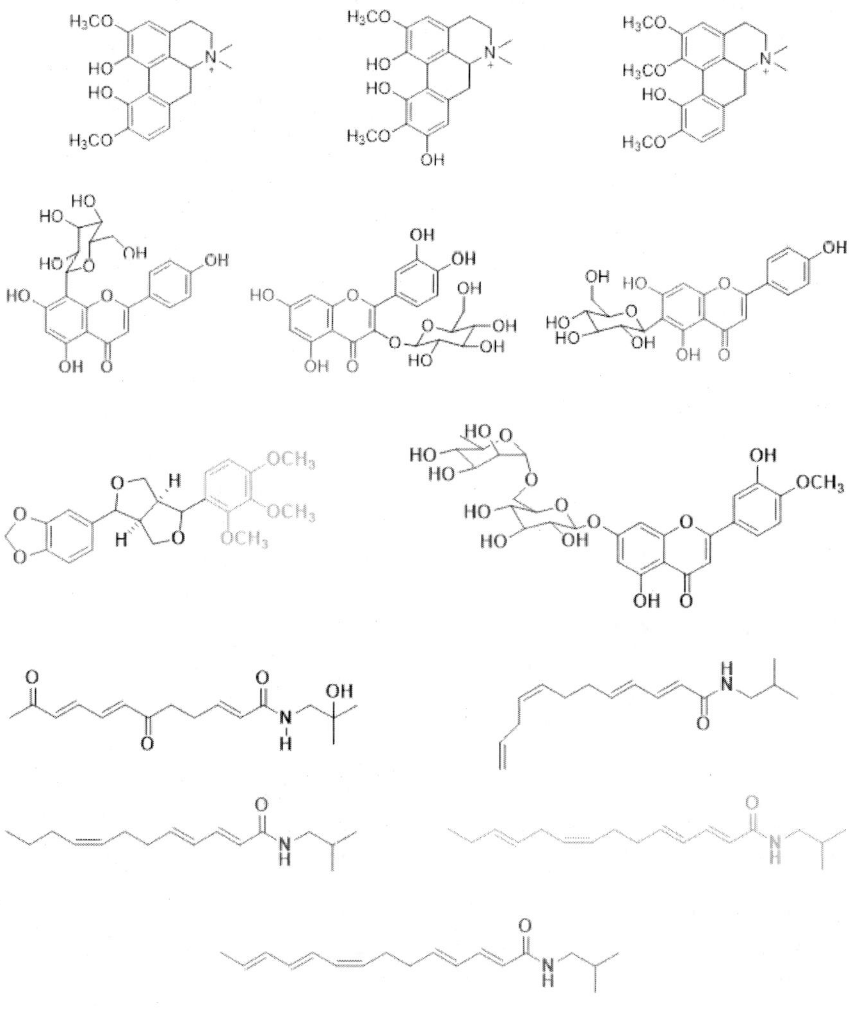

Figure 1. (Continued)

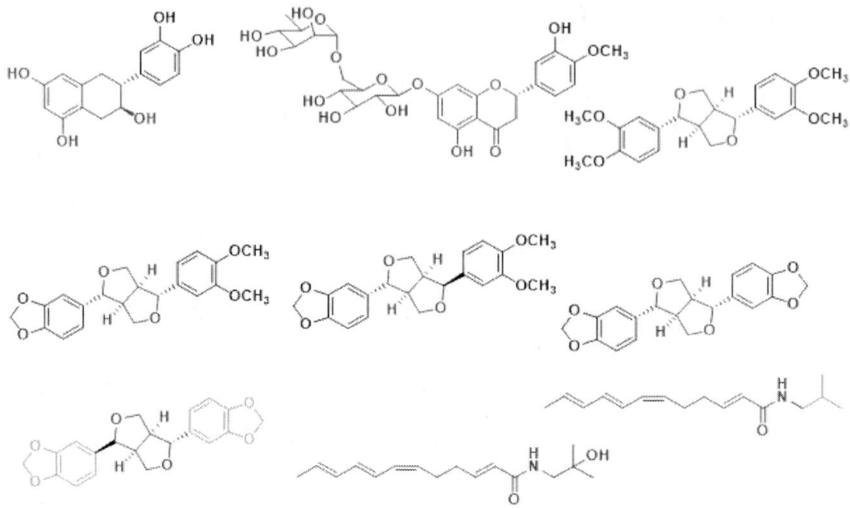

Figure 1. Compounds Identified and Quantified from *Zanthoxylum armatum.*

Pharmacological Profile

Z. armatum is believed to be a magical plant. Traditionally, herbal powder prepared from Zuroor-eQula seeds (Unani formulation) has antimicrobial and anti-inflammatory action (Paridhavi et al., 2007). The twigs of the plant serve as toothbrushes, the fruits are used as spices and the flavouring agents, and bark of the plant is used for dyeing. (Gaur et al., 2007) *Z. armatum* serves as a remedy for many ailments such as diarrhoea, rheumatism, bronchitis, asthma, indigestion, dyspepsia, toothaches, varicose veins, cholera, etc. Different parts of the plant are used for this purpose. Some notable ones are described in the following.

Antioxidative Activity

The fruits of *Z. armatum were* extracted with methanol and ethanol. These extracts exhibit antioxidant activity. This has been established by the DPPH (2,2-diphenyl-1-picrylhydrazyl) scavenging method. The subject animals were albino wistar rats. (Batool et al., 2010, Brijwal et al., 2013, Firake et al., 2014, Akbar et al., 2014, Kanwal et al., 2015)

Anti-Inflammatory Activity

Another finding reports the anti-inflammatory activity of the ethanolic extracts of *Z. armatum*. Swelling was observed in the paws of male wistar rats when ethanolic extract from the bark of the plant was administered. The lignans present in the extract have been reported to have analgesic activity. However, the plant's ethanolic extract of the fruit showed a reduction in carrageenan, which was used as an inducer of edema in the paws of wistar rats (Mehta et al., 2011).

Antimicrobial Activity

Microbial infections can also be treated with *Z. armatum*. In a study, inhibition of *Bacillus subtilis* was reported with an MBC value of 2.5 mg / L was reported. Further toxicity against *Alternaria brassicicola* has also reported from essential oils obtained from *Z. armatum* (Joshi et al., 2009).

Insecticidal and Larvicidal Activity

Many species of mosquitoes were found to be repelled by *Zanthoxylum* sps, viz. *Anopheles stephensi*, *Culex quinquefasciatus*, *Culex pipiens, Aedes aegypti,* and *Aedes albopictus*. This repellent action was found to be comparable with *N, N* diethyl-3 methylbenzamide (DEET). Basically, the larvae of these insect species were found to be killed by seed oil extracts. Both *Z. armatum* and *Z. piperitum* showed insecticidal and larvicidal action (Tiwary et al., 2007, Bachwani et al., 2012; Medhi et al., 2013, Sonu et al., 2015). In another study, mosquito repellents based on coconut oil and mustard oil based mosquito repellents were prepared from *Z. armatum* that gave results comparable and superior results with dimethyl phthalate (DMP). It has also been found to repel leech (Ramanujam et al., 2008).

Piscicide Activity

Z. armatum is used in the management of fish. It is used as a piscicidal agent. The ethanolic extracts of the fruit act in the various tissues of catfish

(*Heteropneustes fossilis*) involving Mg^{2+}, Na^{+}, K^{+}, and ATPase (Verma et al., 2010).

Hepatoprotective Activity

Carbon tetrachloride extracts from *Z. armatum* leaves caused liver toxicity and inflammation (Mehta et al., 2011), while those from bark caused enhancement of the antioxidant enzyme levels. Escalation of these enzymes provided a protective cover for the mice's liver of mice (Ranawat et al., 2009; Barkat et al., 2011).

Antitumor Activity

Z. armatum has the potential to be an anticancer drug. Lupeol, a monoterpene, has shown activity against inflammation and cancer. However, the crude extract of leaves and fruits has been reported to be cytotoxic (Gilani et al., 2010).

Immunomodulation Activity

The crude extracts of *Z. armatum* stimulate the circulatory system and provide a soothing effect for rheumatism and fibrositis. Disorders related to the heart, respiratory system, gut, sodium, and potassium channels can be cured with these extracts.

Antidiabetic Potential

Remarkable anti-diabetic activity has been demonstrated by Tambulin, a flavonol extracted from the fruits of *Z. armatum with* methanol. Tambulin resulted in an increased level of insulin when the mice's islets were stimulated with glucose. However, it did not show any effect on insulin secretion. It does not act directly through the K-ATP channel like tolbutamide, a known drug that belongs to the class of sulfonylureas and was used as a standard. Tambulin works well when glucose concentrations are high. Compared to tolbutamide, tambulin was found to be more active with a lesser toxicity. The other goals for both are different (Hameed et al., 2019).

In another report, aqueous leaf extracts of *Z. armatum* displayed antidiabetic activity in vitro and vivo. The enzymes lipase, -glucosidase, and amylase were inhibited in vitro. Furthermore, low and high doses of extracts were administered in vivo and a hypoglycemic effect was observed (Rynjah et al., 2018).

Conclusion

The promising medicinal property of *Z. armatum* requires in-depth investigation in areas such as anti-diabetic and anticancer. Genetic information about the plant can be helpful in studying its properties. In recent times, the demand for the collection of this plant from the Indian Himalayan region has grown. The plant has proven therapeutic effects and needs to be propagated and conserved.

References

Ahmad, A., Misra, L. N. and Gupta, M. M., 1993. Hydroxyalk-(4Z)-enoic acids and volatile components from the seeds of Zanthoxylum armatum. *Journal of Natural Products*, *56*(4), pp.456-460.

Akbar, S., Majid, A., Hassan, S., Rehman, A. U., Khan, T., Jadoon, M. A. and Rehman, M.U., 2014. Comparative in vitro activity of ethanol and hot water extracts of Zanthoxylum armatum to some selective human pathogenic bacterial strains. *Int. J. Biosci*, *4*(1), pp.285-291.

Bachwani, M., Srivastava, B., Sharma, V., Khandelwal, R. and Tomar, L., 2012. An update review on Zanthoxylum armatum DC. *Am. J. Pharm. Tech. Res*, *2*(1), pp.274-285.

Barkatullah, Ibrar, M. and Muhammad, N., 2011. Evaluation of Zanthoxylum armatum DC for in-vitro and in-vivo pharmacological screening. *African Journal of Pharmacy and Pharmacology*, *5*(14), pp.1718-1723.

Batool, F., Sabir, S. M., Rocha, J. B. T., Shah, A. H., Saify, Z. S. and Ahmed, S. D., 2010. Evaluation of antioxidant and free radical scavenging activities of fruit extract from Zanthoxylum alatum: a commonly used spice from Pakistan. *Pak J. Bot.*, *42*(6), pp.4299-311.

Bhatt, V., Kumar, N., Sharma, U. and Singh, B., 2018. Comprehensive metabolic profiling of Zanthoxylum armatum and Zanthoxylum acanthopodium leaves, bark, flowers and fruits using ultra high performance liquid chromatography. *Separation Science Plus*, *1*(5), pp.311-324.

Brijwal, L., Pandey, A. and Tamta, S., 2013. An overview on phytomedicinal approaches of Zanthoxylum armatum DC.: An important magical medicinal plant. *J. Med. Plants Res*, *7*(8), pp.366-370.

Dweck, A.C., 1995. *The William garden collection of Chinese medicinal plants.*

Gaur, R. D., 2008. *Traditional dye yielding plants of Uttarakhand, India.*

Gilani, S. N., Khan, A. U. and Gilani, A. H., 2010. Pharmacological basis for the medicinal use of Zanthoxylum armatum in gut, airways and cardiovascular disorders. *Phytotherapy Research: An International Journal Devoted to Pharmacological and Toxicological Evaluation of Natural Product Derivatives*, *24*(4), pp.553-558.

Gupta, S., Bhaskar, G. and Andola, H.C., 2011. Altitudinal variation in Essential oil content in leaves of Zanthoxylum alatum Roxb. a high value aromatic tree from Uttarakhand. *Research Journal of Medicinal Plant*, *5*(3), pp.348-351.

Hameed, A., Raza, S.A., Khan, M. I., Baral, J., Adhikari, A., Nur-e-Alam, M., Ahmed, S., Al-Rehaily, A.J., Ashraf, S., Ul-Haq, Z. and Hafizur, R.M., 2019. Tambulin from Zanthoxylum armatum acutely potentiates the glucose-induced insulin secretion via KATP-independent Ca2+-dependent amplifying pathway. *Biomedicine & Pharmacotherapy*, *120*, p.109348.

Joshi, B., Lekhak, S. and Sharma, A., 2009. Antibacterial property of different medicinal plants: Ocimum sanctum, Cinnamomum zeylanicum, Xanthoxylum armatum and Origanum majorana. *Kathmandu university journal of science, engineering and technology*, *5*(1), pp.143-150.

Kala, C. P., Farooquee, N. A. and Dhar, U., 2005. Traditional uses and conservation of timur (Zanthoxylum armatum DC.) through social institutions in Uttaranchal Himalaya, India. *Conservation and Society*, *3*(1), pp.224-230.

Kalia, N. K., Singh, B. and Sood, R. P., 1999. A new amide from Zanthoxylum armatum. *Journal of Natural Products*, *62*(2), pp.311-312.

Kanwal, R., Arshad, M., Bibi, Y., Asif, S. and Chaudhari, S. K., 2015. Evaluation of Ethnopharmacological and Antioxidant Potential of Zanthoxylum armatum DC. *Journal of Chemistry*, *2015*.

Medhi, K., Deka, M. and Bhau, B.S., 2013. The genus Zanthoxylum–a stockpile of biological and ethnomedicinal properties. *Open Access Scientific Reports*, *2*(3), pp.1-8.

Mehta, D. K., Bhandari, A., Satti, N. K., Singh, S., Das, R., Suri, K. A. and Sharma, S. N., 2011. Anti-inflammatory activity of methanolic extract of fruit of Zanthoxylum armatum. *Inventi Rapid: Planta Activa*.

Paridhavi, M. and Agrawal, S. S., 2007. *Safety evaluation of a polyherbal formulation*, Zuroor-E–Qula.

Ramanujam, S. N. and Ratha, B. K., 2008. Effect of alcohol extract of a natural piscicide—Fruits of Zanthoxylum armatum DC. on Mg2+-and Na+, K+-ATPase activity in various tissues of a freshwater air-breathing fish, Heteropneustes fossilis. *Aquaculture*, *283*(1-4), pp.77-82.

Ranawat, L., Bhatt, J. and Patel, J., 2010. Hepatoprotective activity of ethanolic extracts of bark of Zanthoxylum armatum DC in CCl4 induced hepatic damage in rats. *Journal of ethnopharmacology*, *127*(3), pp.777-780.

Rynjah, C. V., Devi, N. N., Khongthaw, N., Syiem, D. and Majaw, S., 2018. Evaluation of the antidiabetic property of aqueous leaves extract of Zanthoxylum armatum DC. using in vivo and in vitro approaches. *Journal of traditional and complementary medicine*, *8*(1), pp.134-140.

Samant, S. S., Dhar, U. and Palni, L. M. S., 1998. Medicinal plants of Indian Himalaya: diversity, distribution. *Potential Value, Gyanodaya Prakashan*.

Sati, S. C., Sati, M. D., Raturi, R., Badoni, P. P. and Singh, H., 2011. A new flavonoidal glycoside from stem bark of Zanthoxylum armatum. *IJPI's J. Pharm. Herb. Form*, *1*(2), pp.29-32.

Sekar, T., Ayyanar, M. and Gopalakrishnan, M., 2010. MEETING REPORT: Medicinal plants and herbal drugs. *Current Science*, *98*(12), pp.1558-1559.

Sonu, B. and Bharat, B., 2015. Phytochemical and pharmacological activities of Zantoxylum armatum. DC.: an overview. *Research Journal of Pharmaceutical, Biological and Chemical Sciences*, *6*(5), pp.1403-1409.

Tiwary, M., Naik, S. N., Tewary, D. K., Mittal, P. K. and Yadav, S., 2007. Chemical composition and larvicidal activities of the essential oil of Zanthoxylum armatum DC (Rutaceae) against three mosquito vectors. *Journal of vector borne diseases*, *44*(3), p.198.

Verma, N. and Khosa, R. L., 2010. *Hepatoprotective activity of leaves of Zanthoxylum armatum DC in CCl 4 induced hepatotoxicity in rats.*

Waheed, A., Mahmud, S., Akhtar, M. and Nazir, T., 2011. Studies on the components of essential oil of Zanthoxylum armatum by GC-MS. *American Journal of Analytical Chemistry*, *2*(2), p.258.

Zhang, Y., Peng, Y., Zeng, D., Chen, F., Qin, Q. and Huang, Y. I., 2010. Insecticidal activity of essential oil from Zanthoxylum armatum fructification against two mosquito species. *Guangxi Zhiwu/Guihaia*, *30*(2), pp.274-279.

Chapter 9

The Pharmaceutical Importance of *Ocimum Sanctum* in Diabetic Management

Satyalakshmi Siragam*
Srinivasa Rao Yerraguntla
Venkata Kamala Kumari Paravastu
and Rama Rao Borra
Department of Pharmaceutics, Vignan Institute of Pharmaceutical Technology, Duvvada, Visakhapatnam, Andhra Pradesh, India

Abstract

Diabetes is the most common metabolic disorder that leads to chronic complications of crucial physiological systems, namely the nervous system, cardiovascular, renal system, and eyes. Resistance to insulin secretion or failure to make enough insulin can lead to the progenesis of type 2 diabetes in adults. In the last 30 years, the frequency of type 2 diabetes has increased rapidly, with about 537 million adults all over the world suffering from diabetes and 6.7 million deaths are directly related to diabetes. The adverse effects of lifelong drug use of oral anti-diabetic drugs of synthetic origin have been tremendously reported and stress the importance of alternative therapies with no side effects. Herbal treatment for chronic disorders has the potential to overcome the challenge of synthetic drug therapy. Tulsi, *Ocimum sanctum,* is an aromatic plant that has been extensively studied for its unique biological activities. Tulsi is regarded as a wonder plant that relieves various stress conditions through a mixture of pharmacological benefits. Tulsi has been studied extensively in the management of blood glucose, hypertension, and blood cholesterol

* Corresponding Author's Email: satyalaxmi148@rediffmail.com.

In: Antidiabetic Plants
Editor: Arpita Roy
ISBN: 979-8-88697-957-2

levels attained due to disturbances in metabolism. Eugenol is one of the main phytoactive principles found in Tulsi to lower blood glucose levels. This chapter provides information on the origin and phytochemical properties of tulsi, biological activities, diabetes statistics, and antidiabetic mechanisms of *O. sanctum*. The published work on the antihyperglycemic activity of *Ocimum sanctum* on animals and humans is summarized. *O. sanctum* nanoparticles therapy for diabetes was incorporated.

Keywords: *Ocimum sanctum*, antihyperglycemic, antidepressant, animal models, clinical studies, nanoparticles

Introduction

The effectiveness of herbs and their related preparations were documented in the ancient system of Indian medicine. Thousands of years ago, the tradition of herbal medicine therapy for obstinate diseases was started and the proofs were incorporated into Vedas. The increase in the use of herbal products is due to their safety and efficacy, and is becoming a part of public health concerns.

Reports have shown that blended herbal formulations are used successfully to heal acute and chronic diseases and disorders associated with the skin, lungs, liver, heart, brain, etc. Ancient civilised places- of few Asian countries-are still applying herbs-based remedies for the treatment of acute and chronic disorders (Mohd and Iqbal, 2019). Statistics from the World Health Organisation (WHO) indicated that 3 out of 4 people around the world practise using conventional medicine. Without proper guidance and scientific knowledge, most people have used herbal products. To date, 170 of the WHO member states have used traditional medicine. Due to the increase in users of traditional drugs users, to provide access to safe and effective treatment, and to obtain more benefits, WHO established the Global Centre for Traditional Medicine at Jamnagar, Gujarat, India (WHO, 2022) to add the essence of science and technical knowledge to make traditional herbal products even more effective.

Plant-derived medicines are significant for the treatment of various conditions because of the rich number of bioactive constituents that play an important role in the development of new drugs. Scientifically evidenced that each plant part is rich in medicinal principles. Not all plants are safe to use because they are toxic and have a negative impact on organs. Therefore, we need a protocol to standardise the extract of plant parts to develop a phytoformulation. In recent years, there has been great interest in investigating herbal treatments for chronic diseases such as diabetes. Currently, many nutraceuticals are commercially available to treat diabetes (Morad *et al.*, 2018). The current chapter aimed to brief on the history, epidemiology, diagnosis, treatment of diabetes, the role of phytochemicals in diabetes treatment, the pharmacognosy of *Ocimum sanctum, the* mechanism of Tulsi in the management of diabetes, and finally the prospects of Tulsi in the control of diabetes were elaborated.

Diabetes

Diabetes mellitus is the most common metabolic disorder and ranks among the leading causes of premature deaths. Globally it is a chronic health issue that can keep the body at a very high risk for other serious health complications (Deshpande et al., 2008, Ghorbani, 2013). Interrupted metabolism of carbohydrates, fats, proteins; loss of insulin secreting capacity of β-cells is the major cause that leads to irregularity in blood glucose (BG) levels (Katzung et al., 2011). Insulin deficiency creates a physiological state in which various tissues, muscles, and liver are unable to take glucose from the blood, resulting in elevated sugar levels in the blood; this status is described as diabetes or hyperglycemia. Diabetes is of three different types, Type 1, Type 2, and gestational diabetes mellitus. Type 1 diabetes occurs due to the loss of β cell of islets of Langerhans functioning. Short-term loss of β cell mass due to genetic predisposition can cause Type 2 diabetes, is commonly described as insulin-dependent diabetes, occurs mostly in people with obesity. People with impaired glucose tolerance (IGT) or defective fasting glycemia (IFG) are more prone to progressing type 2 diabetes. Pregnant women in the 2nd or 3rd trimester are at risk for gestational diabetes-characterised hyperglycemia (Jarald et al., 2008). The clinical conditions of diabetes are poly dipsea, polyurea, poly phagia, fatigue, nausea, vomiting, infertility in men, delayed wound healing, and loss of clarity of vision (Syed and Neetu, 2013, Wannes and Marzouk, 2016). The loss of equilibrium between reactive oxygen species (ROS) production and enzymatic or non-enzymatic antioxidant capacity is known as oxidative stress (OS). OS is also an important cause of the development of diabetes. Any drug that can show antioxidant activity against reactive oxygen species can normalise blood sugar levels (Verma et al., 2018).

Diagnosis and Treatment

The availability of inexpensive test procedures for BG makes early diabetes diagnosis easier. The standard figure to confirm diabetes in healthy man in a fasting state is 80 mg/dl and 160 mg/dl in the postprandial state. Diabetic individuals are identified by finger prick blood sugar test, fasting blood sugar, glucose tolerance test (Myoclinic, 2022). Treatment of diabetes includes BG that reduces oral anti-diabetic drugs, diet, and physical activity.

The reports of different National Health Institutes that investigate the various aspects of diabetes, listed the following complications in diabetic patients (Steinmetz et al., 2021; Saran et al., 2015).

- Adults suffering from diabetes are 2 to 4 times at risk of cardiac arrests and strokes.
- Diabetes with reduced blood flow increases the risk of foot ulcers due to nerve damage to the feet.
- Capillary damage to the retina can lead to diabetic retinopathy, which is the main cause of blindness, and 10 lakh people lost their vision due to diabetes.
- Diabetes predominantly causes kidney failure.
- Diabetes increases the risk of susceptibility to COVID-19.

According to the International Diabetes Federation, the world's diabetics are as follows:

In 2021, confirmed diabetics were 537 million in the age group of 20-79 years. This count will increase to 643 million by 2030 and 783 million by 2045. In undeveloped and developing countries, 3 out of 4 adults were diabetic. 6.7 million deaths were the result of diabetes. Type 1 diabetics are around more than 1.2 million children and adolescents. During pregnancy1, 1 in 6 live births are affected by diabetes. 541 million adults are at risk for type 2 diabetes (International Diabetes Federation, 2021).

Lifelong therapy with oral glycaemic drugs and continuous monitoring is the best treatment for diabetes. The diverse mechanisms of oral anti-diabetic drugs enable them to be used alone or in combination. Regardless of the benefits of BG control, hyperglycemic drugs have severe side effects that are associated with the abdomen, metabolic complications, central nervous system (CNS) symptoms, skeletal muscle, urogenital complications, etc. (Keezhipadathil, 2019).

The side effects of synthetic anti-diabetic drugs, their availability and affordability can be a major concern for acquiring the proper therapy and treatment of diabetes. Low-income countries are shifting from synthetic formulations to traditional herbal medicines to obtain safer and more effective treatment for diabetes management (Raiya et al., 2017).

Numerous proprietary herbs and formulations are in use against diabetes. Plants that were investigated for their antidiabetic properties are listed here. Ash gourd (*Benincasahispida*), *Aloe vera*, neem, church steeples (*Agrimonia eupatoria*), tulsi (*Ocimum sanctum*), mango, mulberry (Babul (Acacia arabica), onion, bitter apple (*Citrullus colocynthis*), eucalyptus, banyan tree (*Ficus benghalenesis*), potato, kiwach (*Mucuna pruriens*), *hibiscus*, ivy gourd, etc. (Jonnalagadd and Selkar 2013).

Anti-diabetic herbal drugs have been shown to improve pancreatic tissue toward insulin production and inhibit the secretion of enzymes responsible for carbohydrate metabolism (Ezeani et al., 2017). Of the several herbs listed above, *Ocimum sanctum* (Tulsi) is one of the best options for the management of diabetes management because of its complex chemical constituents and its diverse pharmacological activities.

Ocimum sanctum (OSM) Holy basil is an everlasting herb that belongs to the *Lamiaceae* family and grows with a square stem. It is straight, hard-branched, strongly odorous, and less hairy. The native place of Tulsi is India and other places in Asian and African countries and grows even at higher altitudes in the mountain regions of the Himalayas (Mondal et al., 2009; Parotta, 2001; World Health Organization, 2002). *Ocimum* means 'fragrant lipped', and *sanctum* means "holy" status of the plant. In India, OSM is most popularly known as Tulsi and is present as the most important holy plant in the Hindu Vedic system. The Ayurvedic system of medicine referred to Tulsi as 'The Queen of Herbs', 'The Incomparable One," and "The Mother Medicine of Nature' due to its medicinal values (Priyabrata et al., 2010). The ancient Vedas described the values of Tulsi and it is the religious worship plant of Hindus. Hindus follow the culture of growing Tulsi plants in or around the home. Ayurveda describes the best ways to take Tulsi for its medicinal benefits in the treatment of multiple health issues.

Tulsi has a complex chemical composition and contains minerals, vitamins, and many more biologically active compounds. The availability of each component differs from plant to plant according to the variety of strains. In addition, growing climatic conditions, collection and processing procedures also greatly influence the proportion of phytochemical constituents.

The interaction between the active phytochemicals leads to synergistic pharmacological benefits, and, traditionally, various systems of medicine have been practising the formulation of poly herbal mixtures for their added effects. However, gross activity cannot be duplicated with extracts of Tulsi. The properties of Tulsi, such as biological inheritance and the existence of complex biological constituents, have unresolved their characterisation and standardization by latest technology until now. The volatile oil of the Tulsi leaf (Kelm et al., 2000) contains the most important chemical principle, eugenol, which is a phenolic compound of essential oil, other constituents are urosolic acid, carvacrol, linalool, limatrol, caryophyllene, methyl carvicol, the volatile oil of seed contains fatty acids and sitosterol; further, the gum of the seed has a small proportion of xylose sugars, and the green leaves contain anthocyans.

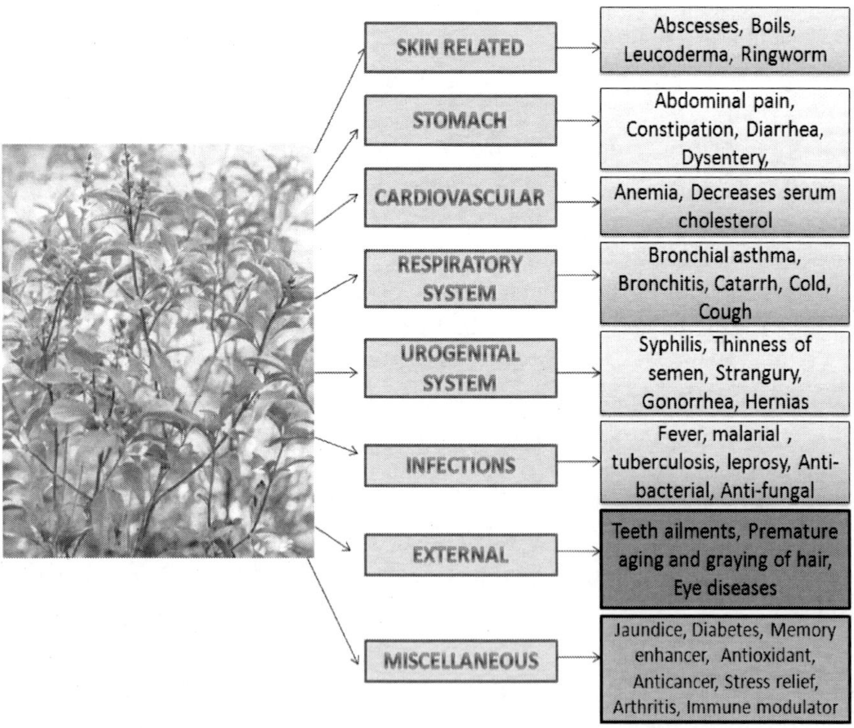

Figure 1. Pharmacological activities of OSM.

Although Tulsi is known for its energy-provider property as a common vitaliser and increases physical tolerance, caffeine and other stimulants are present. The other parts of Tulsi contain phytochemical constituents that show extensive biological activities, including saponins, flavonoids, triterpenoids, and tannins (Jaggi et al., 2003). Furthermore, the phenolic active principles are responsible for acting as antioxidant and anti-inflammatory compounds. The flavonoids-Orientin and Vicenin are aqueous soluble flavonoids that protect the chromosomes of lymphocytes from radiation. The highest proportion of eugenol is present in OSM in comparison to other *Ocimum* species. Eugenol is the essential phytochemical component that is the main component of lowering BG (Singh et al., 2016). An investigation of OSM for the study of anti-diabetic activity was shown reduced BG levels by 38% by blocking α-glucosidase at the same time insulin and glycated hemoglobin (HB) levels remained unchanged. Aqueous extracts of *OSM* leaves with polyphenols, caffeic acid, p-coumaric acid have remarkable anti-diabetic effects (Wongsa et al., 2012; Casanova et al., 2014).

The pharmacological activities of OSM are listed below and are represented in Figure 1.

Antidiabetic Mechanism of OSM

It contains a diverse class of phytoconstituents with extensive therapeutic benefits: in control of BG, blood cholesterol, blood pressure, stress reliever; suppress reactive oxygen functional groups, anticataract, microbicidal, anti-inflammatory, antiarthritic, cardioprotective, hepatoprotective, in the regulation of immunity and healing of wounds, etc. It appears to be an incomparable plant with multiple pharmacological activities that can resolve all the associated complications of diabetes. The phytochemical constituents exhibit synergism to establish normal blood sugar levels. Along with eugenol; carvacrol, linalool, caryophylline, β-sitosterol were determined for hypoglycemic potency (Ngan et al., 2020).

Anti-Diabetic Mechanisms

Figure 2, explains the multiple mechanisms of OSM in the treatment of diabetes (Hannan et al., 2014).

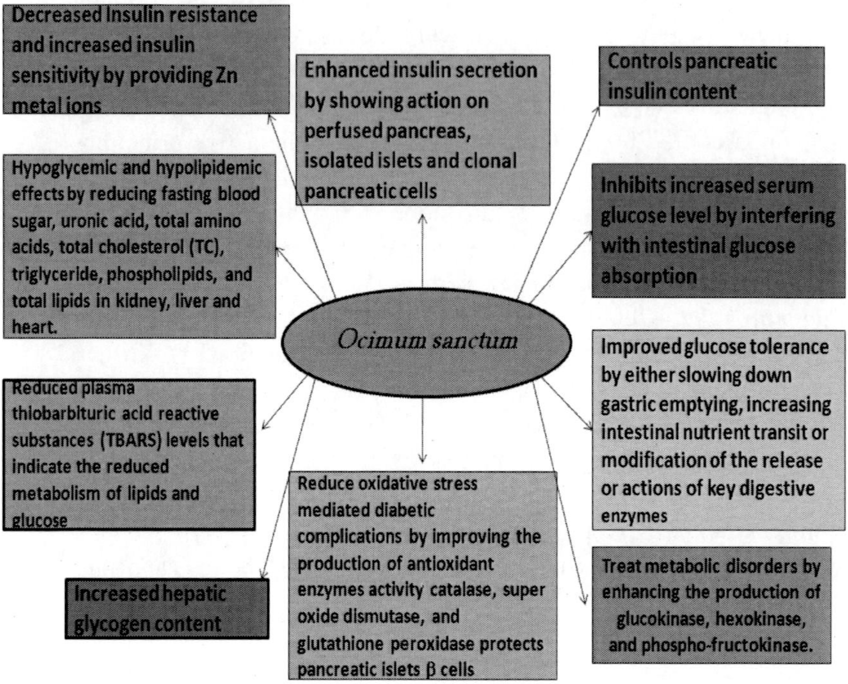

Figure 2. Mechanisms of OSM in the management of diabetes.

Investigation of the Antihyperglycemic Activity of OSM in Animal Models

The insulin production and antioxidant property of the *OSM* water extract in diabetic rats were evaluated. Oxidative stress, BG, lipids, triglyceride, creatinine, and bilirubin content was increased in diabetic rats and decreased insulin secretion compared to the OSM treated group (Shiv Kumar Jayant and Nalini Srivastava, 2016).

Fresh OSM leaves of OSM were supplemented along with 2 g / kg body weight to albino rabbits for 30 days and showed lower levels of BG in the test group. An oxidative enzyme such as superoxide dismutase levels were increased, a significant reduction in glutathione and total thiols and peroxidised fats was diagnosed in the treated group compared to the untreated group. Green leaves of OSM were shown to contain free radical scavenging activity (Jyoti et al., 2004).

The effect of fixed oil from OSM leaves on streptozotocin-induced diabetic rats was determined for the serum lipid profile and blood sugar levels. Various amounts of fatty acids in the oil were estimated by gas chromatography-mass spectrometry). α-linolenic acid was found to be the key fatty compound present in the fixed oil of OSM. Fixed oil was responsible for glucose reduction, lipid reduction, and antifree radical effects in the tested rats. Furthermore, fixed oil protected tested rat kidney tissue from oxidative stress under diabetic conditions (Thamolwan et al., 2016).

Three new bioactive constituents of the alcoholic root extract were selected, elucidated as glucopyranosyloxy benzoate and n-decanoyl-β-D-glucopyranosyl derivatives, along with previously characterised ursolic acid and palmityl glucoside. These active principles may be responsible for the reduction of blood sugar and triglycerides, total fat, and serum insulin levels (Ahmad et al., 2012).

The ethanolic extract of OSM leaves was used to determine antidiabetic activity on diabetes induced rats with alloxan. Sustained oral hypoglycemic activity was obtained in treated animals and this effect was comparable to synthetic hypoglycemic agents-glibenclamide, which belong to the category of sulfonylurea (Abhilash et al., 2013).

The enzymes responsible for carbohydrate metabolism- glucokinase, hexokinase, and phosphofructokinase-were influenced by OSM. This study was carried out in diabetes-induced rats for 1 month. The authors also estimated the content of glycogen in insulin-dependent and non-insulin-dependent tissues. Decreased BG levels from 9.06 to 26.4% were observed in the tested animals. The glucose content increased in insulin independent tissues such as the kidney, on the other hand, decreased glycogen content was observed in insulin dependent tissues such as skeletal muscle and liver (Vats et al., 2004).

The phytochemical components that manage diabetes in induced rats are also responsible for protecting cigarette smoking-induced rats from chronic obstructive pulmonary disease (COPD). Molecular-level coupling studies were employed to determine the strong binding efficiency between the main active principles (eugenol, cyclhexane, and caryophyllene) of leaf extract of OSM and the antioxidant enzymes associated with OSM. The *in vivo* and *in silico* findings support that leaf extract markedly suppressed the diabetes by suppressing oxidative stress through free radical scavenging activity (Srivastava et al., 2023).

Alcoholic and water extracts of eight different Asian basil varieties were tested for type 2 diabetes targeting activity. The total soluble phenolic content

(TSP), phenolic acid profiles, total antioxidant activity (TA), α-amylase, and α-glucosidase enzyme inhibitory activities of -amylase and -glucosidase were higher in basil varieties compared to standard drugs (Mishra et al., 2020).

Eugenol extracted from OSM for its binding efficiency with albumin was studied by the blind docking method. The strong interaction was exhibited by eugenol with surface-exposed lysines. In diabetes-induced rats, eugenol was found to decrease glucose levels by 38% due to inhibition of α-glucosidase inhibition whereas there was no change in the glycated hemoglobin content. A lesser number of AGE (Advanced Glycation End-Products) changed peptides were observed in eugenol-treated mice. The AGE content was determined by the Western blotting technique using anti-AGE antibody. Lesser lesions were observed in mice treated with eugenol, which were relieved by histopathological studies. This study proved that eugenol has a dual action in the management of diabetes (Singh et al., 2016).

The ethanolic extract of OSM markedly decreased diabetic symptoms with a simultaneous improvement in glycogen, HB, and protein in STZ-induced diabetic rats. Enhanced insulin, peptide levels, and glucose tolerance were also observed (Narendhirakannan et al., 2006).

Stimulatory insulin production was observed in OSM-treated diabetic rats (Hannan et al., 2006; Grover et al., 2005). Male rats induced with corticosteroids were diagnosed with regulated BG levels with OSM leaf extract (Gholap and Kar, 2004). Powder form of OSM leaves fed to healthy and diabetic rats for 1 month. The results of the sugar testing showed a significant decrease in BG, urogenic acid, and total amino acid levels (Rai et al., 1997). The antidiabetic activity of OSM in diabetic rats was estimated and reduced BG levels were comparable to Tolbutamide (Chattopadhyay et al., 1993).

Clinical Investigation of OSM for Anti-Diabetic Activity

According to the literature, the first clinical study was conducted in 1964 with 10 diabetic patients who reported that within 3 months, a 14 g Krishna Tulsi plant infusion reversed the diabetic condition (Luthy, 1964).

Almost 30 years later, the first randomised placebo-managed trial was reported; Daily intake of 2.5g of OSM leaves significantly improved urinary fasting and postprandial BG levels in patients with type 2 diabetes 1 month later (Agrawal et al., 1996).

Significant improvement in BG and average BG was reported in type 2 diabetic volunteers who were co-administered with 0.3 g of OSM leaf infusion and glibenclamide anti-antidiabetic drug for 12 weeks, compared to drug treatment alone (Somasundaram et al., 2012).

Significant results were obtained with Tulsi leaves and curry leaves powder compared to Tulsi alone in diabetic patients. After 14 days, a drastic change in BG levels was observed (Venkatesan et al., 2015).

OSM and neem leaf extract in combination reported a drastic reduction in BG in a 12-week randomised trial in patients with type 2 diabetes (Kochhar et al., 2009).

40 volunteers (20 men and 20 women) were randomly selected to determine OSM leaf powder against diabetes. Each subject received a 3 gm powder containing a soft gelatin capsule in the morning on an empty stomach for 45 days. Fasting, postprandial, and average glucose levels were monitored. Compared to female subjects, male subjects have shown a better reduction in glucose levels. The average glucose levels were the same in both patients (Riddhi et al., 2016).

Pharmacokinetics, molecular coupling simulations - molecular dynamics, and binding free energy studies were used to study the antidiabetic potential of OSM for α-glucosidase, α-amylase, aldose reductase, and glycation in multiple stages. Essential oils of OSM are rich in isoeugenol- a phenylpropene, propenyl-substituted principal guaiacol. Through molecular coupling modelling, isoeugenol has greater enzyme targeting efficiency, with binding than standard medicines.

Furthermore, dynamic molecular studies have shown that isoeugenol is more stable at the binding sites than standard drugs used. The researchers succeeded in discovering the single lead molecule; isoeugenol with the dual action of firm binding potential and stability. In silico studies have shown that isoeugenol is a potential inhibitor of α-glucosidase, α-amylase, aldose reductase, and glycation (Reshma et al., 2022).

Nano-Formulations of OSM for Anti-Diabetic Activity

Techniques employed for the preparation of nano-formulations of plants exhibit potential advantages such as easy and fast, economical, ecological, stable for a long period, convenient and reproducible (Siragam, 2022). Very few studies reported the anti-diabetic potential of OSM in nanoformulations.

Stable AgNPs were synthesised in the size range of 3 to 25 nm using aqueous leaf extracts of *O. basilicum*, OSM, and in combination.

The leaf extract of OSM, which reduced the silver nitrate there, led to the rapid formation of AgNPs at room temperature, represented a higher rate of reaction compared to other synthetic methods, and more energy conversion led to rapid synthesis. The AgNPs characterised have exhibited α-amylase and α-glucosidase enzymes that block age there by retarded carbohydrate digestion rate, thus providing an alternative and less evasive strategy in the reduction of postprandial hyperglycemia in diabetic subjects. Furthermore, the bactericidal activity against *Gramme positive and negative microbes*, and other *pathogenic* species was evaluated (Veshara et al., 2017).

The titanium dioxide (TiO_2) nanoparticles enclosed in the OSM leaf extract were synthesised and incorporated into 2% chitosan (CS) gel for diabetic wound healing. The excellent efficacy of *in vivo* wound healing was obtained, which was proved by histopathological studies of healed wounds in diabetic rats (Ahmad et al., 2022). The ursolic acid extracted from OSM was formulated into nanoparticles using nanoprecipitation techniques to overcome the hydrophobicity associated with it. Non-insulin dependent diabetes-induced Wistar albino rats were treated with formulated nanoparticles for 4 weeks. Optimised and characterised ursolic acid nanoparticles have a significant reduction in elevated BG levels in dose-dependent manner with a prominent lipid-lowering and antioxidant effect (Anil Kumar et al., 2022).

Conclusion

Herbal practitioners have been passing instructions on how to prepare herbs medicine verbally, usually do not keep recorded data, but now the WHO has established the Global Centre for Traditional Medicine in India to combine science and technical knowledge to make traditional herbal products even more effective. Many developing countries and nations practising herbal drugs for treatment of clinical conditions are now trying to document medical research data on herbs. It simplifies the validation of scientific data and compares the pharmacological benefits of herbal drugs. Herbs are good for medicinal purposes and serve as a basic source for the isolation of semi-synthetic chemical compounds to prepare cosmetics and nutritional products. The side effects of synthetic formulations and increased health concerns led many people to adopt natural therapies. The demand for phytopharmaceuticals or nutraceuticals can be projected to increase in the coming years, with the expected increased commercialisation of herbal supplements, and for herbal formulations, the business will flourish. It was found that the safety and inexpensiveness of plant products could lead to tremendous manipulation of plants and its parts in the future.

Acknowledgments

The authors are grateful to Dr. L. Rathaiah Chairman of Vignan Group of Institutions for supporting us to complete the present chapter.

References

Agrawal, P., Rai, V. and Singh, R. B., 1996. Randomized placebo-controlled, single blind trial of holy basil leaves in patients with noninsulin-dependent diabetes mellitus. *International journal of clinical pharmacology and therapeutics*, *34*(9), pp. 406-409.

Ahmad, M. Z., Alasiri, A. S., Ahmad, J., Alqahtani, A. A., Abdullah, M. M., Abdel-Wahab, B. A., Pathak, K., Saikia, R., Das, A., Sarma, H. and Alzahrani, S. A., 2022. Green Synthesis of Titanium Dioxide Nanoparticles Using Ocimum sanctum Leaf Extract: *In Vitro* Characterization and Its Healing Efficacy in Diabetic Wounds. *Molecules*, *27*(22), p.7712.

Ahmad, M. Z., Ali, M. and Mir, S. R., 2012. Anti-diabetic activity of Ocimum sanctum L. roots and isolation of new phytoconstituents using two-dimensional nuclear magnetic resonance spectroscopy. *J Pharmacogn Phytother*, *4*, pp. 75-85.

Antora, R. A. and Salleh, R. M., 2017. Antihyperglycemic effect of Ocimum plants: A short review. *Asian Pacific Journal of Tropical Biomedicine*, *7*(8), pp. 755-759.

Benowitz, N. L., Katzung, B. G., Masters, S. B. and Trevor, A. J., 2011. Drugs used in hypertension. *Basic and clinical pharmacology. New York: McGraw-Hill Medical*, pp. 182-4.

Casanova, L. M., Da Silva, D. and Sola-Penna, M., Camargo LMdM., Celestrini DdM, Tinoco L. W., Costa S. S. (2014). Identification of chicoric acid as a hypoglycemic agent from Ocimum gratissimum leaf extract in a biomonitoring *in vivo* study. *Fitoterapia*, *93*, pp. 132-141.

Chattopadhyay, R. R., 1993. Hypoglycemic effect of Ocimum sanctum leaf extract in normal and streptozotocin diabetic rats. *Indian journal of experimental biology*, *31*(11), pp. 891-893.

Deshpande, A. D. and Harris-Hayes, M., 2008. Schootman: Epidemiology of diabetes and diabetes-related complications. *M Phys Ther*, *88*, pp. 1254-1264.

Ezeani, C., Ezenyi, I., Okoye, T. and Okoli, C., 2017. Ocimum basilicum extract exhibits antidiabetic effects via inhibition of hepatic glucose mobilization and carbohydrate metabolizing enzymes. *Journal of intercultural ethnopharmacology*, *6*(1), p. 22.

Federation, I. D., 2021. IDF Diabetes Atlas, tenth. *International Diabetes*.

Gandhi, R., Chauhan, B. and Jadeja, G., 2016. Effect of Ocimum sanctum (Tulsi) powder on hyperglycemic patient. *Indian Journal of Applied Research*, *6*(5).

Gholap, S. and Kar, A., 2004. Hypoglycaemic effects of some plant extracts are possibly mediated through inhibition in corticosteroid concentration. *Die Pharmazie-An International Journal of Pharmaceutical Sciences*, *59*(11), pp. 876-878.

Ghorbani, A., 2013. Best herbs for managing diabetes: a review of clinical studies. *Brazilian Journal of Pharmaceutical Sciences*, *49*, pp. 413-422.

Grover, J. K., Vats, V. and Yadav, S. S., 2005. Pterocarpus marsupium extract (Vijayasar) prevented the alteration in metabolic patterns induced in the normal rat by feeding an adequate diet containing fructose as sole carbohydrate. *Diabetes, Obesity and Metabolism*, *7*(4), pp. 414-420.

Hannan, J., Ojo, O., Rokeya, L., Khaleque, J., Akhter, M., Flatt, P. and Abdel-Wahab, Y., 2014. Actions underlying antidiabetic effects of Ocimum sanctum leaf extracts in animal models of type 1 and type 2 diabetes.

Hannan, J. M. A., Marenah, L., Ali, L., Rokeya, B., Flatt, P. R. and Abdel-Wahab, Y. H. A., 2006. Ocimum sanctum leaf extracts stimulate insulin secretion from perfused pancreas, isolated islets and clonal pancreatic beta-cells. *Journal of Endocrinology*, *189*(1), p. 127.

Jaggi, R. K., Madaan, R. and Singh, B., 2003. Anticonvulsant potential of holy basil, Ocimum sanctum Linn., and its cultures.

Jarald, E., Joshi, S. B. and Jain, D., 2008. Diabetes and herbal medicines.

Jayant, S. K. and Srivastava, N., 2016. Effect of Ocimum sanctum against alloxan induced diabetes and biochemical alterations in rats. *Integr Obesity Diabetes*, *2*(5), pp. 1-4.

Jonnalagadd, V. G. and Selkar, N., 2013. Antidiabetic herbal products marketed in India: An update. *Journal of Medicinal Plants*, *1*(6).

Keezhipadathil, J., 2019. Evaluation of suspected adverse drug reactions of oral anti-diabetic drugs in a tertiary care hospital for type ii diabetes mellitus. *Indian Journal of Pharmacy Practice*, *12*(2).

Kelm, M. A., Nair, M. G., Strasburg, G. M. and DeWitt, D. L., 2000. Antioxidant and cyclooxygenase inhibitory phenolic compounds from Ocimum sanctum Linn. *Phytomedicine*, *7*(1), pp. 7-13.

Khan, M. S. A. and Ahmad, I., 2019. Herbal medicine: current trends and future prospects. In *New look to phytomedicine* (pp. 3-13). Academic Press.

Kochhar, A., Sharma, N. and Sachdeva, R., 2009. Effect of supplementation of Tulsi (Ocimum sanctum) and Neem (Azadirachta indica) leaf powder on diabetic symptoms, anthropometric parameters and blood pressure of non insulin dependent male diabetics. *Studies on Ethno-Medicine*, *3*(1), pp. 5-9.

Luthy, N. and Martinez-Fortun, O., 1964. A study of a possible oral hypoglycemic factor in albahaca morada (Ocimum sanctum L.).

Malapermal, V., Botha, I., Krishna, S. B. N. and Mbatha, J. N., 2017. Enhancing antidiabetic and antimicrobial performance of Ocimum basilicum, and Ocimum sanctum (L.) using silver nanoparticles. *Saudi Journal of Biological Sciences*, *24*(6), pp. 1294-1305.

Martiz, R. M., Patil, S. M., Thirumalapura Hombegowda, D., Shbeer, A. M., Alqadi, T., Al-Ghorbani, M., Ramu, R. and Prasad, A., 2022. Phyto-computational intervention of diabetes mellitus at multiple stages using isoeugenol from Ocimum tenuiflorum: A combination of pharmacokinetics and molecular modelling approaches. *Molecules*, *27*(19), p. 6222.

Mishra, L. K., Sarkar, D., Mentreddy, R. and Shetty, K., 2020. Evaluation of phenolic bioactive-linked anti-hyperglycemic and Helicobacter pylori inhibitory activities of Asian Basil (Ocimum spp.) varieties. *Journal of Herbal Medicine*, *20*, p. 100310.

Mondal, S., Mirdha, B. R. and Mahapatra, S. C., 2009. The science behind sacredness of Tulsi (Ocimum sanctum Linn.). *Indian J Physiol Pharmacol*, *53*(4), pp. 291-306.

Moradi, B., Abbaszadeh, S., Shahsavari, S., Alizadeh, M. and Beyranvand, F., 2018. The most useful medicinal herbs to treat diabetes. *Biomedical research and therapy*, *5*(8), pp. 2538-2551.

Narendhirakannan, R. T., Subramanian, S. and Kandaswamy, M., 2006. Biochemical evaluation of antidiabetogenic properties of some commonly used Indian plants on streptozotocin-induced diabetes in experimental rats. *Clinical and Experimental Pharmacology and Physiology*, *33*(12), pp. 1150-1157.

Pattanayak, P., Behera, P., Das, D. and Panda, S. K., 2010. Ocimum sanctum Linn. A reservoir plant for therapeutic applications: An overview. *Pharmacognosy reviews*, *4*(7), p. 95.

Rai, V. A., Iyer, U. and Mani, U. V., 1997. Effect of Tulasi (Ocimum sanctum) leaf powder supplementation on blood sugar levels, serum lipids and tissues lipids in diabetic rats. *Plant foods for human nutrition*, *50*, pp. 9-16.

Rao, S. A., Vijay, Y., Deepthi, T., Lakshmi, C. S., Rani, V. and Rani, S., 2013. Antidiabetic effect of ethanolic extract of leaves of Ocimum sanctum in alloxan induced diabetes in rats. *Int J Basic Clin Pharmacol*, *2*(5), pp. 613-616.

Rizvi, S. I. and Mishra, N., 2013. Traditional Indian medicines used for the management of diabetes mellitus. *Journal of diabetes research*, *2013*.

Saran, R., Li, Y. and Robinson, B., 2015. US Renal Data System 2014 Annual Data Report: Epidemiology of Kidney Disease in the United States (vol 66, pg S1, 2015). *American Journal of Kidney Diseases*, *66*(3), pp. 545-545.

Sethi, J., Sood, S., Seth, S. and Talwar, A., 2004. Evaluation of hypoglycemic and antioxidant effect of Ocimum sanctum. *Indian Journal of Clinical Biochemistry*, *19*, pp. 152-155.

Singh, A. K., Pandey, H., Ramteke, P. W. and Mishra, S. B., 2019. Nano-suspension of ursolic acid for improving oral bioavailability and attenuation of type II diabetes: A histopathological investigation. *Biocatalysis and Agricultural Biotechnology*, *22*, p. 101433.

Singh, P., Jayaramaiah, R. H., Agawane, S. B., Vannuruswamy, G., Korwar, A. M., Anand, A., Dhaygude, V. S., Shaikh, M. L., Joshi, R. S., Boppana, R. and Kulkarni, M. J., 2016. Potential dual role of eugenol in inhibiting advanced glycation end products in diabetes: proteomic and mechanistic insights. Scientific reports, 6(1), p. 18798.

Siragam, S. L., 2022. Biomedical Applications of Phytonanotechnology. In *Phytonanotechnology* (pp. 77-97). Singapore: Springer Nature Singapore.

Somasundaram, G., Manimekalai, K., Salwe, K. J. and Pandiamunian, J., 2012. Evaluation of the antidiabetic effect of Ocimum sanctum in type 2 diabetic patients. *International journal of life science and pharma research*, *5*, pp. 75-81.

Srivastava, A., Pandey, V., Yadav, V., Singh, S. and Srivastava, R., 2023. Potential of hydroethanolic leaf extract of Ocimum sanctum in ameliorating redox status and lung injury in COPD: an *in vivo* and in silico study. *Scientific Reports*, *13*(1), p. 1131.

Steinmetz, J. D., Bourne, R. R., Briant, P. S., Flaxman, S. R., Taylor, H. R., Jonas, J. B., Abdoli, A. A., Abrha, W. A., Abualhasan, A., Abu-Gharbieh, E. G. and Adal, T. G., 2021. Causes of blindness and vision impairment in 2020 and trends over 30 years, and prevalence of avoidable blindness in relation to VISION 2020: the Right to Sight: an analysis for the Global Burden of Disease Study. *The Lancet Global Health*, *9*(2), pp. e144-e160.

Suanarunsawat, T., Anantasomboon, G. and Piewbang, C., 2016. Anti-diabetic and anti-oxidative activity of fixed oil extracted from Ocimum sanctum L. leaves in diabetic rats. *Experimental and therapeutic medicine*, *11*(3), pp. 832-840.

Tran, N., Pham, B. and Le, L., 2020. Bioactive compounds in anti-diabetic plants: From herbal medicine to modern drug discovery. *Biology*, *9*(9), p. 252.

Vats, V., Yadav, S. P. and Grover, J. K., 2004. Ethanolic extract of Ocimum sanctum leaves partially attenuates streptozotocin-induced alterations in glycogen content and carbohydrate metabolism in rats. *Journal of ethnopharmacology*, *90*(1), pp. 155-160.

Venkatesan, P. and Sengupta, R., 2015. Effect of supplementation of Tulsi leaves or curry leaves or combination of both type 2 diabetes. *International Journal of Pure & Applied Bioscience (IJPAB)*, *3*(2), pp. 331-337.

Verma, S., Gupta, M., Popli, H. and Aggarwal, G., 2018. Diabetes mellitus treatment using herbal drugs. *International Journal of Phytomedicine*, *10*(1), pp. 1-10.

Wannes, W. A. and Marzouk, B., 2016. Research progress of Tunisian medicinal plants used for acute diabetes. *Journal of Acute Disease*, *5*(5), pp. 357-363.

Wongsa, P., Chaiwarit, J. and Zamaludien, A., 2012. *In vitro* screening of phenolic compounds, potential inhibition against α-amylase and α-glucosidase of culinary herbs in Thailand. *Food Chemistry*, *131*(3), pp. 964-971.

Chapter 10

Azadirachta Indica as an Antidiabetic Plant: Current Status and Future Prospects

Noopur Srivastava[1,*]
Nisha Saxena[2]
and Chhaya Dagar[1]

[1]Department of Chemistry and Biochemistry, Sharda School of Basic Sciences and Research, Sharda University, Greater Noida, Uttar Pradesh, India
[2]Department of Chemistry, M. R. M. College, Lalit Narayan Mithila University, Darbhanga, Bihar, India

Abstract

Azadirachta indica popularly known as 'wonder plant' is an evergreen tree, grown in various parts of the Indian subcontinent, one of those plants that has been greatly used in ayurveda, unani, and homoeopathic medicines and has become a focus of today's medicine. Also called 'Neem' in Hindi, NLEs (neem leaf extracts) have shown a reduction in glycogenolytic effect and glucose utilisation by muscles and adipose tissue (peripheral) due to the action of epinephrine. It has been reported to stop the suppressive consequence of serotonin on glucose-induced insulin secretion intervened by glucose. NLEs possess compounds such as rutin ($C_{27}H_{30}O_{16}$) and quercetin ($C_{15}H_{10}O_7$) that show hypoglycemic / antihyperglycemic effects. Meliacinolin, a tetranortriterpenoid isolated from neem leaf, and Azadirachtolide have shown an antidiabetic action. NLEs have also reported showing a wide spectrum of effects on diabetes control. Currently, there are many more challenges in the exploratory study of *A. indica*, such as new compounds and their role in the

* Corresponding Author's Email: noopursriv@gmail.com.

In: Antidiabetic Plants
Editor: Arpita Roy
ISBN: 979-8-88697-957-2

management of lipid metabolism, oxidative stress, insulin resistance, and response to enzymes.

Keywords: diabetes, neem, antidiabetic, hypoglycemia

Introduction

Phytoconstituents are promising leading candidates for antidiabetic pharmacological actions. phytoconstituents, such as flavonoids, glycosides, terpenoids, alkaloids, saponins, and carotenoids, play indispensable roles in antidiabetic regimes. The current chapter describes the ingredients of the antidiabetic components of *A. indica* with insulin mimetic activity. It is a multipurpose plant, known as a divine or miraculous tree, and has its origin in Asia. Research on *A. indica* dates back to the 1920s when an Indian researcher first discovered its insect repellent activity. In developing nations in Asia and Africa, neem enjoys a significant position due to its wide spectrum of medicinal value (Kumar et al., 2011). The name *A. indica* was assigned back in 1830 (De Jussiieu et al., 1830).

Taxonomy and Morphology

A. indica (Neem tree) is found in tropical and semi-tropical regions. It belongs to the Meliaceae family (mahogany family) (Gautam et al., 2021).

The A. indica tree has a height of 15-20 m. It is an evergreen tree. In extreme drought, it may shed most or nearly all of its leaves. The branches are extensive. Almost each part of the neem tree has been reported to have some medicinal property or the other.

It grows where precipitation is as little as 46 cm per year and flourishes in areas that suffer from oppressive heat of up to 49-50°C. It can live up to 200 years (Kirtikar et al., 1975; Thakur et al., 1981, Koul et al., 1990; Pakrashi et al., 1994).

History and Geographical Distribution

A. indica is found to occur in more than 78 countries around the world, mainly in India and neighbouring nations. It adapts to various types of soils such as clay, sandy, saline and soils with pH 4-10. Approximately there are around 20 million trees in India itself, which is 60% of the total population of *A. indica* in the world (Sharma et al., 2022, Kumar et al., 2009, Siddiqui et al., 2004, Akhila et al., 1999, Bhat et al., 2011, Perez-Gutierrez et al., 2012, Pillai et al., 1981, Kumar et al., 2011).

The neem tree is capable of tolerating drought. It dwells in areas that have precipitation between 40 and 120 cm annually. It can grow in locations where annual precipitation is below 40 cm, depending on ground water levels. It cannot tolerate a temperature below 4 ° C (shedding of leaves and death may follow).

Genome

The first attempts at A. indica gene sequencing of *A. indica* were made in 2012 but whole genome sequencing, total expression of ARN, and the metabolite profiling studies were published (Kuravadi et al., 2019). They also reported that 32,278 genes were differentially expressed out of 44,495 genes and 87Mb of repetitive DNA in the neem. In another finding, they reported 267 Mb as the size of the neem genome at 70% (Kurvadi et al., 2015; Bhambani et al., 2017; Bhambani et al., 2017a, Bhambani et al., 2017b). In addition, they reported perfect bonds of AzaA and AzaB with AiCYP16671 and AiCYP16365 in molecular coupling studies. This also indicates that two CYPs are involved in AzaA biosynthesis. There have also been reports on the evaluation of genetic variability using the AFLP marker (Singh et al., 2002). Omic research was carried out on azadirachtin. However, further studies are required to find the biochemical route of the main metabolites. Also, due to the overwhelming medicinal properties, neem plantation should be taken up in large numbers. Treatment of diabetes involves many parameters; several genes control it (Baliga et al., 2011).

Chemical Constitution

It has more than 300 biologically active molecules, although they are not evenly distributed in plant parts. The fruits of the neem plant have higher levels of bioactive phytochemicals than other tissues. Classes of compounds include flavonoids, catechins, gallic acid, saponins, nimbins, limonoids, azadirachtins, and epoxy-azadirodione.

More than 60 constituents have been isolated from Neem leaf extracts (NLEs) The important ones are –Azadirachtin, Ascorbic acid, Chlorogenic acid, Hyperoside, Kaempferol, Kaempferol-3-o-rutinoside, Myricetin, Nimbafalavone, Nimbandial, Nimbin, Nimbin-6-deacetyl, Nimbenene, Nimbocinolide, Nimbocinone, Nimbolide, Nimocin, Nimocinol, Nimocinolide, Quercetin, Quercetin-rhamnoside, Rutin, Scopoletin, Stigmaterol, Valasinin, and Zafaral.(Yadav et al., 2016) Many more components with medicinal value have also been reported Figure 1 (Sharma et al., 2022, Kumar et al., 2009, Chattopadhyay et al., 1999, Siddiqui et al.).

Meliacinolin exhibited repression of α-glucosidase and α-amylase enzyme activities in vitro. In addition to blood glucose level, other variables were also found to be re-established in streptozotocin-induced diabetic mice to normal levels (Perez Gutierrez et al., 2012).

Nimbidin, when administered orally, demonstrated an appreciable hypoglycaemic effect in fasting rabbits (Pillai et al., 1981).

Azadirachtolide (tetranortriterpenoid from *A. indica* leaves) exhibited significant anti-diabetic and hypolipidemic effects by lowering the levels of FBS (fasting blood sugar), TC (total cholesterol), TG (triglycerides), LDL (low-density protein), and VLDL (very low-density lipoproteins) levels; but also with an elevation of HDL (high-density lipoprotein) level in diabetic rats. Azadirachtolide showed appreciable inhibition against α amylase and α glucosidase (Kumar et al., 2011).

Zafaral and *meliacin anhydride of* these two triterpenoids were extracted from neem leaves using methanol. The other two isolated bioactive compounds isolated were nimocinol and isomeldenin (terpenoids) (Siddiqui et al., 2004).

Quercetin $C_{15}H_{10}O_7$, *Myricetin* $C_{15}H_{10}O_8$, *Astragalin* $C_{21}H_{20}O_{11}$, *Quercitrin* $C_{21}H_{20}O_{11}$, *Isoquercitrin* $C_{21}H_{20}O_{12}$, *Nicotiflorin* C27H30O15, and *Rutin* $C_{27}H_{30}O_{16}$ extracted with *A. indica* contribute to its reduction of high blood glucose levels / lower blood glucose levels. These are flavonoids and additionally show antioxidant properties. They provide the possibility of serving as a substitute to check the pathogenesis of diabetes and its related complications (Vergallo et al., 2019).

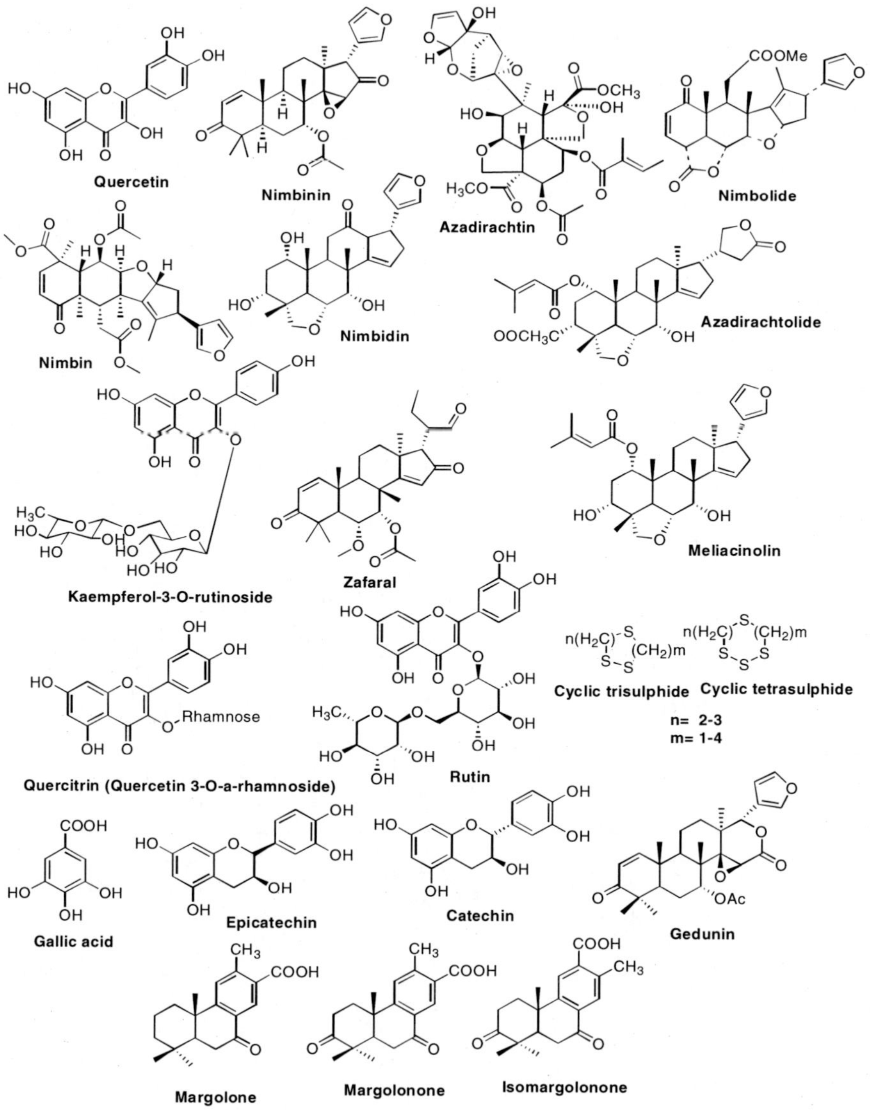

Figure 1. Medicinally important compounds from *A. indica*.

Medicinal Value

Various medicine systems around the world, such as Ayurveda, Chinese medicine, and Unani, have recognised the potential of *A. indica*. The European 'Materia Medica' (early system of medicine) have conferred *A. indica* as the 'Panacea of all diseases'. Indians worship *A. Indica* and call it 'Village Dispensary', 'Divine Tree', 'Nature's Drugstore', 'Heal All', etc. *A. indica* has been used in the treatment of mycobacterial infections (leprosy, tuberculosis), fever, malaria, and ophthalmia in the traditional Ayurveda system. Insecticide, anthelmintic, antifeedant, diuretic, antiseptic, emmenagogue (stimulates menstrual flow), contraceptive, febrifuge (fever control), parasiticide, pediculocide (controlling head lice), and other folk remedies have been reported. It was administered by different routes including oral, vaginal, and topical use. Neem twigs are used to brush your teeth in the Indian subcontinent. Its juice is used to treat skin disorders and keeping *A. indica* leaves in homes helps combat insects.

Table 1. Biological evaluation of different parts of *A. indica*

Pharmacological activity	Part	Chemical constituent
Inhibit Chemiluminescence Generation	Bark	Tannins
Anti-inflammatory and immunomodulatory		(-) epicatechin, gallic acid, Catechin,
Antibacterial		Margolone, Isomargolone, Diterpenoids, Margolonone
Antitumor		Polysaccharides GIaGIb
Anti-inflammatory		Polysaccharide GIIaGIIa
Antiulcer, Antiacid		Glycoside
Diuretic, Spasmolytic, Hypotensive		Ethanolic Extract
Inflammation		Chloroform Extract
Immune stimulant, Anticomplement		Aqueous Extract
Analgesic, alternative and curative fever		Ayurvedic
Antifungal	Leaf	Cyclic Trisulphide
		Tetra sulphide
Hyperglycemic		(Flavonoid)
		Quercetin
Antipyretic and inhibit plaque formation		Methanolic Extract
Immune stimulation, hypoglycemia, antiulcer, antifertility, antiviral, anticarcinogenic, hepatoprotective		Aqueous Extract
CNS depressant		Acetone extract

Pharmacological activity	Part	Chemical constituent
Skin ulcer, Leprosy, ophthalmic problems, anorexia, epistaxis, anorexia, intestinal worms, biliousness		Ayurvedic
Anti-inflammatory and antipyretic	Oil	Nimbidine
Antimalarial and antibacterial		Nimbine
		Nimbolide
Antifeedant and antimalarial		Azadirachtin
Leprosy and intestinal worms		Ayurvedic
antiulcer	Fruit	Phytosterols
Leprosy, wounds, pellets, intestinal worm, epistaxis, phlegm, diabetes, urinary infection		Ayurvedic

The A. indica tree as a whole (including bark, seeds, flowers, and leaves) is used for the preparation of many different medical preparations. Oil from *A. Indica* seeds find utility in cosmetics, such as acne treatment and maintaining skin elasticity. Patients suffering from chicken pox sleep on leaves in India due to its therapeutic value. (Alzohairy et al., 2016, Elakovich et al., 1995). Table 1 illustrates the biological activity reported from different parts of *A. indica* (Biswas et al., 2002).

Antidiabetic Potential

Diabetes is the leading cause of major morbidity and mortality worldwide (Stefan et al., 2003). Three types of diabetes have been reported (Figure 2). The numerous reasons for the increase in the incidence of diabetes are urbanisation, obesity, physical inactivity, and a sedentary lifestyle. The economic consequences of diabetes with its complications and related diseases are large (Wild et al., 2004). Recent reports state that the prevalence of diabetes mellitus is 4% worldwide, approximately 143 million affected persons and is further anticipated to increase to 300 million by 2025 (Mitra et al., 2007). In metropolitan India, death rates are two times higher in people with diabetes compared to healthy individuals (Mohan et al., 2006). Treatment of diabetes with western classical medicines (allopathy) is expensive (Kumar et al., 2009). Therefore, it is necessary to look for herbal alternatives that are comparatively cheaper with fewer side effects.

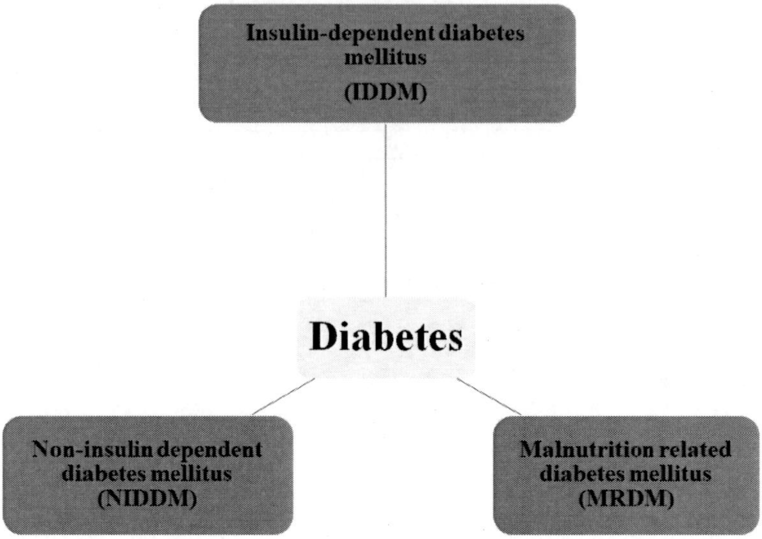

Figure 2. Types of diabetes.

In this regard, some targets have been identified to control diabetes. The first is α-Glucosidase enzyme which is vital in carbohydrate metabolism, as it hydrolyses the terminal glycosidic bonds of saccharides to release α-glucose. Second, some α-glucosidase inhibitors are reported as clinical drugs, eg miglitol and acarbose, these hypoglycemic agents have restrictions and show serious complications (Scott et al., 2000). Third, the decrease in starch digestion by inhibiting the enzyme α-amylase plays a crucial role in the management of diabetes (Eichler et al., 1984).

Exhaustion of peripheral utilisation of glucose and glycogenolytic effect due to the epinephrine action of NLEs of *A. indica* leaf extract has been reported (Chattopadhyay et al., 1999). In another finding, he reported that NLEs blocked the inhibitory effect of serotonin on glucose-mediated insulin secretion (Kumar et al., 2009).

Agunbiade et al., in their findings, administered aqueous plant extract of *A. conyzoides* in an animal model and discovered a reduction in fasting blood glucose of 39.1%. The study led to the indication that the plant extract had less antidiabetic activity than the conventional anti-diabetic drugs (Agunbiade et al., 2012). Interpretations of studies by Nyunai et al. suggest that the leaves of *A. conyzoides leaves* can lower blood glucose levels in normal blood glucose and in streptozotocin-induced hyperglycemic rats (Nyunai et al., 2009).

A hypoglycemic effect was observed in rats after 4 weeks that were induced by alloxan-induced diabetes from leaf extracts of *A. indica.* The results were comparable to those of glibenclamide (oral hypoglycemic drug) (Khosla et al., 2000).

A. indica extracts ($CHCl_3$, CH_3OH and aqueous) were reviewed for diabetes and showed acceptable tolerance for oral glucose and significantly reduced intestinal activity of glucosidase. It also showed an increase in glucose-6-phosphate dehydrogenase activity. The results suggest that the chloroform extracts of *A. indica* and the aqueous extracts are satisfactory aspirants for the treatment of diabetes.

A decrease in serum lipids, blood glucose and serum enzymes and HMG CoA reductase activity was observed in the intestine and liver of alloxan-diabetic rabbits when *A. indica* extracts alone and in combination with glibenclamide (Bopanna et al., 1997).

A decrease in blood glucose was detected in vacuum dried 95% ethanolic vacuum-dried extracts), in albino rats with albino rats with alloxan diabetes. This was repeated once, twice, or three times daily. When evaluating analogous hypoglycaemic activity of the investigational *A. Indica* samples, significant blood glucose-lowering activities are pronounced (Kar et al., 2003).

Gymnema sylvestre and *A. indica* and extracts exhibit hypoglycemic activity irrespective of serum cortisol concentration. Type II diabetes mellitus (NIDDM) may result from chronic elevation of serum corticosteroids (Ganong et al., 1995). Although some plant extracts are known to act as antihyperglycemic and antistressor agents.

Hypoglycaemic effects of *A. indica* are also reported due to inhibition of corticosteroids concentration. Cortisol has been reported to increase gluconeogenesis and decrease peripheral glucose utilisation, leading to diabetes mellitus (Gholap et al., 2004). Excess endogenous or exogenous cortisol results in an increase in serum glucose concentration and potentially induces diabetes mellitus. Therefore, it can be presumed that a plant extract like *A. indica*, which inhibits cortisol secretion, may relieve hyperglycemia (Jeffers et al., 1991).

Two widely used analogues for the induction of diabetes in laboratory animals are alloxan and streptozotocin (Rerup et al., 1970; Mishra et al., 1986). Table 2 summarises the *in vivo* antidiabetic reports for *A. indica.*

Table 2. In vivo Antidiabetic activity reported for *A. indica*

Plant Part	Type of Extract	Dose (mg/kg)	antidiabetic activity	References
Leaves	$CHCl_3$	100/200L	antihyperglycemic	Meenakshi et al., 2011
	Aqueous	500	increased activity of antioxidant enzymes, antihyperglycemic activity, Hb1Ac	Shailey et al., 2012
	Aqueous	250	hypoglycaemic	Kar et 2003
	Aqueous	25-350	hypoglycaemic	Arika et al., 2016
	Aqueous	200	hypoglycaemic	Salehi et al., 2019
	Hot aqueous	-	diabetes wound healing, angiogenesis	Bhagavathy et al., 2016
	Aqueous	200	increased activity of antioxidant enzymes, hypoglycemic effect	Halim et al., 2003
	Aqueous	-	increased activity of antioxidant enzymes, and enzyme inhibitory effects	Christian et al., 2019
	Aqueous	250	hypoglycemic effect	Shori et al., 2013
	Aqueous	250	hypoglycemic effect	Dholi et al., 2011
		500	hypoglycemic effect	Khosla et al., 2000
	Alcoholic	1	hypoglycemic effect	Akter et al., 2013
	Aqueous	620	beta cell regeneration, increase serum	McCalla et al., 2016
	Alcoholic	500	angiogenesis effect, inhibition of hyperglycemia, increased activity of antioxidant enzymes	Gautam et al., 2015
	Aqueous	500		Upreti et al., 2013
	Aqueous	400	Improvement in insulin signalling molecules (*all proteins involved in the action of insulin in the body and the factors that* regulate this pathway) and glucose consumption in the skeletal muscle	Satyanarayana et al., 2015
	Aqueous	400	hypoglycemic effect	Chattopadhyay et al., 1999
	Aqueous alcohol	oral	decline in blood sugar levels	Subapriya et al., 2005
	Aqueous		the equivalent dry leaf in capsules reduced insulin dosage by 30-50%	Shukla et al., 1973
	10% liquid water extract		hypoglycemic effect	Luscombe et al., 1974

Plant Part	Type of Extract	Dose (mg/kg)	antidiabetic activity	References
Flower	Methanol	250	hypoglycemic effect	Ezin et al., 2023
Bark	Aqueous	100	Increased antioxidant enzymes, antihyperglycemic activity, Hb1Ac reduction	Shailey et al., 2012
Stem	Neem sticks (toothbrush)		reduction in serum MCP-1	Anbalagan et al., 2017
Fruit/Seed	Seed oil	5 ml/kg	hypoglycemic effect	Khosla 2005
	Petroleum ether	2	oxidative stress prevention	Gupta et al., 2004
	Petroleum ether	0.9		
Roots	Alcoholic	800	antihyperglycemic and hypoglycemic activity alloxan reduction	Patil et al., 2013
Root & bark	Methanol Methanol		Reduction in triglycerides (32%), creatinine (23%), glucose (18%) cholesterol (15%), lipids (15%), urea (13%)	Patil et al., 2013,
		Glucosidase assay	inhibition by 62.44%	Srivastava et al., 2020
		in mice	41.07%	Srivastava et al., 2020

Controlling Blood Sugar through Antioxidant Properties

G6PD accelerates the reaction of the first pentose phosphate pathway, leading to a decrease in NADPH. Any change in G6PD will alter NADPH levels and negatively impact the entire antioxidant system. Endocrine cells are very sensitive to chemical oxidation and inflammation (Mesgari-Abbasi et al., 2022), which activate the insulin resistance process, leading to diabetes (Shailey et al., 2012; Omóbwálé et al., 2016). *A. indica* leaf and bark extracts have re-established these altered factors very close to the controls.

Conclusion

Anti-diabetic activity is very attractive, which is mainly a result of anti-inflammatory activity. Controlling the generation of reactive oxygen species can be a measure of prevention and intensification of diabetes. Using research-based and technological innovation, we can now use these extracts as current medical supports, understanding their potentials. On the existing knowledge of *A. indica*, further studies and applications of this wonder plant can pave the way for future developments.

References

Agunbiade, O. S., Ojezele, O. M., Ojezele, J. O. and Ajayi, A. Y., 2012. Hypoglycaemic activity of Commelina africana and Ageratum conyzoides in relation to their mineral composition. *African health sciences*, *12*(2), pp.198-203.

Akhila, A., Adam, G., Rani, K., Schmidt, J., Schneider, B., Akhila, A. and Rani, K., 1999. Chemistry of the neem tree (Azadirachta indica A. Juss.). *Fortschritte der Chemie Organischer Naturstoffe/Progress in the chemistry of organic natural products*, pp.47-149.

Akhila, A., Adam, G., Rani, K., Schmidt, J., Schneider, B., Akhila, A. and Rani, K., 1999. Chemistry of the neem tree (Azadirachta indica A. Juss.). *Fortschritte der Chemie Organischer Naturstoffe/Progress in the chemistry of organic natural products*, pp.47-149.

Akter, R., Mahabub-Uz-Zaman, M., Rahman, M. S., Khatun, M. A., Abdullah, A. M., Ahmed, N. U. and Islam, F., 2013. Comparative studies on antidiabetic effect with phytochemical screening of Azadirachta indicia and Andrographis paniculata. *IOSR Journal of Pharmacy and Biological Sciences*, *5*(2), pp.122-128.

Alzohairy, M. A., 2016. Therapeutics role of Azadirachta indica (Neem) and their active constituents in diseases prevention and treatment. *Evidence-Based Complementary and Alternative Medicine*, *2016*.

Anbalagan, R., Srikanth, P., Mani, M., Barani, R., Seshadri, K. G. and Janarthanan, R., 2017. Next generation sequencing of oral microbiota in Type 2 diabetes mellitus prior to and after neem stick usage and correlation with serum monocyte chemoattractant-1. *Diabetes Research and Clinical Practice*, *130*, pp.204-210.

Arika, W. M., Nyamai, D. W., Agyirifo, D. S., Ngugi, M. P. and Njagi, E. N. M., 2016. In vivo antidiabetic effect of aqueous leaf extract of Azardirachta indica, A. juss in alloxan induced diabetic mice. *Journal of Diabetic Complications and Medicine*, *1*(2), pp.1-6.

Baliga, M. S., Bhat, H. P., Pai, R. J., Boloor, R. and Palatty, P. L., 2011. The chemistry and medicinal uses of the underutilized Indian fruit tree Garcinia indica Choisy (kokum): a review. *Food Research International*, *44*(7), pp.1790-1799.

Bhagavathy, S. and Kancharla, S., 2016. Wound healing and angiogenesis of silver nanoparticle from Azadirachta indica in diabetes induced mice. *Int. J. Herb. Med*, *4*, pp.24-29.

Bhambhani, S., Lakhwani, D., Gupta, P., Pandey, A., Dhar, Y. V., Kumar Bag, S., Asif, M. H. and Kumar Trivedi, P., 2017. Transcriptome and metabolite analyses in Azadirachta indica: identification of genes involved in biosynthesis of bioactive triterpenoids. *Scientific reports*, *7*(1), p.5043.

Bhambhani, S., Lakhwani, D., Shukla, T., Pandey, A., Dhar, Y. V., Asif, M. H. and Trivedi, P. K., 2017. Genes encoding members of 3-hydroxy-3-methylglutaryl coenzyme A reductase (HMGR) gene family from Azadirachta indica and correlation with azadirachtin biosynthesis. *Acta Physiologiae Plantarum, 39*, pp.1-13.

Bhat, M., Kothiwale, S. K., Tirmale, A. R., Bhargava, S. Y. and Joshi, B. N., 2011. Antidiabetic properties of Azardiracta indica and Bougainvillea spectabilis: in vivo studies in murine diabetes model. *Evidence-Based Complementary and Alternative Medicine, 2011.*

Bhat, M., Kothiwale, S. K., Tirmale, A. R., Bhargava, S. Y. and Joshi, B. N., 2011. Antidiabetic properties of Azardiracta indica and Bougainvillea spectabilis: in vivo studies in murine diabetes model. *Evidence-Based Complementary and Alternative Medicine, 2011.*

Bhat, M., Zinjarde, S. S., Bhargava, S. Y., Kumar, A. R. and Joshi, B. N., 2011. Antidiabetic Indian plants: a good source of potent amylase inhibitors. *Evidence-Based Complementary and Alternative Medicine, 2011.*

Biswas, K., Chattopadhyay, I., Banerjee, R. K. and Bandyopadhyay, U., 2002. Biological activities and medicinal properties of neem (Azadirachta indica). *Current science*, pp.1336-1345.

Bopanna, K. N., Kannan, J., Sushma, G., Balaraman, R. and Rathod, S. P., 1997. Antidiabetic and antihyperlipaemic effects of neem seed kernel powder on alloxan diabetic rabbits. *Indian journal of Pharmacology*, *29*(3), p.162.

Chatterjee, A. and Pakrashi, S. C., 1994. The treatise of Indian medicinal plants (Publication and information Directorate, CSIR. New Delhi).

Chattopadhyay, R. R., 1999. Possible mechanism of antihyperglycemic effect of Azadirachta indica leaf extract: part V. *Journal of ethnopharmacology*, *67*(3), pp.373-376.

Chattopadhyay, R. R., 1999. Possible mechanism of antihyperglycemic effect of Azadirachta indica leaf extract: part V. *Journal of ethnopharmacology*, *67*(3), pp.373-376.

Christian, E. O., Felicia, E. C., Helen, I. N., Nneka, S. V., Vivian, C. U. and Ogochukwu, A. P., 2019. Antidiabetic property and antioxidant potentials of aqueous extract of Azadirachta indica leaves in streptozotocininduced diabetic rats. *J Med Plants Stud (Internet)*, *7*(6), pp.18-23.

Dholi, S. K., Raparla, R., Mankala, S. K. and Nagappan, K., 2011. Invivo Antidiabetic evaluation of Neem leaf extract in alloxan induced rats. *Journal of applied Pharmaceutical science*, (Issue), pp.100-105.

Eichler, H. G., Korn, A., Gasic, S., Pirson, W. and Businger, J., 1984. The effect of a new specific α-amylase inhibitor on post-prandial glucose and insulin excursions in normal subjects and type 2 (non-insulin-dependent) diabetic patients. *Diabetologia*, *26*, pp.278-281.

Elakovich, S. D., 1996. The Neem Tree: Source of Unique Natural Products for Integrated Pest Management, Medicinal, Industrial, & Other Purposes Edited by Heinrich Schmutterer (Giessen U., FGR). VCH: New York. 1995. xxi+ 680 pp. $125.00. ISBN 3-527-30054-6.

Ezin, V. and Chabi, I. B., 2023. Azadirachta indica: Its Biological, Pharmacological, Antidiabetic Potential, and Omics Applications. In *Antidiabetic Plants for Drug Discovery* (pp. 1-22). Apple Academic Press.

Ganong, W. F., 1995. Review of medical physiology. *Dynamics of blood and lymph flow*, *30*, pp.525-541.

Gautam, M. K., Gangwar, M., Singh, S. K. and Goel, R. K., 2015. Effects of Azardirachta indica on vascular endothelial growth factor and cytokines in diabetic deep wound. *Planta Medica*, *81*(09), pp.713-721.

Gautam, S., Thakur, M., Aggarwal, M. and Vatsa, E., 2021. Azadirachta Indica-A Review as a Potent Anti-Diabetic Drug. *J Sci Aliment Agrícola (Internet)*, *1*(10), pp.1-6.

Gholap, S. and Kar, A., 2004. Hypoglycaemic effects of some plant extracts are possibly mediated through inhibition in corticosteroid concentration. *Die Pharmazie-An International Journal of Pharmaceutical Sciences*, *59*(11), pp.876-878.

Gupta, S., Kataria, M., Gupta, P. K., Murganandan, S. and Yashroy, R. C., 2004. Protective role of extracts of neem seeds in diabetes caused by streptozotocin in rats. *Journal of Ethnopharmacology*, *90*(2-3), pp.185-189.

Halim, M., 2003. Lowering of blood sugar by water extract of Azadirachta indica and Abroma augusta in diabetes rats.

Jeffers, J. G., Shanley, K. J. and Schick, R. O., 1991. Diabetes mellitus induced in a dog after administration of corticosteroids and methylprednisolone pulse therapy. *Journal of the American Veterinary Medical Association*, *199*(1), pp.77-80.

Kar, A., Choudhary, B. K. and Bandyopadhyay, N. G., 2003. Comparative evaluation of hypoglycaemic activity of some Indian medicinal plants in alloxan diabetic rats. *Journal of ethnopharmacology*, *84*(1), pp.105-108.

Khosla, P., Bhanwra, S., Singh, J. and Srivastava, R. K., 2000. Antinociceptive activity of Azadirachta indica (neem) in rats. *Indian Journal of Pharmacology*, *32*(6), p.372.

Khosla, P., Bhanwra, S., Singh, J., Seth, S. and Srivastava, R. K., 2000. A Study of Hypoglycamic Effects Ofzyxwvutsrqponmlkjihgfedcba Azadirachta Indica (Neem) in Normal and Alloxan Diabetic Rabbits. *Indian J Physiol Pharmacol*, *44*(1), pp.69-74.

Kirtikar, K. R. and Basu, B. D., 1975. Medicinal Plants (edsBlatter, E., Cains, JF, Mhaskar, KS). *VivekVihar, New Delhi*, *536*.

Koul, O., Isman, M. B. and Ketkar, C. M., 1990. Properties and uses of neem, Azadirachta indica. *Canadian journal of botany*, *68*(1), pp.1-11.

Kumar, B. D., Mitra, A. and Manjunatha, M., 2009. In vitro and in vivo studies of antidiabetic Indian medicinal plants: A review. *Journal of herbal medicine and toxicology*, *3*(2), pp.9-14.

Kumar, D., Mitra, A. and Manjunatha, M., 2011. Azadirachtolide: An anti-diabetic and hypolipidemic effects from Azadirachta indica leaves. *Pharmacogn. Commun*, *1*, pp.78-84.

Kuravadi, N. A. and Gowda, M., 2019. Phylogeny of neem and related species in the Meliaceae family. *The Neem Genome*, pp.49-51.

Kuravadi, N. A., Yenagi, V., Rangiah, K., Mahesh, H. B., Rajamani, A., Shirke, M. D., Russiachand, H., Loganathan, R. M., Lingu, C. S., Siddappa, S. and Ramamurthy, A., 2015. Comprehensive analyses of genomes, transcriptomes and metabolites of neem tree. *PeerJ*, *3*, p.e1066.

Luscombe, D. K. and Taha, S. A., 1974. Pharmacological studies on the leaves of Azadirachta indica. *Journal of Pharmacy and Pharmacology*, *26*(Supplement_1), pp.110P-111P.

Ma, S., Cutter, J., Tan, C. E., Chew, S. K. and Tai, E. S., 2003. Associations of diabetes mellitus and ethnicity with mortality in a multiethnic Asian population: data from the 1992 Singapore National Health Survey. *American journal of epidemiology*, *158*(6), pp.543-552.

Maithani, A., Parcha, V., Pant, G., Dhulia, I. and Kumar, D., 2011. Azadirachta indica (neem) leaf: A review. *Journal of Pharmacy Research*, *4*(6), pp.1824-1827.

McCalla, G., Parshad, O., Brown, P. D. and Gardner, M. T., 2016. Beta Cell Regenerating Potential of Azadirachta indica (Neem) Extract in Diabetic Rats. *West Indian Medical Journal*, *65*(1).

Mesgari-Abbasi, M., Valizadeh, H., Mirzakhani, N. and Vahdatpour, T., 2022. Protective effects of di-and tri-peptides containing proline, glycine, and leucine on liver enzymology and histopathology of diabetic mice. *Archives of Physiology and Biochemistry*, *128*(1), pp.59-68.

Mishra, G. and Behera, H. N., 1986. Alloxan-induced changes in the collagen characteristics in the skin of male garden lizards, Calotes versicolor, from three age groups. *Archives of gerontology and geriatrics*, *5*(1), pp.11-19.

Mitra, A., Bhattacharya, D. and Roy, S., 2007. Dietary influence on TYPE 2 Diabetes (NIDDM). *Journal of Human Ecology*, *21*(2), pp.139-147.

Mohan, V., Shanthirani, C. S., Deepa, M., Deepa, R., Unnikrishnan, R. I. and Datta, M., 2006. Mortality rates due to diabetes in a selected urban south Indian population-the Chennai Urban Population Study (CUPS-16). *Journal of the Association of Physicians of India*, *54*, pp.113-117.

Nyunaï, N., Njikam, N., Abdenneb, E., Mbafor, J. and Lamnaouer, D., 2009. Hypoglycaemic and antihyperglycaemic activity of Ageratum conyzoides L. in rats. *African Journal of Traditional, Complementary and Alternative Medicines*, *6*(2).

Omóbòwálé, T. O., Oyagbemi, A. A., Adejumobi, O. A., Orherhe, E. V., Amid, A. S., Adedapo, A. A., Nottidge, H. O. and Yakubu, M. A., 2016. Preconditioning with Azadirachta indica ameliorates cardiorenal dysfunction through reduction in oxidative stress and extracellular signal regulated protein kinase signalling. *Journal of Ayurveda and Integrative Medicine*, *7*(4), pp.209-217.

Patil, P., Patil, S., Mane, A. and Verma, S., 2013. Antidiabetic activity of alcoholic extract of neem (Azadirachta indica) root bark. *National Journal of Physiology, Pharmacy and Pharmacology*, *3*(2), p.142.

Perez-Gutierrez, R. M. and Damian-Guzman, M., 2012. Meliacinolin: a potent α-glucosidase and α-amylase inhibitor isolated from Azadirachta indica leaves and in vivo antidiabetic property in streptozotocin-nicotinamide-induced type 2 diabetes in mice. *Biological and pharmaceutical bulletin*, *35*(9), pp.1516-1524.

Pillai, N. R. and Santhakumari, G., 1981. Hypoglycaemic activity of Melia azadirachta Linn (neem). *Indian journal of medical research*.

Pillai, N. R. and Santhakumari, G., 1981. Hypoglycaemic activity of Melia azadirachta Linn (neem). *Indian journal of medical research*.

Rerup, C. C., 1970. Drugs producing diabetes through damage of the insulin secreting cells. *Pharmacological reviews*, *22*(4), pp.485-518.

Salehi, B., Ata, A., V. Anil Kumar, N., Sharopov, F., Ramirez-Alarcon, K., Ruiz-Ortega, A., Abdulmajid Ayatollahi, S., Valere Tsouh Fokou, P., Kobarfard, F., Amiruddin

Zakaria, Z. and Iriti, M., 2019. Antidiabetic potential of medicinal plants and their active components. *Biomolecules*, *9*(10), p.551.

Satyanarayana, K., Sravanthi, K., Shaker, I. A. and Ponnulakshmi, R., 2015. Molecular approach to identify antidiabetic potential of Azadirachta indica. *Journal of Ayurveda and integrative medicine*, *6*(3), p.165.

Scott, L. J. and Spencer, C. M., 2000. Miglitol: a review of its therapeutic potential in type 2 diabetes mellitus. *Drugs*, *59*(3), pp.521-549.

Shailey, S. and Basir, S. F., 2012. Strengthening of antioxidant defense by Azadirachta indica in alloxan-diabetic rat tissues. *Journal of ayurveda and integrative medicine*, *3*(3), p.130.

Sharma, P., Hajam, Y. A., Kumar, R. and Rai, S., 2022. Complementary and alternative medicine for the treatment of diabetes and associated complications: A review on therapeutic role of polyphenols. *Phytomedicine Plus*, *2*(1), p.100188.

Shori, A. B. and Baba, A. S., 2013. Antioxidant activity and inhibition of key enzymes linked to type-2 diabetes and hypertension by Azadirachta indica-yogurt. *Journal of Saudi Chemical Society*, *17*(3), pp.295-301.

Shukla, R., Singh, S. and Bhandari, C. R., 1973. Preliminary clinical trial on antidiabetic actions of Azadirachta indica. *Medicine and surgery*, *13*(11).

Siddiqui, B. S., Afshan, F., Gulzar, T. and Hanif, M., 2004. Tetracyclic triterpenoids from the leaves of Azadirachta indica. *Phytochemistry*, *65*(16), pp.2363-2367.

Singh, A., Chaudhury, A., Srivastava, P. S. and Lakshmikumaran, M., 2002. Comparison of AFLP and SAMPL markers for assessment of intra-population genetic variation in Azadirachta indica A. Juss. *Plant Science*, *162*(1), pp.17-25.

Srivastava, S. K., Agrawal, B., Kumar, A. and Pandey, A., 2020. Phytochemicals of Azadirachta indica source of active medicinal constituent used for cure of various diseases: A Review. *Journal of Scientific Research*, *64*(1), pp.385-90.

Subapriya, R. and Nagini, S., 2005. Medicinal properties of neem leaves: a review. *Current Medicinal Chemistry-Anti-Cancer Agents*, *5*(2), pp.149-156.

Thakur, R. S., Singh, S. B. and Goswami, A., 1981. Biological activities and medicinal properties of neem. *Curr Res Med Aromat Plants*, *3*, pp.135-140.

Upreti, J., Ali, S. and Basir, S. F., 2013. Effect of lower doses of vanadate in combination with Azadirachta indica leaf extract on hepatic and renal antioxidant enzymes in streptozotocin-induced diabetic rats. *Biological trace element research*, *156*, pp.202-209.

Vergallo, C., Panzarini, E. and Dini, L., 2019. High performance liquid chromatographic profiling of antioxidant and antidiabetic flavonoids purified from Azadirachta indica (neem) leaf ethanolic extract. *Pure and Applied Chemistry*, *91*(10), pp.1631-1640.

Wild, S., Roglic, G., Green, A., Sicree, R. and King, H., 2004. Global prevalence of diabetes: estimates for the year 2000 and projections for 2030. *Diabetes care*, *27*(5), pp.1047-1053.

Yadav, D. K., Bharitkar, Y. P., Chatterjee, K., Ghosh, M., Mondal, N. B. and Swarnakar, S., 2016. Importance of Neem Leaf: An insight into its role in combating diseases.

Chapter 11

Conservation Strategies for Antidiabetic Plants: An Overview

Vikram R. Jadhav*
Department of Chemistry, K K W Arts, Science, and Commerce College, Pimpalgaon (B), Maharashtra, India

Abstract

This chapter provides an overview of the conservation strategies for antidiabetic plants that are, which are medicinal plants used to treat diabetes. It examines the methods used in different parts of the world to conserve and sustainably manage these valuable resources. It also identifies potential gaps in current conservation efforts and suggests ways to address them. This chapter discusses the importance of antidiabetic plants and their role in traditional medicine. Then it describes the different strategies used to conserve them, such as in situ and ex situ conservation, germplasm conservation, and biotechnological approaches. It also examines the role of local communities and indigenous peoples in the conservation of these plants and the potential for using participatory approaches to ensure their sustainable use. The chapter then looks at the various challenges that conservation efforts face, including threats from habitat degradation, overexploitation, and climate change. It also discusses the potential of using legal and policy instruments to protect these plants and the need for more research and data collection to understand their ecology and use. It proposes some recommendations to improve conservation strategies for antidiabetic plants. In general, this chapter provides a comprehensive overview of antidiabetic plant conservation strategies and identifies gaps in current

* Corresponding Author's Email: mevikramjadhav@gmail.com.

In: Antidiabetic Plants
Editor: Arpita Roy
ISBN: 979-8-88697-957-2

efforts. It also suggests possible solutions to address these gaps and ensure the sustainable use of these valuable resources.

Keywords: antidiabetic plants, biodiversity, conservation strategies, ecology, traditional medicine

Introduction

Diabetes is a major global health problem, with an estimated 425 million people currently living with the disease, and this number is estimated to increase to more than 629 million by 2045 (Forouhi et al., 2019). Diabetes is a chronic metabolic disorder characterised by elevated blood glucose levels or hyperglycemia. It is estimated that more than 60 million people in India alone suffer from this disease. Antidiabetic plants have been used to prevent and treat diabetes)Avidor et al., 2020). These plants are a potential source of natural therapeutic agents, possessing a variety of biologically active compounds that can be used to regulate blood glucose levels naturally (Roy et al., 2022). Antidiabetic plants are increasingly popular in western and Eastern medicine and their importance in the management of diabetes is growing. Although there is no cure for diabetes, there are treatments available to help manage the condition. One such treatment is the use of antidiabetic plants, which have been found to contain compounds that can help control blood glucose levels)Naidu and Pullaiah, 2003).

This chapter will provide an overview of the available antidiabetic plants and the conservation strategies needed to ensure their continued availability. Antidiabetic plants contain compounds that have been found to have a beneficial effect on blood glucose levels. These plants are generally divided into two categories: medicinal plants and food plants. Medicinal plants contain compounds that act as antidiabetic agents, such as certain herbs, spices, and traditional Indian medicines. Functional food are eaten as part of the diet and contain compounds that can help control blood glucose levels, such as certain fruits, vegetables, grains, and nuts. Antidiabetic plants have long been documented in traditional medicine, and these plants are increasingly being studied and used in modern medicine)Salehi et al., 2019). For example, the plant Gymnema Sylvestre (Figure 1), commonly known as 'the sugar destroyer', has been used in traditional Ayurvedic medicine as an anti-diabetic agent for centuries (Arya et al., 2019). Fenugreek (Trigonella foenum-graecum) (Figure 1) has been used in conventional medicine to treat diabetes and has been found to have significant hypoglycemic effects in animal studies (Bitarafan, Zahra et al., 2019).

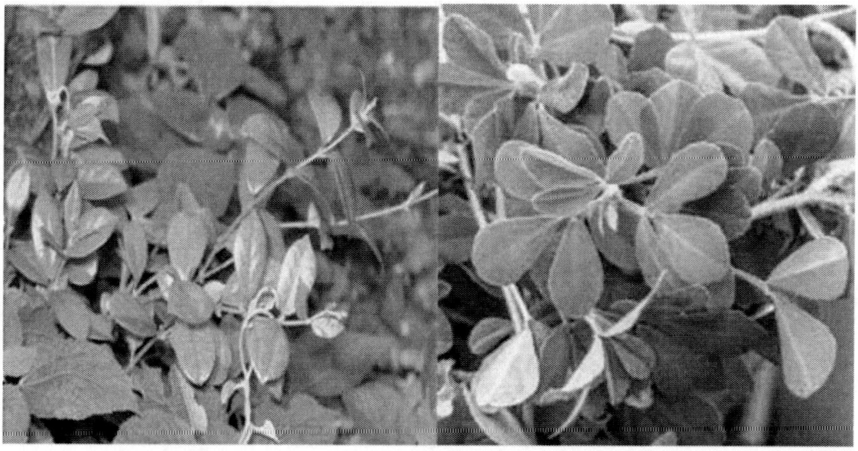

Figure 1. (a) Gudmar plant (*Gymnema Sylvestre)*(b) Methi [Fenugreek (*Trigonella foenum-graecum*)[.

Antidiabetic plants have the potential to offer a variety of benefits to people with diabetes, including improved blood glucose control and reduced risk of long-term complications. However, these plants are increasingly threatened due to habitat destruction, overharvesting, and climate change. To ensure the continued availability of these plants for the treatment of diabetes, it is essential to implement conservation strategies. One of the most effective strategies to conserve antidiabetic plants is to establish protected areas. Protected areas are areas designated for conservation and are managed to ensure the protection of natural habitats. These areas can be established in areas with high biodiversities, such as forests, grasslands, and wetlands, and can protect plants from exploitation and habitat destruction)Rai et al., 2012).

Protected areas can also monitor plants, allowing the detection of potential threats to their survival. Another effective strategy for conserving antidiabetic plants is the use of sustainable harvesting techniques. Sustainable harvesting techniques involve carefully managing the resources of plants, such as their growth and harvesting, to ensure that the plants do not overharvested or their habitats are destroyed. These techniques can help ensure that plants are not overexploited and that their populations remain stable. Finally, education is a crucial strategy for conserving antidiabetic plants (Campbell, 2002). Education about the importance of these plants and their conservation can help raise awareness and encourage people to take action to protect them. Education can be used to promote sustainable harvesting practises and discourage overharvesting of these plants. Antidiabetic plants are a valuable resource for treating and preventing diabetes. It is essential to preserve them to ensure their continued availability)Sharma et al., 2010) (Figure 2). This can be done by establishing protected areas, using sustainable harvesting techniques, and promoting education about the importance of these plants. With these strategies in place, it is possible to ensure the continued availability of antidiabetic plants for the treatment of diabetes.

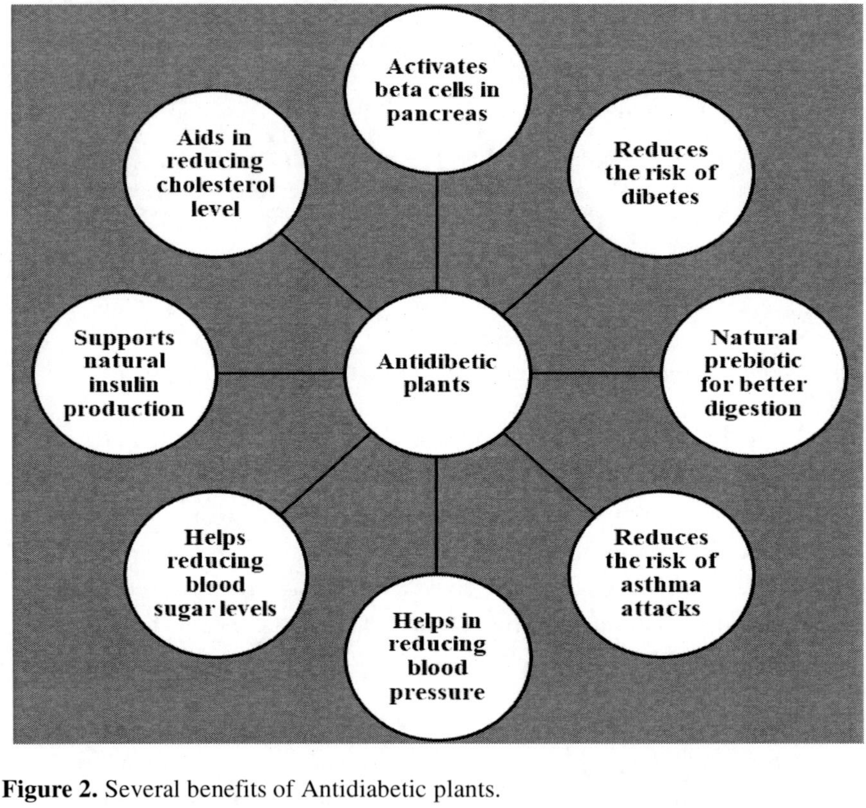

Figure 2. Several benefits of Antidiabetic plants.

Traditional Uses of Antidiabetic Plants

Since antiquity, plants have been used to treat various diseases and diseases and show various benefits (Figure 2). In traditional medicine, plants are a source of potent compounds that can be used to treat and prevent diseases.

Antidiabetic plants have been used in both Western and eastern medicine for centuries. The most common antidiabetic plants in western medicine are ginseng, garlic, and cinnamon (Figure 3). These plants are used for their antioxidant and anti-inflammatory properties and are believed to be effective in regulating blood glucose levels. The most common antidiabetic plants in Eastern medicine are bitter melon, fenugreek, and turmeric (Figure 3). These plants are used for their anti-diabetic effects and their ability to improve insulin sensitivity (Ullah et al., 2022).

In western medicine, antidiabetic plants have been used since ancient times. One of the first known plants used to treat diabetes was the juniper, a native plant of Europe and North America. Juniper berries were used to treat diabetes by ancient Egyptians and Greeks, who believed that the plant had anti-diabetic properties. In the modern era, juniper has been studied for its potential to treat diabetes, but it has not yet been officially approved by the FDA. In Eastern medicine, antidiabetic plants are also widely used. For example, bitter melon, ginseng, and fenugreek are commonly used in Chinese and Ayurvedic medicine to treat diabetes (Keji and Hao 2003; Rutebemberwa et al., 2013).

Bitter melon is believed to be especially effective in lowering blood sugar levels and is often used in combination with other antidiabetic plants (Joseph and Jini, 2013). Ginseng is supposed to help regulate insulin levels, while fenugreek is believed to be effective at controlling blood sugar levels and reducing cholesterol levels. In addition to traditional uses of antidiabetic plants, several conservation strategies are also being used to protect them. Antidiabetic plants are becoming increasingly rare in many parts of the world due to over-harvesting and habitat destruction (Grover et al., 2002). To prevent this, conservationists are working to protect and restore habitats and promote sustainable harvesting practises. In addition, botanicals are being cultivated on farms and gardens, helping to conserve wild plants. This ensures that antidiabetic plants are available for traditional uses and helps create a sustainable source of income for local communities. Finally, antidiabetic plants are being studied for their potential to treat and prevent diabetes in humans (Gantait et al., 2021; Roy et al., 2018). This research helps to ensure that antidiabetic plants remain available for traditional uses, as well as for the development of new treatments and cures for diabetes. Antidiabetic plants have been used for centuries to treat and prevent diabetes in Western and Eastern medicine. As these plants become increasingly rare, conservation strategies are being used to protect and restore wild populations and cultivate them on farms and gardens. Furthermore, research is being conducted to identify new uses for antidiabetic plants, which can lead to new treatments and cures for diabetes (Sood et al., 2005; Mani et al., 2022).

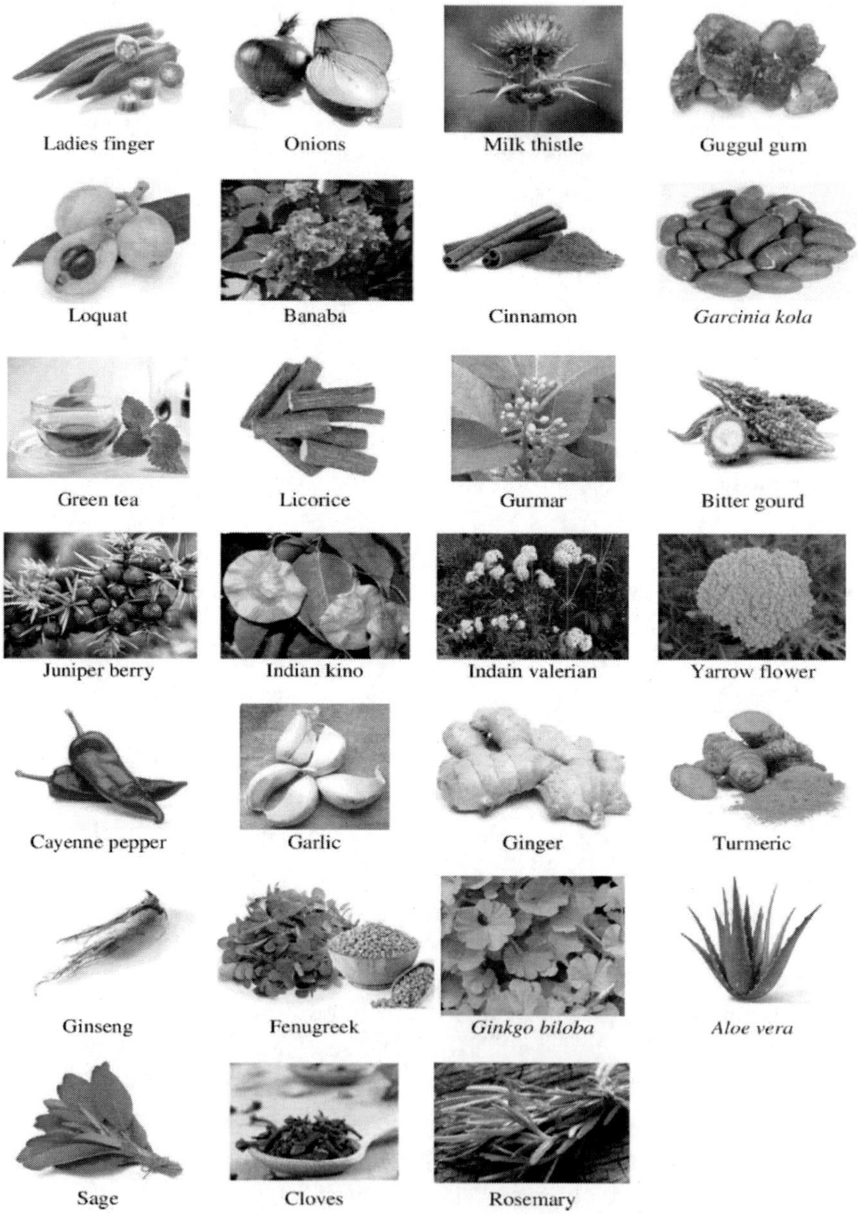
Ladies finger
Onions
Milk thistle
Guggul gum
Loquat
Banaba
Cinnamon
Garcinia kola
Green tea
Licorice
Gurmar
Bitter gourd
Juniper berry
Indian kino
Indain valerian
Yarrow flower
Cayenne pepper
Garlic
Ginger
Turmeric
Ginseng
Fenugreek
Ginkgo biloba
Aloe vera
Sage
Cloves
Rosemary

Figure 3. Some commonly used antidiabetic medicinal plants (Suhani and Khatua, 2018).

Conservation Stratategies

The increasing demand for antidiabetic plants has led to the need for conservation strategies to ensure the sustainability of these species. Antidiabetic plants are used for the treatment of diabetes, a chronic and life-threatening disease that affects millions of people worldwide. The use of antidiabetic plants is becoming increasingly popular because of their effectiveness and cost effectiveness. Conservation of antidiabetic plants is paramount to ensure their continued availability and use (Rohini et al., 2021). Different strategies have been used to conserve these plants, such as habitat protection, ex situ conservation, and the promotion of sustainable harvest practises (Figure 4). Habitat protection involves the safety of the natural habitats of antidiabetic plants to minimise their destruction. Ex situ conservation involves the transfer of antidiabetic plants to a controlled environment, such as a botanical garden, to preserve them. Sustainable harvest practises involve the collection of antidiabetic plants in a way that does not endanger their existence (Ghosh and Chatterjee et al., 2014; Dey et al., 2020; Laleye et al., 2015). However, the increasing demand for these plants is putting pressure on their natural populations and leading to the decline of some species. As such, it is essential to develop strategies to conserve antidiabetic plants.

The most important step toward conserving antidiabetic plants is establishing a clear understanding of the current state of their populations. This involves conducting a population survey to identify threatened species, the extent to which they are threatened, and the factors driving their decline. With this information, it is possible to develop conservation strategies tailored to the specific needs. Once the population survey is completed, the next step is to develop conservation action plans. These plans should include strategies such as habitat protection, species reintroduction, and population monitoring (Ghosh and Chatterjee 2012). Habitat protection is essential for the conservation of antidiabetic plants, as it helps to ensure that plants have the necessary resources to survive and reproduce. Reintroduction of species is also a viable option for threatened species. This involves reintroducing the species into their natural habitats, which can help to restore population size (Annapurna et al., 2013).

Population monitoring is essential to ensure that the population is healthy and that outside factors do not threaten the species. In addition to habitat protection, species reintroduction, and population monitoring, promoting the sustainable use of antidiabetic plants is also essential. This can be done by encouraging the use of sustainable harvesting techniques, such as selective harvesting, and by promoting the development of sustainable farming practises that can help ensure the long-term sustainability. Additionally, it is essential to educate the public about the importance of conserving antidiabetic plants and to create incentives for their conservation (Majid et al., 2017). Finally, it is essential to ensure that conservation strategies are adequately implemented and monitored adequately. This involves establishing an effective monitoring system that can assess effectiveness and identify areas that need improvement (Shori, 2015).

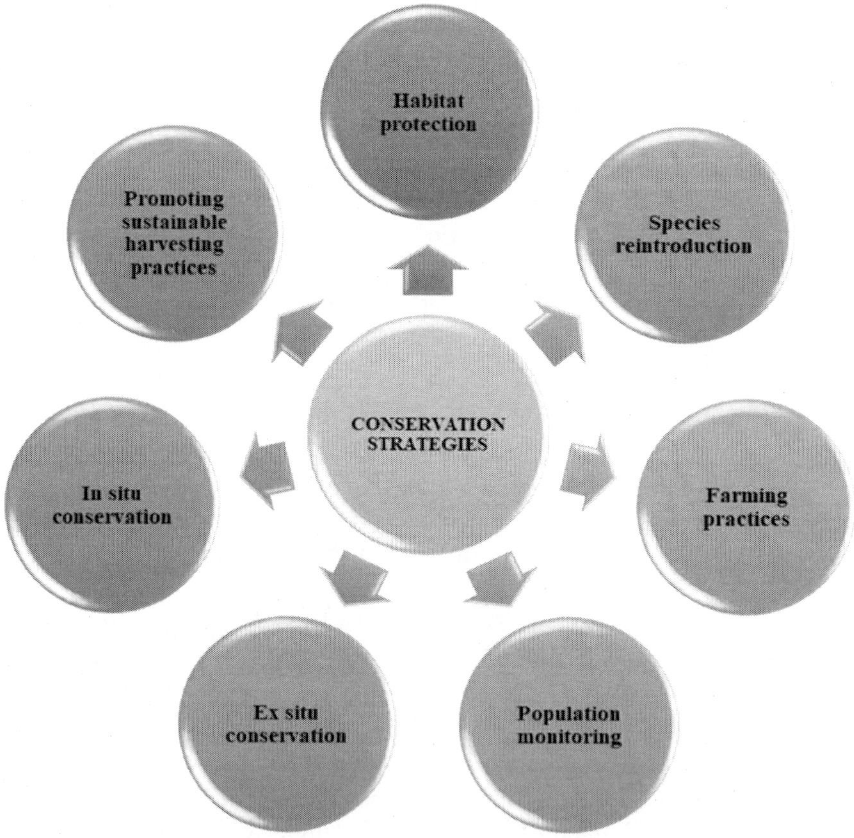

Figure 4. Conservation strategies.

It is important to ensure that the strategies are regularly reviewed and updated as needed. The conservation of antidiabetic plants is an important issue that needs to be addressed. Conservation strategies such as habitat protection, species reintroduction, population monitoring, and sustainable harvesting and farming practises must be implemented to ensure the long-term sustainability of these species. Additionally, effective monitoring and review systems must be established to ensure that the strategies are implemented and monitored. With these strategies in place, it is possible to ensure the conservation of antidiabetic plants and their continued use for the treatment of diabetes (Sharma and Rekha 2016).

Ethnobotanical Studies

Ethnobotanical studies are a type of research that explores the relationships between plants, people, and their environment. Examines traditional knowledge of plant use, often passed down through generations, and is used to identify potential conservation strategies for antidiabetic plants. The conventional understanding of plant use includes medicinal, culinary, agricultural, spiritual and cultural uses, as well as information on the ecology and distribution of plants. Ethnobotanical studies provide crucial information on the medicinal uses of plants, including antidiabetic plants, and can be used to identify potential conservation strategies. The traditional use of antidiabetic plants has been documented in many cultures worldwide (Davids et al., 2016; Bouyahya et al., 2021). For example, in India, the Gymnema Sylvestre medicinal plant has been used for centuries to treat diabetes for centuries (Figure 1). In China, Salvia miltiorrhiza (Figure 5) has been used to treat diabetes since 300 BC. In Mexico, Cinchona officinalis (Figure 5) has been treating diabetes since the 16th century. Ethnobotanical studies can provide valuable information on the traditional use of antidiabetic plants and can be used to inform conservation strategies.

In addition to providing information on traditional uses, ethnobotanical studies can also identify potential threats to the conservation of antidiabetic plants. For example, overharvesting these plants for medicinal purposes can lead to population declines. Ethnobotanical studies can provide information on local harvesting practises and help identify sustainable harvesting strategies. Furthermore, ethnobotanical studies can provide information on the ecology and distribution of antidiabetic plants, which can be used to identify areas that require conservation. Ethnobotanical studies can also identify potential threats to antidiabetic plant populations due to environmental changes. For example, climate change can lead to changes in the availability of resources, such as water, and can affect the habitat of antidiabetic plants.

Ethnobotanical studies can provide information on the impact of climate change on antidiabetic plants, which can be used to identify potential conservation strategies (Das et al., 2016). In addition to providing information on the traditional uses of antidiabetic plants and potential threats to their conservation, ethnobotanical studies can also identify potential research opportunities. For example, ethnobotanical studies can provide information on the chemical constituents of antidiabetic plants, which can be used to develop new treatments for diabetes (Semwal et al., 2007).

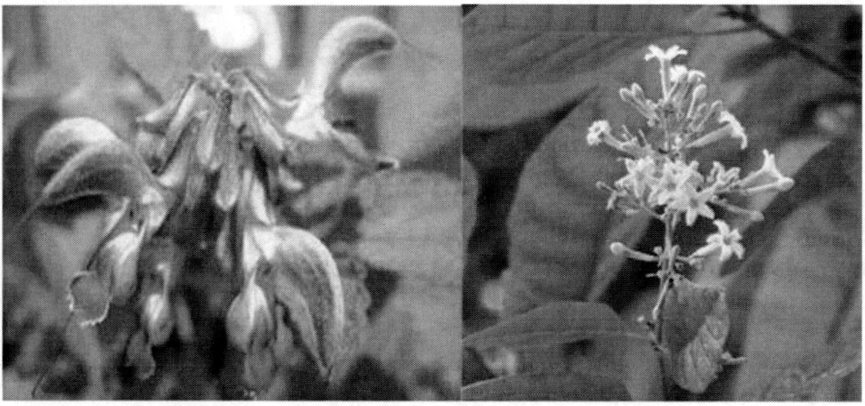

Figure 5. (a) Salvia miltiorrhiza, (b) Cinchona officinalis.

In addition, ethnobotanical studies can provide information on traditional antidiabetic plant cultivation practices of antidiabetic plants, which can be used to develop sustainable cultivation strategies. Ethnobotanical studies are invaluable to understand the conventional uses of antidiabetic plants and develop effective conservation strategies. Ethnobotanical studies can provide information on traditional uses of antidiabetic plants, potential threats to their populations, and potential research opportunities (Chauhan et al., 2010; Grover et al., 2002). Using the insights provided by ethnobotanical studies, conservation efforts for antidiabetic plants can be more effective and sustainable (Dwivedi and Kumar, 2011).

Challenges and Opportunities

Conservation strategies for antidiabetic plants are essential to ensure the survival of medicinal plants and the efficient use of their medicinal properties.

As the demand for these plants and their therapeutic components increases, it is essential to develop strategies that will help them conserve. However, several challenges and opportunities must be addressed to successfully implement these strategies. The first challenge is the lack of information on antidiabetic plants and their medicinal properties. Most of the research on these plants is limited, so it is difficult to determine their exact medicinal properties and ideal growing conditions. Identifying particular plant species and their locations is also a challenge. Without this information, it is not easy to develop accurate conservation strategies. Another challenge is the lack of resources and funding to implement these strategies. Resources must be invested in research, monitoring, and cultivation to effectively conserve these plants. This requires substantial financing, which is often challenging to acquire (Kolhe and Rachh 2018; Rai et al., 2012).

The cost of cultivating and maintaining these plants is often high, making it difficult to sustain their conservation. The third challenge is the lack of awareness about these plants and their medicinal properties. Many people are unaware of the potential uses of these plants, which can lead to their over-harvesting or destruction. Additionally, there is often a lack of knowledge and understanding of the importance of conservation strategies, which can impede their successful implementation. Despite these challenges, there are also numerous opportunities for conservation strategies for antidiabetic plants (Eddouks et al., 2014). An opportunity is to use alternative methods such as in situ conservation, ex situ conservation, and tissue culture to cultivate and preserve these plants. These methods can help to maintain the genetic diversity of plants, reduce the cost of cultivation, and ensure their sustainable use.

The development of integrated management strategies can also be beneficial. This involves coordinating multiple strategies such as cultivation, habitat restoration, and awareness campaigns. This can help ensure the successful conservation of these plants and their medicinal components. Finally, public-private partnerships can also benefit the preservation of these plants. Private sector organisations can provide the necessary resources and funding for research, monitoring, and cultivation. They can also help raise awareness of the importance and medicinal properties of these plants. In general, numerous challenges and opportunities are associated with conservation strategies for antidiabetic plants. It is essential to address these challenges and opportunities to successfully implement these strategies and ensure the successful conservation of these plants. With the right resources and system, antidiabetic plants can be used sustainably and their medicinal properties can be used effectively (Wen et al., 2021; Babu et al., 2013).

Conclusion

The preservation of antidiabetic plants is of great importance, as they provide a natural source of medicine and can be used to treat and prevent diabetes. Various strategies can be used to conserve antidiabetic plants, such as in situ conservation, ex situ conservation, and the use of botanical gardens. In situ conservation is the most preferred method since it ensures that natural habitats and ecosystems are preserved, while ex situ conservation aims to store, grow, and protect plants outside of their natural habitats. Botanical gardens are a valuable tool for conserving antidiabetic plants, as they provide a safe environment for growing and storing them, as well as a place to educate the public about their importance. Long-term monitoring of antidiabetic plants is essential to ensure their health and preservation. Cooperation between governments, local communities, and stakeholders is essential to ensure the success of conservation strategies. In general, conserving antidiabetic plants is necessary to ensure the continued availability of natural medicine and prevent species extinction. Understanding the various conservation strategies available and taking the appropriate measures to implement them can help protect antidiabetic plants and ensure their future for generations to come.

References

Annapurna, D., Srivastava, A. and Rathore, T. S., 2013. Impact of Population Structure, Growth Habit and Seedling Ecology on Regeneration of Embelia ribes Burm. f.—Approaches toward a Quasi in Situ Conservation Strategy.

Arya, S. S., Sonia, N. S. and Nair, D. S., 2021. Functional potential of anti-diabetic medicinal plants. *Journal of Pharmacognosy and Phytochemistry*, *10*(2), pp.1177-1181.

Avidor, D., Loewenstein, A., Waisbourd, M. and Nutman, A., 2020. Cost-effectiveness of diabetic retinopathy screening programs using telemedicine: a systematic review. *Cost Effectiveness and Resource Allocation*, *18*, pp.1-9.

Babu, P. V. A., Liu, D. and Gilbert, E. R., 2013. Recent advances in understanding the anti-diabetic actions of dietary flavonoids. *The Journal of nutritional biochemistry*, *24*(11), pp.1777-1789.

Bitarafan, Z., Asghari, H. R., Hasanloo, T., Gholami, A., Moradi, F., Khakimov, B., Liu, F. and Andreasen, C., 2019. The effect of charcoal on medicinal compounds of seeds of fenugreek (Trigonella foenum-graecum L.) exposed to drought stress. *Industrial Crops and Products*, *131*, pp.323-329.

Bouyahya, Abdelhakim, Nasreddine El Omari, Naoual Elmenyiy, Fatima-Ezzahrae Guaouguaou, Abdelaali Balahbib, Omar Belmehdi, Najoua Salhi, Hamada Imtara,

Hanae Naceiri Mrabti, Mohamed El-Shazly, Youssef Bakri. "Moroccan antidiabetic medicinal plants: Ethnobotanical studies, phytochemical bioactive compounds, preclinical investigations, toxicological validations and clinical evidences; challenges, guidance and perspectives for future management of diabetes worldwide." *Trends in Food Science & Technology* 115 (2021): 147-254.

Campbell, R. K., 2002. Role of the pharmacist in diabetes management. *American Journal of Health-System Pharmacy*, *59*(suppl_9), pp.S18-S21.

Chauhan, A., Sharma, P. K., Srivastava, P., Kumar, N. and Dudhe, R., 2010. Plants having potential antidiabetic activity: a review. *Der Pharmacia Lettre*, *2*(3), pp.369-387.

Das, M., Jain, V. and Malhotra, S., 2016. Impact of climate change on medicinal and aromatic plants. *Indian J. Agric. Sci*, *86*(11), pp.1375-1382.

Davids, D., Gibson, D. and Johnson, Q., 2016. Ethnobotanical survey of medicinal plants used to manage high blood pressure and type 2 diabetes mellitus in Bitterfontein, Western Cape Province, South Africa. *Journal of ethnopharmacology*, *194*, pp.755-766.

Dey, P., Singh, J., Suluvoy, J. K., Dilip, K. J. and Nayak, J., 2020. Utilization of Swertia chirayita plant extracts for management of diabetes and associated disorders: present status, future prospects and limitations. *Natural Products and Bioprospecting*, *10*, pp.431-443.

Dwivedi, P. and Kumar, P., 2011. Anti-diabetic medicinal plants and their conservation: Waging green war on diabetes. *Medicinal Plants-International Journal of Phytomedicines and Related Industries*, *3*(3), pp.181-189.

Eddouks, M., Bidi, A., El Bouhali, B., Hajji, L. and Zeggwagh, N. A., 2014. Antidiabetic plants improving insulin sensitivity. *Journal of Pharmacy and Pharmacology*, *66*(9), pp.1197-1214.

Forouhi, N. G. and Wareham, N. J., 2019. Epidemiology of diabetes. *Medicine*, *47*(1), pp.22-27.

Gantait, S., Verma, S. K. and Sharangi, A. B. eds., 2021. *Biotechnology of Anti-diabetic Medicinal Plants*. Springer.

Ghosh, M. and Chatterjee, S. K., 2012. Medicinal and aromatic plants: Sustainable use, conservation and rural economy. *Planta Medica*, *78*(11), p.PF21.

Ghosh, M. and Chatterjee, S. K., 2014, August. Sustainable development of medicinal and aromatic plants as potential cash crops for the welfare of rural people in eastern India. In *XXIX International Horticultural Congress on Horticulture: Sustaining Lives, Livelihoods and Landscapes (IHC2014): V World 1125* (pp. 201-208).

Grover, J. K., Yadav, S. and Vats, V., 2002. Medicinal plants of India with anti-diabetic potential. *Journal of ethnopharmacology*, *81*(1), pp.81-100.

Joseph, B. and Jini, D., 2013. Antidiabetic effects of Momordica charantia (bitter melon) and its medicinal potency. *Asian pacific journal of tropical disease*, *3*(2), pp.93-102.

Keji, C. and Hao, X.U., 2003. The integration of traditional Chinese medicine and Western medicine. *European Review*, *11*(2), pp.225-235.

Kolhe, S. S. and Rachh, P. R., 2018. Review on potent anti-diabetic plants or herbs from traditional medicine. *Journal of Drug Delivery and Therapeutics*, *8*(5), pp.92-98.

Laleye, F. O. A., Mensah, S., Assogbadjo, A. E. and Ahissou, H., 2015. Diversity, knowledge, and use of plants in traditional treatment of diabetes in the Republic of Benin. *Ethnobotany Research and applications*, *14*, pp.231-257.

Bagnazari, M., Saidi, M., Chandregowda, M. M., Prakash, H. S. and Nagaraja, G., 2017. Phyto-constituents, pharmacological properties and biotechnological approaches for conservation of the anti-diabetic functional food medicinal plant Salacia: A review note. *Applied Food Biotechnology*, *4*(1), pp.1-10.

Mani, S., Bhatt, S. B., Vasudevan, V., Prabhu, D., Rajamanikandan, S., Velusamy, P., Ramasamy, P. and Raman, P., 2022. The updated review on plant peptides and their applications in human health. *International Journal of Peptide Research and Therapeutics*, *28*(5), p.135.

Naidu, K. C. and Pullaiah, T., 2003. *Antidiabetic plants in India and herbal based antidiabetic research*. Regency.

Rai, M. K., Cordell, G. A., Martinez, J. L., Marinoff, M. and Rastrelli, L. eds., 2012. *Medicinal plants: biodiversity and drugs*. CRC Press.

Rohini, M. R., Montero, M. E. M. and Rajasekharan, P. E., 2021. Cryopreservation of Anti-Diabetic Plants. *Biotechnology of Anti-diabetic Medicinal Plants*, pp.437-469.

Roy, A., Khan, A., Ahmad, I., Alghamdi, S., Rajab, B. S., Babalghith, A. O., Alshahrani, M. Y., Islam, S. and Islam, M., 2022. Flavonoids a bioactive compound from medicinal plants and its therapeutic applications. *BioMed Research International, 2022*.

Roy, A., Khan, A., Ahmad, I., Alghamdi, S., Rajab, B. S., Babalghith, A. O., Alshahrani, M. Y., Islam, S. and Islam, M., 2022. Flavonoids a bioactive compound from medicinal plants and its therapeutic applications. *BioMed Research International, 2022*.

Rutebemberwa, E., Lubega, M., Katureebe, S. K., Oundo, A., Kiweewa, F. and Mukanga, D., 2013. Use of traditional medicine for the treatment of diabetes in Eastern Uganda: a qualitative exploration of reasons for choice. *BMC international health and human rights*, *13*, pp.1-7.

Salehi, B., Ata, A., V. Anil Kumar, N., Sharopov, F., Ramirez-Alarcon, K., Ruiz-Ortega, A., Abdulmajid Ayatollahi, S., Valere Tsouh Fokou, P., Kobarfard, F., Amiruddin Zakaria, Z. and Iriti, M., 2019. Antidiabetic potential of medicinal plants and their active components. *Biomolecules*, *9*(10), p.551.

Semwal, D. K., Bamola, A. and Rawat, U., 2007. Chemical constituents of some antidiabetic plants. *Univ. J. Phytochem. Ayur Heig*, *2*(3), pp.40-48.

Sharma, S. and Arya, R., 2016. Biodiversity Conservation with Special Reference to Medicinal Climbers: Present Scenario, Challenges, Strategies, and Policies. *Biotechnological strategies for the conservation of medicinal and ornamental climbers*, pp.23-63.

Sharma, S., Rathi, N., Kamal, B., Pundir, D., Kaur, B. and Arya, S., 2010. Conservation of biodiversity of highly important medicinal plants of India through tissue culture technology-a review. *Agriculture and Biology Journal of North America*, *1*(5), pp.827-833.

Shori, A. B., 2015. Screening of antidiabetic and antioxidant activities of medicinal plants. *Journal of integrative medicine*, *13*(5), pp.297-305.

Sood, S. K., Bhardwaj, R. and Lakhanpal, T. N., 2005. *Ethnic Indian Plants in cure of diabetes*. Scientific publishers.

Suhani, S. and Soubhik, K., 2018. Effects and safety profile of commonly used herbal anti-diabetic preparations. *GSC Biological and Pharmaceutical Sciences*, *4*(2).

Ullah, M., Mehmood, S., Khan, R. A., Ali, M., Fozia, F., Waqas, M., Ullah, R., Alotaibi, A. and Sultan, M. A., 2022. Assessment of antidiabetic potential and phytochemical profiling of viscum album, a traditional antidiabetic plant. *Journal of Food Quality*, *2022*.

Wen, Y., Gao, L., Zhou, H., Ai, C., Huang, X., Wang, M., Zhang, Y. and Zhao, C., 2021. Opportunities and challenges of algal fucoidan for diabetes management. *Trends in Food Science & Technology*, *111*, pp.628-641.

Chapter 12

Conservation Strategies of Antidiabetic Plants

M. Kanthimathi[1]
and S. Kanimozhi[2,*]

[1]Sri Paramakalyani Centre for Environmental Sciences,
Manonmaniam Sundaranar University, Azhwarkurichi, India
[2]Department of Industrial Biotechnology,
Bharath Institute of Higher Education and Research, Selaiyur, Chennai, India

Abstract

Most people in developing countries such as India rely on conventional medical practises like Siddha, Ayurveda, and herbal treatments for primary healthcare treatments. Diabetes mellitus is one of the most prevalent metabolic diseases that affects 2.8% of people worldwide and is expected to reach 5.4% by 2025. Medicinal plants have been used to treat diabetes in traditional medicine throughout the world, and these plants are commonly called antidiabetic plants. Parts of these antidiabetic plants are used to lower blood glucose, and they have active phytoconstituents with the activity of insulin mimetics. The occurrence of flavonoids, coumarins, polyphenols, terpenoids, and other compounds in medicinal plants is assumed to be responsible for the antidiabetic properties. Considering herbal remedies for diabetes, which have been an extremely respected source of medicine, they are now a growing component of contemporary advanced medicine. Most of these antidiabetic plants belong to the families Araliaceae, Moraceae, Cucurbitaceae, Lamiaceae, Asteraceae, Liliaceae, Rosaceae, and Leguminoseae, which have hypoglycemic potential. These antidiabetic plants are the world's most significant sources of diabetes treatment, and

---

* Corresponding Author's Email: kanimozhi.vs@gmail.com

In: Antidiabetic Plants
Editor: Arpita Roy
ISBN: 979-8-88697-957-2

they are drastically depleting. To provide a reliable resource for diabetes treatment, we emphasise the sustainable utilization of these antidiabetic medicinal plants through conservation strategies (such as conservation and cultivation practises *in situ* and *ex situ*) and resource management (such as good agricultural practices). To increase the production and alter the potency of these antidiabetic plants, we advise the application of biotechnological approaches (such as tissue culture, seed technology, and micropropagation). This chapter aims to review the methodologies and approaches for the conservation and sustainable use of these antidiabetic medicinal plants.

Keywords: antidiabetic plants, conservation, diabetes mellitus, sustainable utilization

Introduction

Diabetes mellitus (DM) is the third leading cause of death in humans, along with cancer, cerebrovascular, and cardiovascular diseases. Currently, it is one of the most difficult disorders to treat for medical specialists. DM has been classified as an epidemic by the World Health Organisation (WHO) and is actively spreading. DM complications are expensive to treat for affected persons. In recent decades, numerous medicinal plants have been the subject of intensive research on the screening for antidiabetic phytochemicals. The last two decades have seen a huge increase in the number of people diagnosed with DM worldwide. The latest data from the International Diabetes Federation (IDF) and the World Health Organisation (WHO) claim that DM now affects246 million people worldwide. Among those affected, 46% of those impacted were between the ages of 40 and 59, which is, when they are economically most productive and it is expected to rise to nearly 784 million by the year 2045 (IDF, 2021; Saeedi et al., 2019). Various factors, including social differences, population growth, ageing, urbanisation, lifestyle changes, physical inactivity, psychological trauma, obesity, hormonal disorder, and inheritance, are promoting the spread of the DM pandemic. Although several drugs are available to treat DM, some can cause serious side effects, such as gastrointestinal, liver, and kidney problems. The demand for novelmethods to cure or reduce the effects of this diabetes is growing. As drugs have their own side effects, for the treatment and prevention of diabetes, today DM patients are increasingly using medicinal plants as an alternative source of medications. Approximately 50% of current medications are manufactured from natural components, which have long been a significant source of drugs. The foundation of ancient medical practises has always been plants, which have provided constant relief for thousands of years, especially for DM. Tropical countries such as India have an abundance of antidiabetic (AD) medicinal plants due to their appropriate geoclimatic conditions. The ethno-medical survey among the tribal community may help identify AD plants, dosage, and its parts used for the preparation of herbal medicine against DM. The anti diabetic drug industries are solely dependent on the wild population of AD plants. Overexploitation, habitat destruction, and urbanisation are the primary cause of biodiversity loss of several anti-diabetic plants. The disappearance of many AD plants could imply the loss of lifesaving treatments for DM and also involve the loss of certain plant metabolites.

Antidiabetic (AD) Plants

Many plants used as antidiabetic drugs have been shown to have a hypoglycemic effect, and researchers are currently investigating how these plants work. There are several plant items with the potential to treat diabetes that work through the characteristics of insulin mimetic or secretagogue. In recent times, certain medicinal plants have been used experimentally in antidiabetic and therapies and have been shown to be helpful in treating DMglobally. The primary mechanisms through which plants have an antihyperglycemic action are their ability to stimulate insulin secretion, restrict glucose absorption from the intestine, or facilitate metabolites in insulin-dependent activities.

Although more than 400 plant species have been identified in the literature as having a hypoglycemic effect, finding novel anti-diabetic medications derived from plants is still appealing, since they include compounds that have different and harmless effects on DM. Leaves, stems, roots, barks, and flowers of some AD plants were the part of the plant for the DM treatment in traditional medicine and also for the synthesis of secondary metabolites used in DM treatments. Several *in vivo* studies conducted in alloxan and streptozotocin (STZ) with active phytochemical ingredients such as flavonoids, alkaloids, saponins, ferulic acid, carbohydrates, nutrients, amino acids and their derivatives, phenolic compounds, benzoic acid and their derivative products, and some secondary metabolites that are believed to have antidiabetic properties (Thenmozhi and Subramanian, 2011; Chao et al., 2014).

Ethnobotanical information from some AD plants provides information on these metabolic compounds and their derivatives in the DM treatment mechanism. For example, alkaloids are used for insulin production, polysaccharides lower blood glucose levels while raising serum insulin levels;dietary fibres aid in reducing the concentration of blood glucose level concentration during preoccupation and post-cibal blood glucose; ferulic acid induces the release of insulin and saponins; and flavonoids are antidiabetic mediators that lower glucose levels and increase insulin from beta islets in the pancreas (Chauhan et al., 2010; Przeor et al., 2022). The list of some AD plants, along with its family and parts that have antidiabetic potential, is presented in the following table (Table 1).

Clinical studies show that plant extracts from the Rosaceae family have been shown to improve insulin production and repair beta islets of the pancreas in STZ-induced mice with STZ. Herbal extract has been shown to lower blood sugar levels in control and treated (alloxan-induced diabetic) mice (Bahrami et al., 2021). Khan et al. (2021) studied the effect from *Prunus persic*a extracts of the Rosaceae family in STZ-induced diabetic rats and found that the extract dramatically lowers blood glucose levels due to increased insulin secretion of insulin by regeneration of beta islets in the pancreas. Singh et al. (2013) observed that *Allium hookerii* leaf significantly decreases the triglycerides, cholesterol, and total protein level, and also it has substantial anti-diabetic effects in STZ-induced diabetic rats. *The extracts of Allii sativi bulbusa* and *Allium sativum* L. contain active constituents of S-allyl cysteine sulfoxide and diallyl disulphide oxide that reduce blood glucose level by increasing insulin secretion. (Sheela et al. 1992). *Gymnema sylvestre* from the Asclepiadaceae family is a prospective plant for the production of a novel diabetes treatment drug. Several studies have been conducted on the mechanism and active ingredients of *Gymnema sylvestre*. The active components were identified as gymnemic acids III, IV, V, VII, and gymnemosides b (Miyatake et al., 1994 and Tan et al., 2000).

Dichloromethane-methanol leaf extracts of *Catharanthus roseus* dramatically lowered blood sugar levels and enhance the enzyme activity of succinate coenzyme Q reductase, glucose 6-phosphate-dehydrogenase, glycogen synthase, and malic dehydrogenase in STZ-induced diabetic mice (Singh et al., 2001). The glucose transport system in the liver was maintained for almost four weeks using ethanolic *Catharanthus roseus* extracts in STZ-induced diabetic rats. Furthermore, the expression of the GLUT gene increased (Al-Shaqha et al., 2015).

Table 1. List of some AD plants with antidiabetic activity

S. No	Anti-diabetic plants	Family	Parts of plants with AD ingredients
1.	*Aegle marmelos*	Rutaceae	Tender leaves
2.	*Artemisia pallens*	Asteraceae	Aerial parts
3.	*Andrographis paniculata*	Acanthaceae	Leaf and root
4.	*Azadirachta indica*	Meliaceae	Tender leaves
5.	*Bacopa monnieri*	Scrophulariaceae	Leaves
6.	*Bidens Pilosa*	Asteraceae	Aerial parts
7.	*Bixa Orellana*	Bixaceae	Aerial parts
8.	*Boerhavia diffusa*	Nyctaginaceae	Leaves and tender branches
9.	*Butea monosperma*	Fabaceae	Leaves
10.	*Carica papaya*	Caricaceae	unripen fruits
11.	*Cassia auriculata*	Caesalpiniaceae	Leaves, flowers
12.	*Catharanthus roseus*	Apocynaceae	Leaf buds and tender twigs
13	*Cinnamomum zeylanicum*	Lauracae	Bark
14.	*Cissampelos pareira*	Menispermaceae	Roots
15.	*Coccinia grandis*	Cucurbitaceae	Flowers, unripen fruits, twigs
16.	*Cressa cretica*	Convolvulaceae	Whole plant
17.	*Croton cajucara*	Euphorbiaceae	Bark
18.	*Cucumis sativus*	Cucurbitaceae	Seeds, unripen fruits
19.	*Curcuma longa*	Zingiberaceae	Rhizome
20.	*Ficus benghalensis*	Moraceae	Bark, tree sap
21.	*Ficus racemose*	Moraceae	unripen fruits
22.	*Gmelina arborea*	Verbenaceae	Young leaves
23.	*Gymnema sylvestre*	Asclepiadaceae	Leaves
24.	*Gynura procumbens*	Asteraceae	Leaves
25.	*Helicteres isora*	Sterculiaceae	Roots and bark
26.	*Hemidesmus indicus*	Asclepiadaceae	Roots, fruits and leaves
27.	*Hybanthus enneaspermus*	Violaceae	Whole plant
28.	*Ichnocarpus frutescens*	Apocynaceae	Leaves and fruits
29.	*Lawsonia inermis*	Lythraceace	Flowers and seeds
30.	*Luffa acutangula*	Cucurbitaceae	Fruit peel and roots
31.	*Madhuca indica*	Sapotaceae	Bark
32.	*Momordica charantia*	Cucurbitaceae	Fruits
33.	*Moringa oleifera*	Moringaceae	Fruits and leaves
34.	*Murraya koenigii*	Rutaceae	Leaves

Table 1. (Continued)

S. No	Anti-diabetic plants	Family	Parts of plants with AD ingredients
35.	*Paspalum scrobiculatum*	Poaceae	Grains
36.	*Phyllanthus emblica*	Euphorbiaceae	Leaves and fruits
37.	*Pistia stratiotes*	Araceae	Young plant
38.	*Plumbago indica*	Plumbaginaceae	Roots
39.	*Portulaca quadrifida*	Portulacaceae	Seeds
40.	*Psoralea corylifolia*	Fabaceae	seeds
41.	*Pterocarpus marsupium*	Fabaceae	Seeds, bark and heart wood
42.	*Punica granatum*	Punicaceae	Root bark and fruit rind
43.	*Sida acuta*	Malvaceae	Roots
44.	*Sphaeranthus indicus*	Asteraceae	whole plant
45.	*Swertia chirayita*	Gentianaceae	Whole plant
46.	*Syzygium cumini*	Myrtaceae	fruits and seeds
47.	*Teramnus labialis*	Fabaceae	Aerial parts
48.	*Tinospora cordifolia*	Menispermaceae	stem
49.	*Tribulus terrestris*	Zygophyllaceae	Leaves, fruits and roots
50.	*Xanthium strumarium*	Asteraceae	Fruits

The chloroform extracts of *Acacia arabica* were tested on albino rats. The findings of this investigation demonstrated that serum glucose levels decreased while low-density lipoprotein (LDL) and high-density lipoprotein (HDL) levels increased. Chloroform extracts of *Beninca sahispida* fruit, *Tinispora cordifolia* stem, aerial parts of *Ocimum sanctum* and *Jatropha curcus* leaves are also used to reduce blood glucose level. In another study, the extract of *Acacia arabica* shows similar results in STZ-induced diabetic mice (Patil et al., 2011 and Hegazy et al., 2013). Agarwal et al. (2012) investigated the effects of chloroform, ethanol, and aqueous extracts of *Citrullus colocynthis* on control and test (alloxan-induced diabetic) rats. Compared to ethanol, root chloroform and root water extracts substantially reduce blood sugar (Amin et al., 2017).

STZ-induced mice fed 100 to 200 mg/kg aerial extracts of *Cucumis maderaspatanus and Coccinia indica showed a decreased level of blood sugar* (Balaraman et al., 2010). *The extracts of Musa paradisiaca and Coccinia indica were found to be effective in the treatment of protein metabolic abnormalities in STZ-induced diabetes. The composite extract has a preventive therapeutic effect against diabetes due to its ability to regenerate cells* (Mallick et al. 2009). *The extract of the stem of Tinospora Cordifolia* improves lipid metabolic derangements in DM of STZ-induced diabetic mice (Nagaraja et al., 2008). Oral administration of hexane, methanol and ethyl acetate extracts of its stem at a dose of 250 mg / kg was reported to have effective antidiabetic properties by lowering blood glucose levels (Rajalakshmi et al., 2009). In STZ-induced diabetic mice, the combination of different herbs such as *E. officinalis, S. cumini, A. indica, G. sylvestre, J. curcus, T. cordifolia, M. charantia, E. littorale,* and *C. longa* drastically reduces lipid peroxidation and increases antioxidant activity (Patel et al., 2009; Chougale et al., 2009 and Patil et al., 2011).

Loss of Biodiversity

Destructive harvesting has resulted in depletion and scarcity. The loss of habitat caused by the export of AD plants taken from natural sources; many of these species have suffered a large and irreparable loss of genetic stock. One of the most serious hazards to AD medicinal plants is forest degradation. The decline in biodiversity of AD plants is mainly due to habitat loss, overexploitation of natural resources, climate change, human population, natural or man-made environmental disasters, environmental pollution, industrialisation, and modern civilisation (Ajay kumar et al., 2017). The extinction of so many AD plants is attributed to the overexploitation of forest areas. Accessibility to forest areas and overexploitation by human overexploitation could cause the extinction of certain AD plants. The serious threat to AD plants is their medicinal value. Unfortunately, many beneficial plants are being lost due to rapid forest deforestation (Sen et al., 2011). Based on the criteria of the International Union for the Conservation of Nature (IUCN) red list criteria, along with other medicinal plants, AD plants are classified at regional and global levels as vulnerable, extinct, endangered, least concerned, and threatened at the regional and global levels. To protect medicinal plants, it is essential to reduce the depletion of natural resources, prevent deforestation, cultivate AD plants and develop morecell culture methods (Sen et al., 2015). To prevent future depletion of antidiabetic herbal riches, efforts must be made to protect, preserve (both *in situ* and *ex situ* methods of conservation) and grow AD plants.

Table 2. Conservation status of anti-diabetic plants

IUCN status	Anti-diabetic plants
NT	*Aegle marmelos, Pterocarpus marsupium,*
LC	*Andrographis paniculate, Azadirachta indica*, Bacopa monnieri, Butea monosperma *, C, arica papaya*, Catharanthus roseus*, Cissampelos pareira, Cressa cretica, Ficus racemose, Gmelina arborea, Ichnocarpus frutescens, Lawsonia inermis, Momordica charantia*, Moringa oleifera*, Paspalum scrobiculatum, Phyllanthus emblica*, Pistia stratiotes, Punica granatum*, Sphaeranthus indicus, Syzygium cumini, Tribulus terrestris*
DD	*Boerhavia diffusa, Cassia auriculata, Curcuma longa*,*
NE	*Coccinia grandis, Cucumis sativus, Ficus benghalensis, Helicteres isora, Hybanthus enneaspermus, Luffa acutangular, Murraya koenigii*, Plumbago indica, Portulaca quadrifida, Sida acuta, Tinospora cordifolia, Citrulluscolocynthis, Coccinia indica.*
EN	*Gymnema sylvestre, Psoralea corylifolia*
R	*Hemidesmus indicus, Benincasahispida,*
CE	*Madhuca indica*
VU	*Swertia chirayita*

NT – Near Threatened, LC – Least Concern, DD – Data Deficient, NE – Not Evaluated, EN – Endangered, R – Rare, VU – Vulnerable, CE – Critically Endangered, * - Species under cultivation.

Conservation Status of Anti-Diabetic Plants

Many studies have been conducted on the preservation and sustainable usage of AD plants (Larsen et al., 2007; Uprety et al., 2012) (Table 2). The conservation status of some of the AD plants is listed in Table 2. A seriesof suggestions have been made about their protection, including the necessity for integrated conservation measures based on both *in situ* and *ex situ* approaches in addition to the creation of platforms for the estimation of biodiversity and making reliable observations (Hamilton 2004). The following conservation methods for AD plant resources are worth considering: The government should promote traditional forest conservation approaches. Conservation *in situ* through the creation of natural biosphere reserves. *Ex situ* conservation is accomplished by establishing AD plants and trees arboretum, restoration of landscapes and botanical gardens, and also by other means such as – Establishment of an AD plant gene bank- Appropriate evaluation of population estimation, mapping, taxonomy and biology of endangered AD plants – to raise awareness of the possible commercial production of therapeutic AD plants among local farmers - To hold frequent farmer training camps for cultivation, harvesting, and long term usage - Print and electronic media should be used to disseminate all pertinent knowledge regarding the conservation of AD plants (Nishteshwar, 2014).

Conservation Strategies

Traditional health care practises for diabetic treatment depend mainly on medicinal plants and therapeutic herbs grown in the wild. Indigenous knowledge associated with the conservation and utilisation of AD plants is little. Due to this, the biodiversity of AD plants is being depleted due to exploitation. Scientific methods and social initiatives can both be used to address the conservation of AD plants. The genetic diversity of these plants may be preserved using the following fourmethods, viz., *in situ* conservation, *Ex-situ* conservation, cultivation practices, and Legislation.

In-Situ Conservation

Most AD plants fall into the least concern categories; some are not evaluated. Few AD plants such as *Gymnema sylvestre* and *Psoralea corylifolia* are endemic species, their therapeutic benefits are mostly due to the existence of specialised metabolites that react to stimuli in their wild habitats, but may not manifest themselves in a culture background (Figuèiredo and Grèlle, 2009; Coley et al., 2003). We can preserve natural communities and native plants while preserving their complex web of interactions through *in situ* community conservation (Gepts 2006). Furthermore, *in situ* conservation reinforces the relationship between resource protection, management, and long-term use (Long et al., 2003) and expands the variety of plants that can be preserved (Forest et al., 2007). Over worldwide, *in situ* conservation efforts have been concentrated on creating conservation zones and employing an ecosystem and biosphere-orientated approach rather than a species-orientated approach (Ma et al., 2012). Effective *in situ* conservation depends on regulations, restrictions, and probable adherence ofAD plants to their growing environments (Volis et al., 2010).

Natural Reserves

The decline in AD plant resources is mostly due to habitat deterioration and destruction (Camm et al., 2002). To maintain and restore biodiversity, natural reserves were established as protected areas for significant wild resources

(Rodriguez et al., 2007). And more than 12,700 protected nature forest reserve areas have been established worldwide, covering 13.2 million km2 or 8.81% of the planet's surface area (Huang et al., 2002). It is necessary to evaluate the beneficiation and ecological services of each habitat if we want to conserve AD medicinal plants through the protection of important natural habitats (Liu et al., 2011).

Wild Nurseries

Due to financial constraints and conflicting land uses, it is difficult to designate every natural environment as a protected area (Kramer and Havens, 2009). A wild nursery can be built in a protected region, natural habitat, or a place that is within a small distance of where plants normally occur for the regular growth, development, and restraint domestication of rare, endemic, threatened, vulnerable, and endangered AD plants (Strandby and Olsen, 2008). Although overexploitation, habitat destruction, and invasive species have severely harmed the number of wild species populations, wild nurseries can offer a practical solution for the *in situ* conservation of rare, vulnerable and endangered ADplants (Liu et al., 2011).

Ex - In Situ Conservation

The *ex situ* conservation method is an excellent supplement to *in situ* methods, particularly for the conservation of AD medicinal plants, which have been overused and at risk of extinction and have sluggish development, low species richness, and high vulnerability to infectious diseases that impair replanting (Yu et al., 2010). *Ex situ* conservation, is frequently an urgent action done to conserve AD plants, strives to nurture and naturalise vulnerable species to ensure their continuous existence and occasionally to generate significant amounts of seeding, transplanting, or replanting material required in the production of medications (Swarts Dixon, 2009). In addition to maintaining greater efficacy when cultivated in gardens removed from their original habitats, several species of formerly wild AD plants can also have their reproductive components carefully selected and stored in seed banks for future restoration.

Botanic Gardens

Botanic gardens can preserve the biosphere to increase the survival rate of vulnerable and threatened AD plants (Havens et al., 2006) and also play a significant role in *ex situ* conservation (Huang et al., 2002). Notwithstanding the fact that live collections typicallyincludea small number of specimens fromeach species and are therefore of limited utility for gene conservation for the preservation of genetic diversity (Yuan et al., 2010), botanicalgardens contain a number of distinctive qualities. They frequently contain a taxonomically and environmentally varied flora and incorporate a wide range of plants that are cultivated under comparable conditions and similar circumstances (Primack et al., 2009). Botanical gardens can contribute to the preservation of AD medicinal plants by creating certainguidelines for their proliferation and culture and initiatives for adoption, incorporation, domestication, and selective breeding.

Seed Banks

Seed banks are usedto maintain the physiological and genomic variety of indigenous plants, especially endangered or threatened AD plants, since they provide a superior means of conserving and a superior means of maintaining the genetic variability of many ADplantsthan in botanical gardens (Li, Pritchard, 2009). The Millennium Seed Bank at the Royal Botanic Gardens, London, is the renowned seed bank. Accessing plant specimens for the evaluation of its traits is made relatively fast because ofseed banks, which helps inpreservingthe surviving natural populations (Schoen and Brown, 2001). Recovery and regeneration of AD plant species in their natural environment andeffectively supportingthe rehabilitation of wild populations are the tough issues associated withseed banking technology (Li and Pritchard, 2009).

Cultivation Practices

Domestic cultivation is a common and widely accepted method, although the resources of AD medicinal plants collected in the wild are often thought to be more effective than those grown. Due to pesticide contamination, low concentrations of active substances, and incorrect botanical provenance, cultivation offers the opportunity to employ innovative ways to address issues that arise in the development of AD plants. The yields of active phytochemicals, i.e., the secondary metabolite compounds, which may be increased by cultivation under regulated growth circumstances, and production stability are guaranteed. Optimal amounts of water, minerals, nutrients, optional supplements, and ecological factors such as weather, temperature, sunlight, moisture, and rainfall are provided throughout the cultivation processes in order to increase the yield of the secondary bioactive compound that cures DM.

Good Agricultural Practices

To manage high quality and superior yield, as well as to enable the standardisation of AD plant pharmaceuticals, good agricultural practises (GAP) of ADplants have been developed (Chan et al., 2012). Using available information to solve numerous problems, a GAP method provides high-quality, safe, and non-polluting herbal medications(Muchugi et al., 2008). The GAP covers a broad spectrum of topics, including the environment of manufacturing sites, gene bank maintenance, culture, collection, environmental monitoring, visible or microscopic authentication, biochemical analyses of phytochemical constituents, metal element inspection, etc. (Makunga et al., 2008). The adoption of GAP is actively supported by several nations. For example, Chinese government officials have encouraged good agricultural practises for the development of regularly administered medicinal herbs in areas where such ADplants are commonly grown (Ma et al., 2012).

Organic Farming

The capacity of organic farming to provide integrated, compassionate, economical and environmentally sustainable production methods for ADplants has drawn growing attention (Rigby and Cáceres, 2001). The objectives of organic ADplant cultivation includethe conservation, sustainable long-term use of such plants, and the creation of pharmaceutical materials, especially secondary metaboliteswith improved quality and greater yield. The absence of artificial fertilisers, insecticides and weedicides—many of them are now prohibited by organic certification requirements in certain countries of Europe and in North America, which is the distinguishing aspect of organic farming (Rigby and Cáceres, 2001). Theecological balances of habitats are maintained by sustainable agriculture and organic farming, which is beneficial to the ecosystem and biosphere (Rigby and Cáceres, 2001). The emergence, growth, development, and maintenance of ADmedicinal plants and the production of importantphytochemical compounds of pharmaceutical importance are substantially affected by the application of organic fertilisers, which continuously supply nutrients and enhance soil stabilisation. Long-term growth, development, productivity, viability, and sustainability of AD plants are becoming more dependent on organic farming (Macilwain, 2004).

Legislation

In certain countries like India, there are no specific laws or rules for protecting AD plants that thrive in forests. Some forest-related regulations in place that address the conservation of these plants. Forest Protection Act, Wildlife Protection Act, Forest Conservation Act, Environment Protection Act, and National Biodiversity Act are some of the regulations created by those governments for the preservation of forests, which directly or indirectly protect wild flora, including the AD plants.

Sustainable Utilization

Sustainable use is theguiding principle for how humans must use nature and natural products. Only sustainable development may be considered real development. It is certain that continuing to collect medicinal plants will restrict the limits of future generations if doing so decreases the natural population. Several communities in the past used intricate and frequently unwritten laws to regulate the exploitation of the natural environment. A legal framework is required to replace these traditions now that they have crumbled.The government should control the harvesting and exploitation of therapeutic herbs in the wild. Endangered medicinal plant harvesting in the wild should be restricted to propagation alone. The trade in medicinal plants and their products should be regulated by the government through conventions such as CITES (Convention on International Trade in Endangered Species). A programme to improve methods for the harvest and preservation of medicinal plants and the processing of their products should be developed and coordinated by the Ministries of Agriculture, Health and Trade (Santosh and Ashalata, 2020).

Conclusion

The demand for ADplants is dwindling because an exponential daily demand for medicinal plants is dwindling away at an exponential daily demand for medicinal plant resources are being used. Therefore, it is vital to concentrate on the conservation of medicinal plants to compensate for the loss of wild plant sources and meet the demand for medical plants. Conservation approaches can start and support the management of conservation and sustainable use of ADplants for healthcare requirements. Making sure that populations of plant species continue to expand and change in the wild, in their native habitats, is the best way to promote conservation.

References

Agarwal, V. I. P. I. N., Sharma, A. K., Upadhyay, A. N. S. H. U., Singh, G. O. P. E. N. D. R. A., and Gupta, R. A. J. I. V. (2012). Hypoglycemic effects of *Citrullus colocynthis* roots. *Acta Pol Pharm*, 69(1), pp. 75-9.

Al-Shaqha, W. M., Khan, M., Salam, N., Azzi, A., and Chaudhary, A. A. (2015). Anti-diabetic potential of *Catharanthus roseus* Linn. and its effect on the glucose transport gene (GLUT-2 and GLUT-4) in streptozotocin induced diabetic wistar rats. *BMC complementary and alternative medicine*, 15(1), pp. 1-8.

Amin, A., Tahir, M., and Lone, K. P. (2017). Effect of *Citrullus colocynthis* aqueous seed extract on beta cell regeneration and intra-islet vasculature in alloxan induced diabetic male albino rats. *JPMA*, 67(715).

Bahrami, G., Izadi, B., Miraghaee, S. S., Mohammadi, B., Hatami, R., Sajadimajd, S., and Batooie, N. (2021). Antidiabetic potential of the isolated fractions from the plants of Rosaceae family in streptozotocin-induced diabetic rats. *Research in pharmaceutical sciences*, 16(5), p. 505.

Balaraman, A. K., Singh, J., Dash, S., and Maity, T. K. (2010). Antihyperglycemic and hypolipidemic effects of *Melothria maderaspatana* and *Coccinia indica* in Streptozotocin induced diabetes in rats. *Saudi Pharmaceutical Journal*, 18(3), pp. 173-178.

Camm, J. D., Norman, S. K., Polasky, S., and Solow, A. R. (2002). Nature reserve site selection to maximize expected species covered. *Operations Research*, 50(6), pp. 946-955.

Chan, K., Shaw, D., Simmonds, M. S., Leon, C. J., Xu, Q., Lu, A., Sutherland, I., Ignatova, S., Zhu, Y. P., Verpoorte, R., and Williamson, E. M. (2012). Good practice in reviewing and publishing studies on herbal medicine, with special emphasis on traditional Chinese medicine and Chinese materia medica. *Journal of Ethnopharmacology*, 140(3), pp. 469-475.

Chao, C. Y., Sung, P. J., Wang, W. H., and Kuo, Y. H. (2014). Anti-inflammatory effect of *Momordica charantia* in sepsis mice. *Molecules*, 19(8), pp. 12777-12788.

Chauhan, A., Sharma, P. K., Srivastava, P., Kumar, N., and Dudhe, R. (2010). Plants having potential antidiabetic activity: a review. *Der Pharmacia Lettre*, 2(3), pp. 369-387.

Chougale, A. D., Ghadyale, V. A., Panaskar, S. N., and Arvindekar, A. U. (2009). Alpha glucosidase inhibition by stem extract of *Tinospora cordifolia*. *Journal of Enzyme Inhibition and Medicinal Chemistry*, 24(4), pp. 998-1001.

Chunlin, L., Heng, L., Zhiqin, O., Xiangyun, Y., Qin, L., and Bruce, T. (2003). Strategies for agrobiodiversity and promotion: a case study from Yunnan, China. *Biodiversity and conservation*, 12(6), pp. 1145-1156.

Coley, P. D., Heller, M. V., Aizprua, R., Araúz, B., Flores, N., Correa, M., Gupta, M., Solis, P. N., Ortega-Barría, E., Romero, L. I., and Gómez, B. (2003). Using ecological criteria to design plant collection strategies for drug discovery. *Frontiers in Ecology and the Environment*, 1(8), pp. 421-428.

Federation, I. D. (2021). *IDF Diabetes Atlas*, tenth. International Diabetes.

Figueiredo, M. S., and Grelle, C. E. V. (2009). Predicting global abundance of a threatened species from its occurrence: implications for conservation planning. *Diversity and Distributions*, 15(1), pp. 117-121.

Forest, F., Grenyer, R., Rouget, M., Davies, T. J., Cowling, R. M., Faith, D. P., Balmford, A., Manning, J. C., Procheş, Ş., van der Bank, M., and Reeves, G. (2007). Preserving the evolutionary potential of floras in biodiversity hotspots. *Nature*, 445(7129), pp. 757-760.

Gaonkar, V. P., and Hullatti, K. (2020). Indian Traditional medicinal plants as a source of potent Anti-diabetic agents: A Review. *Journal of diabetes & metabolic disorders*, 19, pp. 1895-1908.

Gepts, P. (2006). Plant genetic resources conservation and utilization: the accomplishments and future of a societal insurance policy. *Crop science*, 46(5), pp. 2278-2292.

Hamilton, A. C. (2004). Medicinal plants, conservation and livelihoods. *Biodiversity & Conservation*, 13, pp. 1477-1517.

Havens, K., Vitt, P., Maunder, M., Guerrant, E. O., and Dixon, K. (2006). *Ex situ* plant conservation and beyond. *Bioscience*, 56(6), pp. 525-531.

Hegazy, G. A., Alnoury, A. M., and Gad, H. G. (2013). The role of *Acacia Arabica* extract as an antidiabetic, antihyperlipidemic, and antioxidant in streptozotocin-induced diabetic rats. *Saudi Med J*, 34(7), pp. 727-733.

Huang, H., Han, X., Kang, L., Raven, P., Jackson, P. W., and Chen, Y. (2002). Conserving native plants in China. *Science*, 297(5583), pp. 935-936.

Kadam, S. T., and Pawar, A. D. (2020). Conservation of medicinal plants: A review. *Int. Ayurvedic Med. J*, 8, pp. 3890-3895.

Khan, N. U., Qazi, N. G., Khan, A. U., Ali, F., Hassan, S. S. U., and Bungau, S. (2022). Anti-diabetic Activity of Brucine in Streptozotocin-Induced Rats: In Silico, *In Vitro*, and *In Vivo* Studies. *ACS omega*.

Kramer, A. T., and Havens, K. (2009). Plant conservation genetics in a changing world. *Trends in plant science*, 14(11), pp. 599-607.

Kumar, A., and Verma, A. K. (2017). Biodiversity loss and its Ecological impact in India. *International Journal on Biological Sciences*, 8(2), pp. 156-160.

Larsen, H. O., and Olsen, C. S. (2007). Unsustainable collection and unfair trade? Uncovering and assessing assumptions regarding Central Himalayan medicinal plant conservation. *Biodiversity and Conservation*, 16, pp. 1679-1697.

Li, D. Z., and Pritchard, H. W. (2009). The science and economics of *ex situ* plant conservation. *Trends in plant science*, 14(11), pp. 614-621.

Liu, C., Yu, H., and Chen, S. L. (2011). "Framework for sustainable use of medicinal plants in China", *Plant diversity*, 33, 65–68.

Ma, J., Rong, K., and Cheng, K. (2012). Research and practice on biodiversity *in situ* conservation in China: progress and prospect. *Biodiversity Science*, 20(5), pp. 551-558.

Macilwain, C. (2004). Organic: is it the future of farming? *Nature*, 428(6985), pp. 792-794.

Makunga, N. P., Philander, L. E., and Smith, M. (2008). Current perspectives on an emerging formal natural products sector in South Africa. *Journal of Ethnopharmacology*, 119(3), pp. 365-375.

Mallik, C., and De D, G. D. (2009). Correction of protein metabolic disorders by composite extracts of *Musa paradisiaca* & *Coccinia Indica* in stz induced diabetic albino rats: an approach through the pancreas. *Pancreas*, 38(3), pp. 322-329.

Miyatake, K., Kensho, G., Fujimoto, T., Noguchi, E., Shinohara, M., Takenaka, S., Taira, T., Priya Upadhaya, S., Ichimoto, I., and Nakano, Y. (1994). Effect of conduritol A, a polyol from *gymnema sylvestre*, on the development of diabetic cataracts in streptozotocin-treated rats and on aldose reductase. *Bioscience, biotechnology, and biochemistry*, 58(4), pp. 756-757.

Muchugi, A., Muluvi, G. M., Kindt, R., Kadu, C. A., Simons, A. J., and Jamnadass, R. H. (2008). Genetic structuring of important medicinal species of genus *Warburgia* as revealed by AFLP analysis. *Tree Genetics & Genomes*, 4, pp. 787-795.

Nagaraja Puranik, K., Kammar, K. F., and Devi, S. (2008). R, Efficacy of *Tinospora cordifolia* (Wild.) extracts on blood lipid profile in streptozotocin diabetic rats. Is it beneficial to the heart. *Biomedical research*, 19(2), pp. 92-96.

Nishteswar, K. (2014). Depleting medicinal plant resources: A threat for survival of Ayurveda. *Ayu*, 35(4), p. 349.

Patil, R. N., Patil, R. Y., Ahirwar, B., and Ahirwar, D. (2011). Evaluation of antidiabetic and related actions of some Indian medicinal plants in diabetic rats. *Asian Pacific Journal of Tropical Medicine*, 4(1), pp. 20-23.

Primack, R. B., and Miller-Rushing, A. J. (2009). The role of botanical gardens in climate change research. *New Phytologist*, 182(2), pp. 303-313.

Przeor, M. (2022). Some common medicinal plants with antidiabetic activity, known and available in Europe (A Mini-Review). *Pharmaceuticals*, 15(1), p. 65.

Rajalakshmi, M., Eliza, J., Priya, C. E., Nirmala, A., and Daisy, P. (2009). Anti-diabetic properties of Tinospora cordifolia stem extracts on streptozotocin-induced diabetic rats. *Afr J Pharm Pharmacol*, 3(5), pp. 171-180.

Rigby, D., and Cáceres, D. (2001). Organic farming and the sustainability of agricultural systems. *Agricultural systems*, 68(1), pp. 21-40.

Rodríguez, J. P., Brotons, L., Bustamante, J., and Seoane, J. (2007). The application of predictive modelling of species distribution to biodiversity conservation. *Diversity and Distributions*, pp. 243-251.

Saeedi, P., Petersohn, I., Salpea, P., Malanda, B., Karuranga, S., Unwin, N., Colagiuri, S., Guariguata, L., Motala, A. A., Ogurtsova, K., and Shaw, J. E. (2019). Global and regional diabetes prevalence estimates for 2019 and projections for 2030 and 2045:

Results from the International Diabetes Federation Diabetes Atlas. *Diabetes research and clinical practice*, 157, p. 107843.

Schoen, D. J., and Brown, A. H. (2001). The conservation of wild plant species in seed banks: attention to both taxonomic coverage and population biology will improve the role of seed banks as conservation tools. *Bioscience*, 51(11), pp. 960-966.

Sen, S., and Chakraborty, R. (2015). Toward the integration and advancement of herbal medicine: a focus on traditional Indian medicine. *Botanics: Targets and Therapy*, 5, pp. 33-44.

Sen, S., Chakraborty, R., and De, B. (2011). Challenges and opportunities in the advancement of herbal medicine: India's position and role in a global context. *Journal of Herbal medicine*, 1(3-4), pp. 67-75.

Sheela, C. G., and Augusti, K. T. (1992). Antidiabetic effects of S-allyl cysteine sulphoxide isolated from garlic *Allium sativum Linn.Indian journal of experimental biology*, 30(6), pp. 523-526.

Singh, K. D., Chetia, D., and Mazumdar, S. (2013). Anti-diabetic activity of methanolic extract of *Allium hookeri* leaves. *Indo Am J Pharm Sci*, 3, pp. 4098-104.

Singh, S. N., Vats, P., Suri, S., Shyam, R., Kumria, M. M. L., Ranganathan, S., and Sridharan, K. (2001). Effect of an antidiabetic extract of *Catharanthus roseus* on enzymic activities in streptozotocin induced diabetic rats. *Journal of Ethnopharmacology*, 76(3), pp. 269-277.

Snehal, S. P., Rajendra, S. S., and Ramesh, K. G. (2009). Antihyperglycemic, antihyperlipidemic and antioxidant effects of dihar, one kind of tea were flushed with boiling water for drinking among the folk and had been used as an antidiabetic medicinal herb. *Indian J Exp Bio*, 47, pp. 564-70.

Strandby, U., and Olsen, C. S. (2008). The importance of understanding trade when designing effective conservation policy–The case of the vulnerable Abies guatemalensis Rehder. *Biological Conservation*, 141(12), pp. 2959-2968.

Swarts, N. D., and Dixon, K. W. (2009). Terrestrial orchid conservation in the age of extinction. *Annals of botany*, 104(3), pp. 543-556.

Tan, J. J., Zhen, H. S., and Fang, H. (2000). Studies on anti-hyperglycaemic activity of gymnemic acid. *Chinese Journal of Information on Traditional Chinese Medicine*, 7(1), pp. 28-30.

Thenmozhi, A. J., and Subramanian, P. (2011). Antioxidant potential of *Momordica charantia* in ammonium chloride-induced hyperammonemic rats. *Evidence-Based Complementary and Alternative Medicine*, 2011.

Uprety, Y., Asselin, H., Dhakal, A., and Julien, N. (2012). Traditional use of medicinal plants in the boreal forest of Canada: review and perspectives. *Journal of ethnobiology and ethnomedicine*, 8, pp. 1-14.

Volis, S., and Blecher, M. (2010). Quasi *in situ*: a bridge between *ex situ* and *in situ* conservation of plants. *Biodiversity and conservation*, 19, pp. 2441-2454.

Yu, H., Xie, C., Song, J., Zhou, Y., and Chen, S. (2010). TCMGIS-II based prediction of medicinal plant distribution for conservation planning: a case study of *Rheum tanguticum*. *Chinese Medicine*, 5, pp. 1-9.

Yuan, Q. J., Zhang, Z. Y., Hu, J., Guo, L. P., Shao, A. J., and Huang, L. Q. (2010). Impacts of recent cultivation on genetic diversity pattern of a medicinal plant, *Scutellaria baicalensis* (Lamiaceae). *BMC genetics*, 11(1), pp. 1-13.

Index

H

I

L

M

N

O

P

S

T

W

Z

α

Editor Contact Information

Dr. Arpita Roy
Assistant Professor
Department of Biotechnology
School of Engineering & Technology
Sharda University
Greater Noida, India
Email: arbt2014@gmail.com